1995
YEAR BOOK OF
HEMATOLOGY®

Statement of Purpose

The YEAR BOOK Service

The YEAR BOOK series was devised in 1901 by practicing health professionals who observed that the literature of medicine and related disciplines had become so voluminous that no one individual could read and place in perspective every potential advance in a major specialty. In the final decade of the 20th century, this recognition is more acutely true than it was in 1901.

More than merely a series of books, YEAR BOOK volumes are the tangible results of a unique service designed to accomplish the following:

- to *survey* a wide range of journals of proven value
- to *select* from those journals papers representing significant advances and statements of important clinical principles
- to provide *abstracts* of those articles that are readable, convenient summaries of their key points
- to provide *commentary* about those articles to place them in perspective.

These publications grow out of a unique process that calls on the talents of outstanding authorities in clinical and fundamental disciplines, trained literature specialists, and professional writers, all supported by the resources of Mosby, the world's preeminent publisher for the health professions.

The Literature Base

Mosby subscribes to nearly 1,000 journals published worldwide, covering the full range of the health professions. On an annual basis, the publisher examines usage patterns and polls its expert authorities to add new journals to the literature base and to delete journals that are no longer useful as potential YEAR BOOK sources.

The Literature Survey

The publisher's team of literature specialists, all of whom are trained and experienced health professionals, examines every original, peer-reviewed article in each journal issue. More than 250,000 articles per year are scanned systematically, including title, text, illustrations, tables, and references. Each scan is compared, article by article, to the search strategies that the publisher has developed in consultation with the 270 outside experts who form the pool of YEAR BOOK editors. A given article may be reviewed by any number of editors, from one to a dozen or more, regardless of the discipline for which the paper was originally published. In turn, each editor who receives the article reviews it to determine whether or not the article should be included in the YEAR BOOK. This decision is based on the article's inherent quality, its probable usefulness to readers of that YEAR BOOK, and the editor's goal to represent a balanced picture of a given field in each volume of the YEAR BOOK. In addition, the editor indicates when to include figures and tables from the article to help the YEAR BOOK reader better understand the information.

Of the quarter million articles scanned each year, only 5% are selected for detailed analysis within the YEAR BOOK series, thereby assuring readers of the high value of every selection.

The Abstract

The publisher's abstracting staff is headed by a physician-writer and includes individuals with training in the life sciences, medicine, and other areas, plus extensive experience in writing for the health professions and related industries. Each selected article is assigned to a specific writer on this abstracting staff. The abstracter, guided in many cases by notations supplied by the expert editor, writes a structured, condensed summary designed so that the reader can rapidly acquire the essential information contained in the article.

The Commentary

The YEAR BOOK editorial boards, sometimes assisted by guest commentators, write comments that place each article in perspective for the reader. This provides the reader with the equivalent of a personal consultation with a leading international authority—an opportunity to better understand the value of the article and to benefit from the authority's thought processes in assessing the article.

Additional Editorial Features

The editorial boards of each YEAR BOOK organize the abstracts and comments to provide a logical and satisfying sequence of information. To enhance the organization, editors also provide introductions to sections or individual chapters, comments linking a number of abstracts, citations to additional literature, and other features.

The published YEAR BOOK contains enhanced bibliographic citations for each selected article, including extended listings of multiple authors and identification of author affiliations. Each YEAR BOOK contains a Table of Contents specific to that year's volume. From year to year, the Table of Contents for a given YEAR BOOK will vary depending on developments within the field.

Every YEAR BOOK contains a list of the journals from which papers have been selected. This list represents a subset of the nearly 1,000 journals surveyed by the publisher and occasionally reflects a particularly pertinent article from a journal that is not surveyed on a routine basis.

Finally, each volume contains a comprehensive subject index and an index to authors of each selected paper.

The 1995 Year Book Series

Year Book of Allergy and Clinical Immunology: Drs. Rosenwasser, Borish, Gelfand, Leung, Nelson, and Szefler

Year Book of Anesthesiology and Pain Management: Drs. Tinker, Abram, Chestnut, Roizen, Rothenberg, and Wood

Year Book of Cardiology®: Drs. Schlant, Collins, Engle, Gersh, Kaplan, and Waldo

Year Book of Chiropractic: Dr. Lawrence

Year Book of Critical Care Medicine®: Dr. Parrillo

Year Book of Dentistry®: Drs. Meskin, Berry, Currier, Kennedy, Leinfelder, Roser, and Zakariasen

Year Book of Dermatologic Surgery: Drs. Swanson, Glogau, and Salasche

Year Book of Dermatology®: Drs. Sober and Fitzpatrick

Year Book of Diagnostic Radiology®: Drs. Federle, Clark, Gross, Latchaw, Madewell, Maynard, and Young

Year Book of Digestive Diseases®: Drs. Greenberger and Moody

Year Book of Drug Therapy®: Drs. Lasagna and Weintraub

Year Book of Emergency Medicine®: Drs. Wagner, Dronen, Davidson, King, Niemann, and Roberts

Year Book of Endocrinology®: Drs. Bagdade, Braverman, Horton, Kannan, Landsberg, Molitch, Morley, Nathan, Odell, Poehlman, Rogol, and Ryan

Year Book of Family Practice®: Drs. Berg, Bowman, Davidson, Dietrich, and Scherger

Year Book of Geriatrics and Gerontology®: Drs. Beck, Reuben, Burton, Small, Whitehouse, and Goldstein

Year Book of Hand Surgery®: Drs. Amadio and Hentz

Year Book of Hematology®: Drs. Spivak, Bell, Ness, Quesenberry, and Wiernik

Year Book of Infectious Diseases®: Drs. Keusch, Barza, Bennish, Gelfand, Klempner, Snydman, and Skolnik

Year Book of Infertility®: Drs. Mishell, Lobo, and Sokol

Year Book of Medicine®: Drs. Bone, Cline, Epstein, Greenberger, Malawista, Mandell, O'Rourke, and Utiger

Year Book of Neonatal and Perinatal Medicine®: Drs. Fanaroff and Klaus

Year Book of Nephrology®: Drs. Coe, Favus, Henderson, Kashgarian, Luke, Myers, and Curtis

Year Book of Neurology and Neurosurgery®: Drs. Bradley and Wilkins

Year Book of Neuroradiology: Drs. Osborn, Eskridge, Grossman, Hudgens, and Ross

Year Book of Nuclear Medicine®: Drs. Gottschalk, Blaufox, McAfee, Zaret, and Zubal

Year Book of Obstetrics and Gynecology®: Drs. Mishell, Kirschbaum, and Morrow

Year Book of Occupational and Environmental Medicine: Drs. Emmett, Frank, Gochfeld, and Hessl

Year Book of Oncology®: Drs. Simone, Bosl, Glatstein, Longo, Ozols, and Steele

Year Book of Ophthalmology®: Drs. Cohen, Laibson, Augsburger, Benson, Eagle, Flanagan, Nelson, Rapuano, Sergott, Tasman, Tipperman, and Wilson

Year Book of Orthopedics®: Drs. Sledge, Poss, Cofield, Dobyns, Frymoyer, Griffin, Springfield, Swionkowski, and Wilson

Year Book of Otolaryngology–Head and Neck Surgery®: Drs. Paparella and Holt

Year Book of Pain: Drs. Gebhart, Haddox, Jacox, Janjan, Marcus, Rudy, and Shapiro

Year Book of Pathology and Laboratory Medicine®: Drs. Mills, Bruns, Gaffey, and Stoler

Year Book of Pediatrics®: Dr. Stockman

Year Book of Plastic, Reconstructive, and Aesthetic Surgery: Drs. Miller, Cohen, McKinney, Robson, Ruberg, and Whitaker

Year Book of Podiatric Medicine and Surgery®: Dr. Kominsky

Year Book of Psychiatry and Applied Mental Health®: Drs. Talbott, Ballanger, Breier, Meltzer, Tasman, Schowalter, and Frances

Year Book of Pulmonary Disease®: Drs. Bone and Petty

Year Book of Rheumatology: Drs. Sergent, LeRoy, Meenan, Panush, and Reichlin

Year Book of Sports Medicine®: Drs. Shephard, Drinkwater, Eichner, Torg, Col. Anderson, and Mr. George

Year Book of Surgery®: Drs. Copeland, Bland, Deitch, Eberlein, Howard, Luce, Seeger, Souba, and Sugarbaker

Year Book of Thoracic and Cardiovascular Surgery: Drs. Ginsberg, Lofland, and Wechsler

Year Book of Transplantation®: Drs. Sollinger, Eckhoff, Hullett, Knechtle, Longo, Mentzer, and Pirsch

Year Book of Ultrasound®: Drs. Merritt, Babcock, Carroll, Goldstein, and Mittelstaedt

Year Book of Urology®: Drs. Howards and deKernion

Year Book of Vascular Surgery®: Dr. Porter

1995

The Year Book of HEMATOLOGY®

Editor
Jerry L. Spivak, M.D.
Professor of Medicine and Oncology, Division of Hematology, Department of Medicine, The Johns Hopkins University School of Medicine, Baltimore, Maryland

Associate Editors
William R. Bell, M.D.
Professor of Medicine, Radiology, and Nuclear Medicine; Clinical Director, Division of Hematology, Department of Medicine, The Johns Hopkins University School of Medicine, The Edythe Harris Lucas–Clara Lucas Lynn Professor in Hematology, Baltimore, Maryland

Paul M. Ness, M.D.
Director, Transfusion Medicine, Department of Pathology, The Johns Hopkins University School of Medicine; Principal Officer, American Red Cross Blood Services, Greater Chesapeake and Potomac Regions

Peter J. Quesenberry, M.D.
Director, Cancer Center, University of Massachusetts, Worcester

Peter H. Wiernik, M.D.
Professor of Medicine, Montefiore Medical Center and Albert Einstein College of Medicine, Bronx, New York

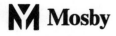 Mosby

St. Louis Baltimore Boston Chicago London Madrid Philadelphia Sydney Toronto

Vice President and Publisher, Continuity Publishing: Kenneth H. Killion
Director, Editorial Development: Gretchen C. Murphy
Developmental Editor: Kris Baumgartner, R.N.
Acquisitions Editor: Shelley Scott
Illustrations and Permissions Coordinator: Bernadette R. Bauer
Director of Editorial Services: Edith M. Podrazik, R.N.
Senior Information Specialist: Terri Santo, R.N.
Information Specialist: Nancy Dunne, R.N.
Senior Medical Writer: David A. Cramer, M.D.
Senior Project Manager: Max F. Perez
Senior Production Editor: Wendi Schnaufer
Production Coordinator: Sandra Rogers
Editing Coordinator: Rebecca Nordbrock
Proofroom Supervisor: Barbara M. Kelly
Vice President, Professional Sales and Marketing: George M. Parker
Marketing and Circulation Manager: Barry J. Bowlus
Marketing Coordinator: Lynn Stevenson

1995 EDITION
Copyright © December 1994 by Mosby-Year Book, Inc.

Printed in the United States of America
Composition by International Computaprint Corporation
Printing/binding by Maple-Vail

Mosby-Year Book, Inc.
11830 Westline Industrial Drive
St. Louis, MO 63146

Editorial Office:
Mosby-Year Book, Inc.
200 North LaSalle St.
Chicago, IL 60601

International Standard Serial Number: 0912-5998
International Standard Book Number: 0-8151-8128-0

Table of Contents

Mosby Document Express

Copies of the full text of the original source documents of articles abstracted or referenced in this publication are available by calling Mosby Document Express, toll-free, at **1 (800) 55-MOSBY.**

With Mosby Document Express, you have convenient, 24-hour-a-day access to literally every article on which this publication is based. In fact, through Mosby Document Express, virtually any medical or scientific article can be located and delivered by FAX, overnight delivery service, international airmail, electronic transmission of bitmapped images (via Internet), or regular mail. The average cost of a complete, delivered copy of an article, including up to $4 in copyright clearance charges and first-class mail delivery, is $12.

For inquiries and pricing information, please call the toll-free number shown above. To expedite your order for material appearing in this publication, please be prepared with the code shown next to the bibliographic citation for each abstract.

Journals Represented

Mosby subscribes to and surveys nearly 1,000 U.S. and foreign medical and allied health journals. From these journals, the Editors select the articles to be abstracted. Journals represented in this YEAR BOOK are listed below.

American Heart Journal
American Journal of Clinical Pathology
American Journal of Emergency Medicine
American Journal of Epidemiology
American Journal of Hematology
American Journal of Infection Control
American Journal of Medicine
American Journal of Obstetrics and Gynecology
American Journal of Pathology
American Journal of Pediatric Hematology/Oncology
American Journal of Surgery
Anesthesiology
Angiology
Annals of Internal Medicine
Annals of Surgery
Annals of Thoracic Surgery
Archives of Disease in Childhood
Archives of Pathology and Laboratory Medicine
Archives of Surgery
Artificial Organs
Australasian Radiology
Blood
Bone Marrow Transplantation
British Heart Journal
British Journal of Cancer
British Journal of Surgery
Cancer
Cancer Research
Cardiovascular Research
Chest
Circulation
Clinical Nuclear Medicine
Critical Care Medicine
European Journal of Cancer
European Journal of Haematology
Experimental Hematology
Gynecologic and Obstetric Investigation
International Journal of Cancer
International Journal of Epidemiology
International Journal of Radiation, Oncology, Biology, and Physics
Investigative Radiology
Israel Journal of Medical Sciences
Journal of Clinical Investigation
Journal of Clinical Microbiology
Journal of Clinical Oncology
Journal of Clinical Pathology
Journal of Experimental Medicine
Journal of Immunology
Journal of Internal Medicine
Journal of Laboratory and Clinical Medicine

Journal of Pathology
Journal of Pediatric Orthopedics
Journal of Pediatrics
Journal of Rheumatology
Journal of Trauma
Journal of Urology
Journal of Vascular Surgery
Journal of the American Academy of Child Adolescent Psychiatry
Journal of the American College of Cardiology
Journal of the American Medical Association
Journal of the American Society of Nephrology
Journal of the National Cancer Institute
Kidney International
Lancet
Leukemia
Medicine
Modern Pathology
Nature
New England Journal of Medicine
Pediatric Radiology
Pediatric Research
Proceedings of the National Academy of Sciences
Science
Southern Medical Journal
Stroke
Surgery
Thrombosis and Haemostasis
Thyroid
Transfusion
Transplantation
Transplantation Proceedings
Vox Sanguinis

STANDARD ABBREVIATIONS

The following terms are abbreviated in this edition: acquired immunodeficiency syndrome (AIDS); central nervous system (CNS); colony-forming unit (CFU); colony-stimulating factor (CSF); computed tomography (CT); electrocardiography (ECG); erythropoietin (EPO); granulocyte colony-stimulating factor (G-CSF); granulocyte-macrophage colony-stimulating factor (GM-CSF); human immunodeficiency virus (HIV); human T-cell lymphotropic virus (HTLV); interleukin (IL); magnetic resonance (MR) imaging (MRI); red blood cell (RBC); von Willebrand's factor (vWF); white blood cell (WBC).

Introduction

Spring came gently to Baltimore this year, benefiting not only its citizens but also its birds, including our Orioles. I do not make this comment randomly or merely from civic pride. Rather, I do so as both a point of information because I saw so few of you at the spring clinical meeting (AFCR, ASCI, AAP) in Baltimore last April and as a follow-up to my opening remarks in these pages last year about those who consider Hematology a dying subspecialty. I started attending the spring clinical meetings just after residency when they were still held in Atlantic City. Attendance was high and the atmosphere charged, not only with regard to the transfer and critique of scientific information, but also because of the posturing so integral to the human condition, as it was at these meetings that academic reputations were made and careers enhanced. In Baltimore this spring, the clinical meetings, like the weather, were more inviting because the atmosphere was subdued. Even the format was different. Platform sessions were abolished and every abstract was presented as a poster. In place of the former, the participants of each poster session and a preselected group of experts convened in a conference room where most abstracts were briefly presented and discussed in the context of the particular scientific discipline. This approach proved very effective for information exchange as long as abstract groupings were appropriate and the "experts" did their homework.

In spite of the attractive new format and atmosphere, attendance struck me as disappointingly low, and to recapitulate on last year's theme where I found that the volume of the ASH abstract book approximated that of the greater metropolitan Baltimore telephone directory, I decided to do another geometric analysis. Between 1974 and 1994, whilst the size of the ASH abstract book increased 2.3-fold, the spring clinical meetings' abstract book shrank by 42%. Having been raised in an era when the spring clinical meetings were the jewel in the crown of academic medicine, I found this observation most telling. Clearly, in an era when generalists are in demand more than ever, the research base has shifted to the subspecialty societies. Not only is Hematology, along with other subspecialties, thriving, but elitism has given way to egalitarianism, which is the proper setting for the conduct and presentation of research. More importantly, however, I foresee a potential problem. If the government favors generalists in medicine and the bulk of the seminal research is conducted at the subspecialty level, how will the necessary transfer of information occur? This is not meant to imply that we must keep alive traditions that are no longer useful or perpetuate inappropriate values, but rather that as in all things, a balance is always desirable. The rush to generalism prompted purely by suspect economic motives should be tempered.

Year books such as this one, of course, provide a fallback position, and, once again, hematologists and oncologists continue to push forward the frontiers of knowledge. With respect to recombinant EPO, there may be some relief on the horizon for our anemic myelodysplastic patients. Recombinant EPO has not had a record of accomplishment in these patients. By my calculation, of 240 anemic myelodysplastic patients described in the literature treated with EPO alone, only 15% had a satisfactory response with respect to a hemoglobin increase, even with a dose escalation to 2,000 units/kg. In contrast, when EPO was combined with G-CSF, a response rate of 42% was achieved (Abstract 116-95-1-7). Importantly, age, gender, French-American-British subtype, duration of disease, and cytogenetic abnormalities did not impact negatively on responsiveness, but high pretreatment EPO levels did. Now, this is not inexpensive therapy, and, of course, it is unclear how durable the responses will be or whether such therapy will influence survival. If, however, the quality of life is enhanced, this approach could prove to be of major benefit in this troubled group of patients. Bench also met bedside with respect to secondary erythrocytosis because a mutant EPO receptor with a truncated cytoplasmic domain in a pedigree with familial erythrocytosis recapitulated the behavior observed in tissue culture cells transfected with an EPO receptor with an intentionally truncated cytoplasmic domain (Abstract 116-95-1-19). This is the type of correlation that gives basic science a good name. Those of you who are interested in paroxysmal nocturnal hemoglobinuria will also be in for a treat as we present two articles (Abstracts 116-95-1-10 and 116-95-1-11) defining the molecular basis for this disorder. Now, we just need a cure.

With respect to WBCs, inhibitors of progenitor cell proliferation are under active investigation (Abstracts 116-95-2-2 and 116-95-2-10) because of their potential for myeloprotection during radiotherapy. Furthermore, although previous dogma held that myeloid growth factors acted locally, newer data (Abstract 116-95-2-12) suggest that GM-CSF may circulate physiologically.

I have been following Dr. David Roodman's work with great interest for many years. Actually, we started out with back-to-back articles in *Experimental Cell Research* and eventually collaborated on a research project. However, David has gone on to better things, in particular, the osteoclast, and I thought it would be timely for him to bring us up to date on this fascinating cell, which we occasionally encounter in the bone marrow and which as hematologists we should know more about. He has provided us with a superb review in his special article.

The chapter on coagulation factors and platelets compiled by my colleague, Dr. William Bell, is also as usual very informative. Dipyridamole should no longer be in our anticoagulant formula (Abstract 116-95-3-8), but a very useful study defining the risks of warfarin anticoagulation (Abstract 116-95-3-57) should be on everyone's reading list. Drs. Burrows and Kelton have done us a real service in their analysis of antenatal thrombocytopenia (Abstract 116-95-3-16); it appears that only those infants suffering from alloimmune thrombocytopenia are at risk of hemorrhage. This should reduce the incidence of cesarean sections. As usual, the literature continues to be flooded with studies comparing recombinant tissue plasminogen activator with streptokinase and claiming superiority for the former. I tend to side with the cogent comments of William Bell with regard to tissue plasminogen activator. Interestingly, fibrinogen is once again a matter of scrutiny with respect to atherosclerotic disease (Abstracts 116-95-3–52 to 116-95-3–55). Iron briefly held the stage last year. However, because fibrinogen is an acute-phase reactant, it would be worthwhile to determine whether it is a surrogate marker for some other process as opposed to representing a risk in its own right. It was also of interest to learn how quickly subclinical vitamin K deficiency develops (Abstract 116-95-3–26), because bleeding due to vitamin K deficiency is fairly common in chronically ill hospitalized patients but is often overlooked. Although low-molecular-weight heparin has been quickly and widely embraced for its apparent convenience and safety, Abstract 116-95-3–64 suggests that some caution be exercised in the employment of this agent. In this regard, I hope that everyone will read Abstract 116-95-3–58. Finally, I think that there are few indications for inserting Dr. Greenfield's filter, and Trousseau's syndrome certainly is not one of them (Abstract 116-95-3–66).

Dr. Peter Wiernik has assembled an interesting chapter on hematologic malignancies. The β_2-microglobulin appears to correlate with tumor stage in Hodgkin's disease (Abstract 116-95-4–3), adding another prognostic indicator for that disorder, and Burns and Schiffman remind us to think of thymic hyperplasia when assessing tumor regression after therapy for mediastinal disease (Abstract 116-95-4–6)—a small point that can make a big difference for the patient. For our pediatric colleagues, there are many important articles on childhood Hodgkin's disease (Abstracts 116-95-3–48, 116-95-4–7, 116-95-4–8, 116-95-4–10 to 116-95-4–12, 116-95-4–16, and 116-95-4–17. The results of therapy for HIV-associated lymphoma are improving (Abstract 116-95-4–29), and it appears that the debate over cyclophosphamide, doxorubicin, vincristine, and prednisone (CHOP) vs. more intensive chemotherapy regimens for non-Hodgkin's lymphoma is over—CHOP wins (Abstract 116-95-4–30). Unfortunately, the progress with lymphomas has not been mirrored by progress in the therapy for multiple myeloma.

Interestingly, the biochemical mechanism for myelofibrosis in hairy-cell leukemia appears to be the synthesis of fibronectin by these cells (Abstract 116-95-4–44). Fludarabine is receiving much attention in the treatment of chronic lymphocytic leukemia (Abstracts 116-95-4–47 and 116-95-4–48). We badly need more therapeutic options for this disease, but whether we really need these options for early-stage chronic lymphocytic leukemia is, to my mind, questionable. Unfortunately, many patients who are resistant to alkylating agents are also resistant to fludarabine. It must not be forgotten, of course, that fludarabine causes profound immunosuppression with the attendant infectious risks, but the M.D. Anderson experience suggests that the incidence of severe infections is low. Certainly, it was not surprising to learn that prednisone added nothing to fludarabine therapy; it added nothing in the past to chlorambucil therapy either. The observation that some patients who are refractory to fludarabine are also refractory to 2-chlorodeoxyadenosine was disappointing (Abstract 116-95-4–49), but this issue is not fully resolved.

I was very interested in the data of Robertson et al. on the effectiveness of low-dose cytosine arabinoside in chronic-phase chronic myelocytic leukemia (Abstract 116-95-4–51). Interferon, although effective in chronic myelocytic leukemia, does not give durable remissions in many patients, and cytosine arabinoside alone or in combination with it would be a useful addition to the management of patients unsuitable for marrow transplantation. In the chapter on bone marrow transplantation, I was also intrigued with the observations of Carmel and his associates (Abstract 116-95-5–27) on the use of nitrous oxide anesthesia in bone marrow donors. Nitrous oxide is known to inactivate vitamin B_{12}, and its use during marrow harvest appears to be inappropriate (just another small point). In this regard, the possible relationships between magnetic fields and childhood acute leukemia (Abstract 116-95-4–73) raise questions about the effects of MRI in this age group. This situation is reminiscent of when fluoroscopy was employed for fitting children's shoes. I remember the fascination of seeing my metatarsals, as well (fortunately) as my annoyance at the resistance of the salesman in letting me linger too long over the view. When I grew older (fortunately) and smarter, I went back to visit this gentleman and his machine, but both were gone! Finally, once again, for our pediatric colleagues, the section on acute lymphocytic leukemia is large and informative.

My colleague, Dr. Paul Ness, has, as usual, not only selected a provocative cohort of articles dealing with the controversial issues in transfusion medicine, but has also provided lucid and thoughtful critiques. There has been intense scrutiny of autologous blood donation and the role of recombinant EPO. With respect to the prospects of infection or immunomodulation, blood appears safer than ever before, and there now may be a greater risk from undertransfusion than from overtransfusion (Abstract 116-95-6–40). Certainly, a rigid hemoglobin threshold should not be adhered to blindly (Abstracts 116-95-6–24 and 116-95-6–32). Cancer recurrent rates are not affected by allogeneic blood (Abstract 116-95-6–37), and although recombinant EPO can enhance blood donation, in nonanemic donors, it provided no advantage to aggressive phlebotomy with respect to allogeneic blood exposure (Abstract 116-95-6–14). Recombinant EPO is effective given perioperatively to anemic patients for elective hip replacement without autologous donation (Abstract 116-95-6–25), but the cost-benefit ratio needs to be better defined. The issue of waste in autologous blood donation is now as important as those of infection reduction or immunomodulation. The mechanism for HLA-antibody–associated platelet transfusion failure appears at hand (Abstract 116-95-6–8); evidently these antibodies efficiently activate platelets. Unfortunately, filtration of platelet concentrates (Abstract 116-95-6–9) does not prevent this problem. Last year, in these pages, the potentiating effects of platelet-activating factor on blood component toxicity was featured (p 348). This year, potential new villains, namely, inflammatory cytokines generated in platelet concentrates (Abstract 116-95-6-10), have been identified, including IL-8 (neutrophil-activating factor). There is a certain symmetry to this and also a potential remedy—leukodepletion—if a cause-and-effect relationship can be established. Finally, I want to call your attention to Abstract 116-95-6-27, which concerns aprotinin. It is now available and will be used perisurgically, but we still do not understand how it works and when it will be most beneficial.

Finally, faithful readers will note a departure this year from our usual organization. I have organized all articles on bone marrow transplantation into a separate chapter. This was not done randomly, but rather in anticipation of next year when Dr. Karl Blume will join the editorial board with responsibility for the literature concerning bone marrow transplantation. Given the importance of the subject and the scope of the literature, this is probably a long-overdue move. I am delighted that Dr. Blume agreed to join us, and I thank our publishers for agreeing to increase the size of the YEAR BOOK OF HEMATOLOGY for this purpose. In closing, I want to wish all of you a good year. Nashville will be the venue for the next ASH meeting, and I look forward to seeing you there.

Jerry L. Spivak, M.D.

1 Red Blood Cells

Introduction

To paraphrase Mark Twain, reports of the death of hematology are greatly exaggerated, and anyone who requires proof of this need only review the chapter on red blood cells that follows. I have opened with the first reported example of nonathletic abuse of EPO (Abstract 116-95-1-1). As my comments indicate, suspicion and proof differ in their requirements, but the report is, nevertheless, interesting. Abuse notwithstanding, evidence continues to accumulate about the safety of recombinant EPO. In the nondialysis population (see Abstract 116-95-1-2), hypertension is not a serious issue, but sufficient anecdotal reports of its occurrence mandate blood pressure monitoring during the initial phase of therapy, particularly in hypertensive patients. The issues involving EPO therapy in anemic premature infants are slowly being resolved (see Abstract 116-95-1-4,) and an even more recent report (1) further defines the patient population most likely to benefit. The EPO receptor belongs to the hematopoietic growth factor receptor superfamily, and many of the other membrane-bound receptors in this family have soluble analogs. As is demonstrated in Abstract 116-95-1-6, the EPO receptor is no different, but the biological significance of soluble EPO receptors remains to be determined. Perhaps the most important contribution with respect to EPO therapy this year is a clinical trial of recombinant EPO and G-CSF (Abstract 116-95-1-7) in anemic myelodysplastic patients that demonstrates for the first time a substantial response rate (42%) with respect to alleviation of anemia. In spite of the high cost and lack of evidence of any impact on survival, alleviation of transfusion-dependent anemia is still a major accomplishment in this disease. In the area of hemolytic anemia, this year's literature provided some useful reminders about transplantation-induced hemolysis (Abstract 116-95-1-8) and the hematologic toxicity of lead (Abstract 116-95-1-9). Paroxysmal nocturnal hemoglobinuria is rapidly shedding its mysteries such that we now understand both the biochemical defect (Abstract 116-95-1-10) and its genetic locus (Abstract 116-95-1-11). The propensity for thrombosis in this disorder appears to be partly explainable by complement-induced platelet membrane changes (Abstract 116-95-3-11). The ambiguities of parvovirus B19 tropism (Abstract 116-95-1-17) and infection (Abstract 116-95-1-13) are also being resolved, and a new and promising therapeutic approach for treating end-stage patients with thalassemia has been described (Abstract 116-95-1-14). The first molecular lesion accounting for familial erythrocytosis has been defined (Abstract 116-95-1–19) and appropriately involves a cytoplasmic segment of the EPO receptor that was previously identified as having a negative regulatory influence. Finally, a follow-up on the treatment of polycythemia vera using α-interferon has been published (Abstract 116-95-1–20). I am a devoted believer in phlebotomy, but there are, of course, situations where other remedies are required, i.e., pruritus, *symptomatic* thrombocytosis (the italics are mine), and organomegaly. Organomegaly is the most difficult to treat, and if α-interferon can correct organomegaly in polycythemia vera, this benefit will surely outweigh its many toxicities.

J.L. Spivak, M.D.

Reference

1. Maier RF, et al: N Engl J Med 330:1173, 1994.

Erythropoietin

Recombinant Erythropoietin Overdose

Brown KR, Carter W Jr, Lombardi GE (St Luke's-Roosevelt Hosp Ctr, New York; Albert Einstein College of Medicine, New York)
Am J Emerg Med 11:619–621, 1993   116-95-1–1

Background.—No cases of nonanemic patients deliberately self-administering recombinant human EPO (rHuEPO) have been documented. One delusional, critically ill patient surreptitiously injected this drug, causing a dangerous increase in hematocrit.

Case Report.—Man, 62, was seen in the emergency department with a 3-day history of worsening shortness of breath and a nonproductive cough. High-concentration oxygen was administered in the ambulance on the way to the hospital. The patient was a retired biomedical engineer and had a medical history that included chronic obstructive lung disease, hypertension, and chronically low hematocrit. He reported using only an aerosolized bronchodilator and antibiotics for a respiratory infection. On physical examination, he was noted to be thin and anxious, with labored breathing and cyanotic, cool, moist skin. He was alert and oriented but agitated. The hemoglobin level was 23.4 g/dL; the hematocrit was 70.4; leukocytes, 12,000; and platelets, 256,000/mm³. The partial pressure of arterial oxygen was 83 mm Hg and the partial pressure of carbon dioxide in arterial blood was 73 mm Hg. Chest radiography showed infiltrates in the right lower lobe and left lingula. The patient was ventilated mechanically, and antibiotics and vasopressor treatment were begun. The patient, communicating by writing, repeatedly reported that his "intravascular volume was low" and that he had hematuria and a "renin defect and fluid problems." He often demanded a transfusion to "correct anemia." His private physician was contacted and reported that this patient had a history of somatic delusions and practiced self-medication. The patient was confronted with this information and he admitted that he had been injecting himself daily with rHuEPO for several months. He had also been taking penicillin, metronidazole, norfloxacin, and ciprofloxacin for 1 week before his hospitalization. With serial phlebotomy and intravenous hydration, his hematocrit gradually returned to 48%. His course was complicated by several episodes of angina, hypertension, and a barotrauma-related pneumothorax that required continued endotracheal intubation. His pneumonia and angina responded quickly to standard therapy. He was eventually transferred to a psychiatric hospital for further care.

Conclusion.—This patient, who had worked in an allied health-care field and had access to rHuEPO, caused his hematocrit to increase to a dangerously high level. The unusual possibility of EPO abuse should be considered in patients with unexplained erythrocytosis.

▶ Given the widespread allegations of EPO abuse by athletes, it was inevitable that abuse would occur under other circumstances. Unfortunately, the case described here is not as straightforward as the authors imply, and their argument is not helped by the omission of relevant data. First, this patient clearly had significant obstructive airway disease, otherwise he could not have achieved a partial pressure of carbon dioxide in arterial blood of 73 mm Hg together with a partial pressure of arterial oxygen of 83 mm Hg and a pH of 7.01 (H_2CO_3, 18 mEq/L) on "high-concentration" oxygen. Although he was said to have a "chronically low hematocrit," the authors (and their reviewers) have done us no service by not providing the actual values. Furthermore, we are also not provided with either the red cell mean corpuscular volume, follow-up blood gases, or serum EPO levels. Thus, more appears to be going on here than simple EPO intoxication, and the possibility of diuretic abuse in this hypertensive patient was also not excluded. As an aside, contrary to the authors' contention, erythrocytosis per se does not comprise pulmonary function. It is also worth noting that if, indeed, the patient truly injected substantial quantities of recombinant EPO, there was no change in his platelet count. I make that point for those who still cling to the notion that EPO can elevate the platelet count. Finally, the patient's delusions are worth mentioning. Like the anorexic who has a body image of obesity, this plethoric fellow considered himself to be anemic. As a corollary, the induction of iron deficiency by phlebotomy would, therefore, serve as a permanent prevention for a recurrent episode. Given the current cost of recombinant EPO, the fact that the patient had a "friend" in the pharmaceutical industry, and the particular delusional system, the possible abuse described in this report, in contrast to that practiced by athletes, is unlikely to be commonly encountered.—J.L. Spivak, M.D.

Adverse Events of Subcutaneous Recombinant Human Erythropoietin Therapy: Results of a Controlled Multicenter European Study

Klinkmann H, Wieczorek L, Scigalla P (Univ of Rostock, Germany; Boehringer Mannheim, Germany)

Artif Organs 17:219–225, 1993   116-95-1–2

Objective.—Many patients with anemia resulting from renal failure have benefited greatly from recombinant human EPO (rHu-EPO). The clinical tolerance of subcutaneously administered rHu-EPO was examined in 362 hemodialysis patients at 16 European centers. All were adults with end-stage renal disease who had been in a dialysis program for at least 6 months.

Methods.—Half of the patients entered the treatment group and received rHu-EPO from the outset, whereas the rest served as a control group for 1 year and then received rHU-EPO in the second year. An initial dose of 3 × 20 units/kg weekly was administered until the target hematocrit of 30–35 volume percent was reached. The total observation time was 266 days.

Findings.—Of a total of 837 adverse effects, 277 were considered serious. Eighteen control patients and 14 in the treated group died. Deaths related to cerebral and pulmonary edema or hyperkalemia were more frequent in treated patients. No tendency toward more frequent hypertension or serious cardiovascular symptoms was evident in patients receiving rHu-EPO. Gastrointestinal and respiratory side effects were less prevalent in the treatment group than in control.

Conclusion.—Subcutaneous treatment with rHu-EPO proved to be safe in this multicenter survey, and it may be even safer than intravenous treatment.

▶ This study documents the adverse effects encountered after EPO therapy in a large number of anemic hemodialysis patients followed longitudinally for 2 years. It differs from previous studies because a more gradual approach to raising the hematocrit was employed. Erythropoietin was administered subcutaneously at 20 units/kg 3 times per week initially, a much lower dose than generally employed but not a more cost-effective dose because it took more than twice as long to reach the target hematocrit. From the perspective of adverse events as compared with a control population, rHu-EPO was remarkably nontoxic except for the expected effects on blood pressure; no increase in vascular access thrombosis was noted. Given the low dose of EPO employed, the occurrence of hypertensive encephalopathy is of interest. Unfortunately, the temporal relationship of this to treatment duration was not provided. Interestingly, except for its effect on blood pressure, EPO had a protective effect with respect to adverse cardiovascular events in this group of patients.—J.L. Spivak, M.D.

Effect of Erythropoietin Therapy and Withdrawal on Blood Coagulation and Fibrinolysis in Hemodialysis Patients

Taylor JE, Belch JJF, McLaren M, Henderson IS, Stewart WK (Ninewells Hosp and Med School, Dundee, Scotland)
Kidney Int 44:182–190, 1993   116-95-1–3

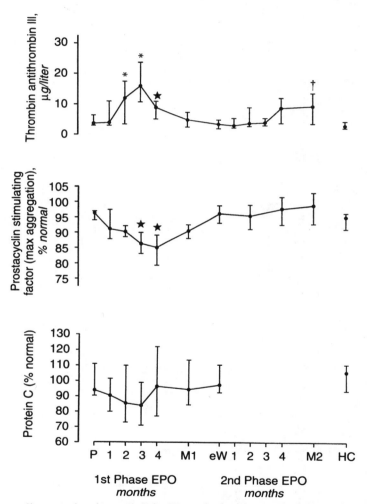

Fig 1–1.—Changes in thrombin-antithrombin III complex (μg/L), prostaglandin I$_2$ stimulating factor (% normal), and protein C (% normal) during EPO therapy. The normal range of thrombin-antithrombin III complex is 1 to 4.1 μg/L. *$P < .01$; ☆$P < .02$; †$P < .05$. (Courtesy of Taylor JE, Belch JJF, McLaren M, et al: *Kidney Int* 44:182–190, 1993.)

Changes in Tissue Plasminogen Activator Antigen, Plasminogen Activator Inhibitor, D-dimer, Erythrocyte Deformability, and Granulocyte Aggregation in Study Patients

	Pre-EPO	1st Maintenance phase (end)	End of washout	2nd Maintenance phase (end)	Controls
Tissue plasminogen activator antigen *% normal*	72 (34–169)	74 (11–251)	129 (29–263)	100 (11–321)	142[a] (82–298)
Plasminogen activator inhibitor *AU/ml*	5.5 (1.0–23.4)	10.9[b] (2.2–25.8)	10.0 (1.0–96,2)	6.5 (0.9–12.4)	15.5[a] (7.6–32.4)
D-dimer *ng/ml*	719 (247–1000)	718 (111–1239)	916[a] (258–1547)	670 (245–2184)	527 (200–1000)
Granulocyte aggregation %	62 (28–86)	57 (27–69)	62 (40–78)	ND	52 (41–59)
Erythrocyte deformability (IRFP)	1.35 (1.27–1.54)	1.36 (1.25–1.50)	1.36 (1.27–1.42)	ND	1.34 (1.27–1.41)

Abbreviation: ND, not done.
Note: Normal ranges are: plasminogen activator inhibitor, 6.7 (2–40) AU/mL; D-dimer, < 400 ng/mL; erythrocyte deformability, 1.11–1.38.
[a] $P < .01$.
[b] $P < .02$ vs. pre-EPO.
(Courtesy of Taylor JE, Belch JJF, McLaren M, et al: *Kidney Int* 44:182–190, 1993.)

Background.—Recombinant human EPO therapy is highly effective in hemodialysis, but its use may enhance the risk of vascular access and extracorporeal thrombosis. To assess these changes and their effect, blood coagulation and fibrinolysis were monitored monthly in patients undergoing hemodialysis during treatment with EPO and after EPO withdrawal.

Methods.—Twenty-one patients undergoing hemodialysis and treated with EPO for anemia solely attributable to renal failure were included. Blood coagulation and fibrinolysis were assessed monthly in the patients treated with EPO and in 4 iron-deficient patients treated with iron dextran infusions alone. Seventeen patients receiving EPO were monitored after a transfusion-free period, and 16 of those patients were also monitored during a second subsequent phase of treatment in which EPO was administered using an alternative route from the first course of treatment. Ten untreated hemodialysis patients with intrinsically high hemoglobin served as controls.

Findings.—The EPO-treated patients had significant increases in the endothelial product factor VIIIvWF antigen (FVIIIvWFAg) and plasma fibrinogen. Levels were similar to those in untreated controls. Levels of FVIIIvWFAg and fibrinogen remained significantly elevated when EPO was withdrawn. Spontaneous, collagen, and adenosine diphosphate-induced platelet aggregation increased after EPO by comparison to normal controls. After EPO withdrawal, there was increased platelet aggregability to collagen and ADP and increased D-dimer. During the first phases of EPO treatment, there were transient but significant changes in plasma measures of the thrombin-antithrombin III complex, prostacyclin-stimulating factor, and protein C. The changes persisted in the thrombin-antithrombin III complex during the second treatment phase (Fig 1–1, table). The route of administration and the dose of EPO had no effect on any parameters. The 4 patients treated with iron dextran had increased platelet aggregation and tissue plasminogen activator antigen in association with a smaller amount of hemoglobin.

Conclusion.—Erythropoietin therapy improves the bleeding tendency of patients undergoing hemodialysis primarily by the influence of red cells on platelet function. The increased red cell mass may be associated with an enhanced risk of vascular access and extracorporeal thrombosis. Monthly monitoring of blood coagulation and fibrinolysis in EPO-treated patients demonstrated that EPO may produce transient changes during the initial months of therapy, after correction of anemia, and after withdrawal. The route of EPO administration and dosage do not appear to influence coagulation changes. Changes in blood coagulation and fibrinolysis during EPO therapy may influence the risk of thrombosis.

▶ The data in this report indicate that EPO induces significant elevations that persist for prolonged periods in plasma proteins including vWF fibrinogen and decreases in antithrombin III, prostacyclin, and protein C. These changes are indicative of a hypercoagulable state. However, in this study, no patient was found to experience either venous or arterial thromboses. Thus, one cannot be certain as to whether these changes actually manifest the thrombotic state. However, these observations should make people aware of this potential problem.

This study unfortunately employed the wrong controls, and the dose of EPO used in the target hemoglobins was also larger than the normal in this situation. The increments in the various coagulant proteins were not impressive, and for the most part, the clotting problems were typical and not unexpected in this patient population.—W.R. Bell, M.D.

Erythropoietin, Protein, and Iron Supplementation and the Prevention of Anaemia of Prematurity

Bechensteen AG, Hågå P, Halvorsen S, Whitelaw A, Liestøl K, Lindemann R, Grøgaard J, Hellebostad M, Saugstad OD, Grønn M, Daae L, Refsum H, Sundal E (Univ of Oslo, Norway)
Arch Dis Child 69:19–23, 1993   116-95-1-4

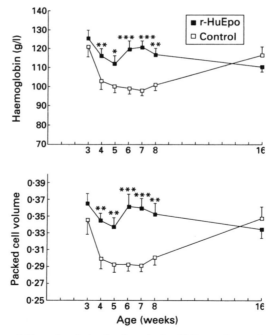

Fig 1-2.—Hemoglobin and packed cell volume in the rHuEpo and control groups. Mean values; *bars* represent standard error. Significant difference between treatment groups and controls: *P < .05; **P < .01, ***P < .001. (Courtesy of Bechensteen AG, Hågå P, Halvorsen S, et al: *Arch Dis Child* 69:19–23, 1993.)

Background.—The decrease in hemoglobin concentration seen in all infants is intensified in preterm infants, mainly as a result of inadequate erythropoiesis. Several studies of the effects of treatment with recombinant human EPO (rHuEPO) have yielded conflicting results. Other studies have shown the importance of nutrition, especially human milk protein and iron, in potentiating erythropoiesis. Protein, rHuEPO, and iron supplementation were combined for the treatment of preterm infants, and the erythropoietic response was observed.

Methods.—Twenty-nine healthy preterm infants, each with a birth weight of 900–1400 g, which was appropriate for gestational age, were entered in a randomized, open, 4-center trial. All infants were breast-fed, and they received oral iron supplements as necessary and human breast milk protein supplements from ages 3–8 weeks. The treatment group of 14 were also treated with subcutaneous rHuEPO 3 times a week from ages 3–7 weeks; 15 infants were in the control group.

Results.—Reticulocytes increased rapidly and significantly in the first 3 weeks of rHuEPO treatment. In the control group, reticulocytes increased normally. The hemoglobin concentration was significantly increased after 1 week of treatment and was sustained throughout treatment (Fig 1-2). Serum iron decreased significantly in the first week of rHuEPO treatment; thereafter iron levels in both groups were equivalent. There were no unexpected findings or significant differences between groups for serum ferritin, total WBC counts, neutrophil counts, or growth. There were no adverse reactions to treatment and no blood pressure differences between groups.

Conclusion.—Preterm infants responded dramatically to exogenous EPO with increased RBC production. The nadir of hemoglobin concentration was similar to that seen in full-term infants. The use of protein and iron supplements explains the clear success of this trial compared with previous studies. Hypertension, neutropenia, and thrombocytosis have been postulated as possible side effects of rHuEPO; these data refute this. Further research should determine the efficacy of this treatment combination on smaller or sick infants.

▶ I was premature in selecting this article for abstraction (no pun intended), but I was searching for some positive data in this area. The pathophysiology of the anemia of prematurity has been well studied, and given the observation that EPO production is reduced in the setting of a full complement of normally responsive erythroid progenitor cells, it was expected that rHuEPO would correct anemia in premature infants. Reality clashed with expectations, however, and it quickly became apparent that the situation was more complex than initially appreciated. To date, there have been 10 published trials of rHuEPO in anemic premature infants, and better definition of the inherent problems is now available. Given an adequate dose of EPO and adequate quantities of supplemental iron and milk proteins, Bechensteen and colleagues have demonstrated that in "healthy, orally fed, well nourished infants" with birth weights greater than 900–1400 g, rHuEPO prevents significant anemia. Unfortunately, given current conservative transfusion practices and advances in neonatal care, infants such as those studied by Bechensteen et al. are not only unlikely to receive blood, but given the improved safety of blood products, their risks from transfusion are now low. The type of infant studied by Bechensteen et al. is also the most likely to respond to EPO. The experience in this regard with smaller, sicker infants is less compelling. On the subject of my premature action, a much larger study has just been published (1) that further defines the benefits of therapy, and I also recommend Dr. Strauss's editorial comments in the same issue (2). You can be sure that both will make an appearance next year.—J.L. Spivak, M.D.

References

1. Maier RF, et al: N Engl J Med 330:1173, 1994.
2. Strauss RG: N Engl J Med 330:1227, 1994.

Erythropoietin Increases Cytosolic Free Calcium Concentration in Vascular Smooth Muscle Cells

Neusser M, Tepel M, Zidek W (Med Univ-Poliklinik, Münster, Germany)
Cardiovasc Res 27:1233–1236, 1993   116-95-1–5

Background.—When EPO is used to treat renal anemia, hypertension is a common side effect. The mechanism by which EPO causes hypertension is not well understood but may be a result of direct vasopressor effects of EPO, which have recently been demonstrated. As calcium concentration is 1 factor that determines vascular tone in smooth muscle cells, the effect of EPO on calcium concentration was investigated in these cells.

Methods.—Primary cultures of vascular smooth muscle cells were obtained from male Wistar-Kyoto rat aortas. Calcium concentration and the effect of EPO were measured with the fluorescent dye, fura2.

Results.—The mean resting calcium concentration was 90.8 nM. Addition of 100 units of EPO per mL significantly increased the calcium concentration to 112.3 nM, and addition of 250 U/mL significantly increased the calcium concentration to 128.4 nM. Preincubation with EPO caused a dose-dependent increase in angiotensin II–induced changes in calcium concentration.

Conclusion.—One cause of EPO-induced hypertension may be an increased peripheral vascular resistance resulting from an increase in calcium concentration in vascular smooth muscle cells.

▶ Given the relatively restricted action of EPO to erythroid and possibly megakaryocyte lineages, this is a surprising article. These calcium effects could explain alterations in vascular smooth muscle tone and hypertension, and they certainly suggest that vascular smooth muscle must respond to EPO, presumably via ligand receptor interactions. Clearly, the next step will be a demonstration of EPO receptors on these cell types.—P.J. Quesenberry, M.D.

Serum Form of the Erythropoietin Receptor Identified by a Sequence-Specific Peptide Antibody

Baynes RD, Reddy GK, Shih YJ, Skikne BS, Cook JD (Kansas Univ, Kansas City)

Blood 82:2088–2095, 1993   116-95-1–6

Background.—Several receptors in the hemopoietin superfamily have been found to have naturally occurring alternatively spliced messenger RNA encoding for potentially secreted soluble forms. These include IL-4, IL-5, IL-6, IL-7, G-CSF, and GM-CSF. Soluble forms of the EPO receptor were searched for in human serum.

Methods.—Polyclonal antibody against an amine-terminal peptide sequence was used in the extracellular domain. Serum samples were obtained from healthy volunteers and patients with various hematologic disorders, including patients with iron deficiency anemia, those with chronic renal failure receiving maintenance dialysis, and those with chronic inflammatory disease, sickle cell anemia, β-thalassemia major, or meagaloblastic anemia from vitamin B_{12} deficiency.

Findings.—Western blotting revealed a protein with a molecular mass of 34 Kd in sera from patients with enhanced erythropoiesis, including sickle cell anemia, thalassemia, and megaloblastic anemia. The protein was rarely found in normal sera. However, it appeared when normal participants were treated with recombinant EPO and disappeared after full treatment of patients with megaloblastic anemia from vitamin B_{12} deficiency. It was not found after myeloablation for bone marrow transplantation but was detected with marrow engraftment (Fig 1–3).

Conclusion.—A 34-Kd protein that highly correlated with enhanced erythropoiesis was found in human sera. The protein could be detected using antibody against a sequence of the amino-terminus of the receptor ectodomain in the area most remote from the cell membrane. This antibody is specific for EPO receptors.

▶ The EPO receptor is a member of the hematopoietic growth factor receptor superfamily, a receptor family that is characterized by the presence in the N-terminal domain of 4 closely spaced cysteine residues and a Trp-Ser Xaa-Trp-Ser motif that is adjacent to the transmembrane domain (1). Other members of this family include the receptors for IL-2, IL-3, IL-4, IL-6, IL-7, GM-CSF, G-CSF, leukocyte inhibitory factor, growth hormone, and prolactin. Soluble forms of a number of these receptors including those for IL-2, IL-4, IL-6, IL-7, leukocyte inhibitory factor, GM-CSF, G-CSF, growth hormone, and prolactin have been identified, and studies of EPO receptor messenger RNA expression have identified a soluble and potentially secretable form of this re-

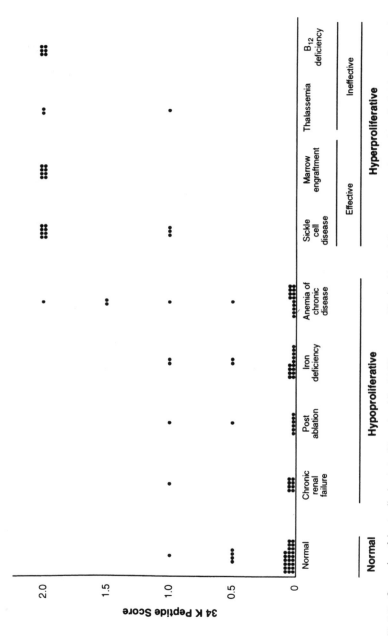

Fig 1-3.—Scatterplot of the visually determined intensity of the 34-Kd protein on Western blot with S25 amino-terminal peptide antibody of sera of normal research subjects and those with a number of conditions featuring altered erythropoietic activity. (Courtesy of Baynes RD, Reddy GK, Shih YJ, et al: *Blood* 82:2088–2095, 1993.)

ceptor. Now Baynes and colleagues, who previously provided data on soluble transferrin receptors, have identified a soluble EPO receptor in human serum with a molecular weight that approximates that of the extracytoplasmic domain of the full-length EPO receptor. The presence of the soluble form of the EPO receptor in the circulation correlated with enhanced erythropoiesis because the protein was easy to detect in patients with sickle cell disease, thalassemia, or megaloblastic anemia, and during marrow engraftment or treatment with recombinant EPO, and it disappeared after vitamin B_{12} therapy in patients with B_{12}-deficient anemia. Since the publication of this paper, Baynes and colleagues have developed an enzyme-linked immunosorbent assay using a more informative antibody and were easily able to detect soluble EPO receptors in normal individuals with levels that were about one third as high as those found in patients with sickle cell anemia but 10-fold greater than after myeloablation for marrow transplantation.

The function of soluble growth factor receptors is not understood (IL-6 possibly being the exception), and recent data from Dr. Winkelmann's (2) laboratory indicate that the putative form of the soluble EPO receptor, based on amplified receptor transcripts, does not bind EPO. Corroboration, of course, will require the isolation of these receptors from the plasma. The presence of circulating soluble EPO receptors could potentially interfere with EPO immunoassays unless the antibody recognized a nonfunctional epitope, in which case total, not free, EPO would be measured. This would also apply to EPO bioassays without the exception of a distinction between total and free hormone. It is now tempting to speculate that the extremely high EPO levels associated with marrow aplasia, which were once erroneously thought to be due to reduced intracellular degradation of the hormone, actually reflect the absence of soluble receptor production. Because the metabolic fate of circulating EPO is unknown, it is possible that binding to soluble receptors could facilitate EPO degradation or even transport through endothelial barriers. In this regard, a more rapid decline in serum EPO is seen in anemic, iron- or B_{12}-deficient patients after nutrient replacement than can be accounted for by the change in red cell mass; this might be explained by enhanced soluble receptor production. Whatever the situation, it will be interesting to learn about the behavior of these receptors in polycythemia vera and other perturbations of erythropoiesis and to determine whether immunoprecipitates of circulating soluble receptors contain EPO.—J.L. Spivak, M.D.

References

1. Bazan JF: *Biochem Biophys Res Commun* 164:788, 1989.
2. Harris EW, Winkelmann JC: *Blood* 80:341a, 1992.

Treatment of the Anemia of Myelodysplastic Syndromes Using Recombinant Human Granulocyte Colony-Stimulating Factor in Combination With Erythropoietin

Negrin RS, Stein R, Vardiman J, Doherty K, Cornwell J, Krantz S, Greenberg PL (Stanford Univ, Calif; Vanderbilt Med Ctr, Nashville, Tenn; Univ of Chicago; et al)
Blood 82:737–743, 1993   116-95-1–7

Background.—The myelodysplastic syndromes (MDSs) are characterized by chronic cytopenias. Patients are predisposed to symptomatic anemias necessitating RBC transfusions, infection, bleeding, and a conversion to acute myeloid leukemia. The results of treatment of 28 patients with MDS with recombinant human G-CSF and recombinant human EPO were evaluated.

Methods.—Of 28 patients beginning the protocol, 24 completed it and were evaluable for erythroid responses. The treatment began with G-CSF, 1 µg/kg in daily subcutaneous injections, and was adjusted to normalize or double neutrophil counts. While continuing G-CSF treatment, EPO was administered in daily subcutaneous injections at 100 units/kg and escalated to 150 and 300 units/kg every 4 weeks.

Findings.—Forty-two percent of the patients had erythroid responses. All had neutrophil responses. Six patients previously undergoing RBC transfusions no longer needed them during the treatment period. Erythroid responses were independent of patient age, French-American-British subtype, disease duration, previous RBC transfusion requirements, or cytogenetic abnormalities at initial evaluation. Pretreatment serum EPO levels were lower in patients with erythroid responses than in patients not responding. Generally, the combined treatment was well tolerated.

Conclusion.—It is possible to administer 2 cytokines together without a negative interaction. This combination of G-CSF and EPO produced erythroid and myeloid responses in a substantial proportion of patients with MDS.

▶ This is an important and long-awaited study. Judging from our outpatient hematology clinic experience as well as the published literature, the anemic patients who are the most difficult to manage are those with myelodysplasia. They are the patients who are not only the most likely to require chronic transfusion therapy, but also the least likely to derive substantial benefit from such therapy. Based on a recent literature survey, recombinant EPO was immediately widely embraced for its potential to alleviate transfusion requirements in anemic patients. Unfortunately, it has proved to be less effective in myelodysplasia than virtually any other situation. To date, experience with over 300 patients has been reported, with an overall response rate of approximately 20% (range 0% to 42%). It is difficult to compare different studies because of the variation in dose and route for EPO as well as the variation in patient population composition. An unexplained feature of myelodysplasia is that serum EPO levels can be either inappropriately elevated or inappropriately reduced and, as has been observed in a number of studies, the higher the serum EPO level, the less likely it is that a response will be obtained. French-American-British classification also seems to have a role because those most likely to respond to EPO alone have the milder forms of myelodysplasia, refractory anemia, or refractory sideroblastic anemia. The possibility that growth factor combinations might be effective was suggested in an earlier study by this same group employing G-CSF alone in myelodysplastic patients. Of course, G-CSF is preferable to GM-CSF because its toxicity is less and because the combination of G-CSF and EPO did not enhance leukemic blast colony formation more than that observed with G-CSF alone, in contrast to its effect in combination with GM-CSF or IL-3 (1). In the study abstracted here, a response rate (42%) much greater than that obtained with EPO alone was achieved without any negative effects. Interestingly, age, gender, French-American-British subtype, duration of disease, and cytogenetic abnormalities did not affect responsiveness, but pretreatment serum EPO levels were a prognostic indicator. The dose of EPO was fairly substantial (100 units/kg daily escalating to 300 units/kg). Splenic pain was the major toxicity in 3 patients; 2 patients progressed to acute leukemia, but a relationship to therapy is uncertain.

These are highly encouraging results, but obviously more data are necessary to determine whether the observed responses are durable and whether there will be a positive influence on overall survival. However, even if survival is not prolonged, assuming it is not reduced, an improvement in the quality of life would make such combination therapy worth the expense. Hopefully, such information will be forthcoming soon.—J.L. Spivak, M.D.

Reference

1. Asano Y, et al: *Blood* 72:1682, 1988.

Hemolytic Anemias

Immune Hemolytic Anemia After Renal Transplantation Secondary to ABO-Minor-Mismatch Between the Donor and Recipient
Gregoire JR (Mayo Clinic, Rochester, Minn)
J Am Soc Nephrol 4:1122–1126, 1993   116-95-1–8

Background.—A patient experiencing immune hemolytic anemia after renal transplantation was described. Hemolysis was caused by an ABO-minor-mismatch between the donor and recipient.

Case Report.—Man, 52, with end-stage renal disease secondary to IgA nephropathy was evaluated for renal transplantation. Hemoglobin was 12.4 g/dL, WBC count was 5.5×10^9/L, and creatinine was 8.6 mg/dL. Both a direct antiglobulin test and an antibody screen test were negative. The patient received a

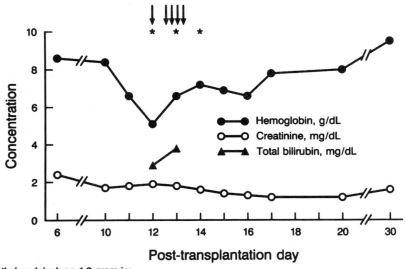

Fig 1–4.—Course of events. (Courtesy of Gregoire JR: *J Am Soc Nephrol* 4:1122–1126, 1993.)

1-haplotype, living-donor kidney from his brother. However, an ABO-mismatch existed, as the recipient was A_1 Rhesus-positive, whereas the donor was O Rhesus-positive. Intraoperative or immediate postoperative transfusions were not administered. Triple-drug immunosuppression with cyclosporine, prednisone, and azathioprine was administered, and after an uneventful hospitalization, the patient was discharged on postoperative day 5. On day 6, the patient was readmitted because of severe, diffuse, lower abdominal pain. Treatment with cyclosporine, prednisone, azathioprine, extended-release nifedipine, clonidine, trimethoprim-sulfamethoxazole, acyclovir, nystatin suspension, and ferrous sulfate was begun. Physical examination revealed moderate to severe abdominal tenderness in both lower quadrants. Hemoglobin was 8.9 g/dL; WBC, 8.5 × 10⁹/L; platelets, 312 × 10⁹/L; and creatinine, 2.4 mg/dL. On day 10, hemoglobin was 8.4 g/dL, which decreased to 5.1 g/dL by day 12, and total bilirubin was 2.9 mg/dL. A blood smear revealed moderate polychromasia and spherocytes and slight anisocytes, poikilocytes, microcytes, macrocytes, and RBC stippling. On days 12–14, methylprednisone, 1 g/day, was administered intravenously. During the ensuing week, a tapering dose of prednisone was administered, ranging from 100 to 40 mg/day. The prednisone dose was adjusted to protocol thereafter. Trimethoprim-sulfamethoxazole was discontinued. On day 12, the patient received 1 unit of group A Rhesus-positive blood, and on day 13 he received 4 units of group O Rhesus-positive blood. These were the only transfusions he received. On day 15, an antibody screen indicated the presence of antibody against panel A_1 cells. The patient was started with oral folate, 2 mg/day, and was discharged on day 16. At discharge, hemoglobin was 6.6 g/dL, increasing to 9.5 g/dL by day

30 (Fig 1-4). On day 93 post-transplantation, no evidence of hemolysis was noted. Hemoglobin was 12.2 mg/dL, direct and indirect antiglobulin tests were negative, reticulocytes, bilirubin, and lactate dehydrogenase were normal, and creatinine was 1.9 mg/dL. A blood smear revealed slight rouleaux formation only.

Conclusion.—This type of hemolysis generally occurs 1–2 weeks post-transplantation, is limited in duration, and can be severe. If transfusions are necessary, blood of the donor's type should be used.

▶ I chose this case report as a reminder because we have recently seen this complication. It is not common; therefore, the cause of the anemia is frequently missed. It was missed in our case (which was why we were consulted) and in this report, where the patient was given the wrong type of blood initially. Of course, in the post-transplantation setting, there are many suspects in addition to graft-vs.-host disease as a cause for anemia, including the immunosuppressive drugs cyclosporine and azathioprine, other drugs such as the sulfonamide derivative employed, parvovirus B19, other viruses, hematophagic histiocytosis, and allograft rejection. In our renal transplant patient, to speed the process along, we reinstituted EPO therapy. This might have accelerated the recovery of the patient described here.—J.L. Spivak, M.D.

Hemolytic Anemia Associated With Lead Poisoning From Shotgun Pellets and the Response to Succimer Treatment
Aly MH, Kim HC, Renner SW, Boyarsky A, Kosmin M, Paglia DE (Univ of Medicine and Dentistry of New Jersey, New Brunswick; West Los Angeles VA Med Ctr; Univ of California, Los Angeles)
Am J Hematol 44:280–283, 1993   116-95-1-9

Background.—A patient with symptomatic lead poisoning and severe hemolytic anemia caused by retained shot gun pellets was described. There is a misconception that retained lead pellets will not result in toxicity when lodged in soft tissue; however, soft tissue retention may facilitate lead absorption more so than lead retained in hard surfaces such as bone. This fallacy resulted in a 4-month diagnostic delay in a patient, despite several clinical indications of lead toxicity.

Case Report.—Man, 37, experienced a shotgun injury to the chest, managed by wound débridement and chest tube insertion. The patient was discharged with a hemoglobin of 9 g/dL. The lead pellets remained lodged on the inner and outer chest wall. Seven weeks later, the patient was readmitted because of abdominal pain, generalized weakness, and weight loss. The hemoglobin level had decreased to 7.2 g/dL, and the reticulocyte count was 13%. Other than intense erythroid hyperplasia, a bone marrow examination was normal. The patient was treated with 4 units of RBC and discharged to outpatient follow-up.

Course of Lead Poisoning From Shotgun Pellet

Date of admission	Reasons for admission	Hb (g%)	Blood lead level (<15 μg/dl)	Comments
6/1/91 1st admission	Shotgun injury to the chest	14.0	Not done	Wound debridement and chest tube; 2 unit RBC
7/22/91 2nd admission	Abdominal pain Anemia	7.2	ND	Reticulocyte 13%; transfused 4 units of RBC
8/9/91 3rd admission	Removal of subcutaneous pellets	9.3	ND	4 units of RBC
10/11/91 4th admission	Recurrent anemia	9.6→5.7	300→79	4 unit RBC transfusion; chelation therapy with DMSA
11/21/91 5th admission	Removal of pellets from the pleura	14.1	ND	
12/4/91	2nd chelation therapy	14.1	90→15	Resolution of lead poisoning symptoms
1/19/92	Symptom free	15.0	>15	Regained weight; 5' pyrimidine nucleotidase level normal

(Courtesy of Aly MH, Kim HC, Renner SW, et al: *Am J Hematol* 44:280–283, 1993.)

Nine weeks after the accident, the patient was readmitted for removal of lead pellets causing discomfort with friction on his back. Approximately 50% of the pellets were removed, and the patient again received 4 units of RBC before discharge. Two months later, the patient reported recurrent and severe abdominal pain, night sweats, increased fatigue, and a total weight loss of 60 lb. Hemoglobin was 9.6 g/dL on admission, and the reticulocyte count was 20.1%. Repeat bone marrow examination revealed intense erythroid hyperplasia, abundant ringed sideroblasts, and normal storage iron. Lead levels were obtained and were well above normal limits. Treatment with Succimer, a new chelating agent, was initiated at 10 mg/kg orally 3 times daily for 5 days and tapered to 10 mg/kg twice daily for the subsequent 14 days. By the third day of treatment, symptoms had improved. Hemoglobin increased from 8 to 12 g/dL by the end of treatment, with normalization of bilirubin, lactic dehydrogenase, and reticulocyte count. After the first course of treatment, retained pellets were removed from the pleura and subcutaneous tissue. A second course of chelation therapy was completed, and the patient experienced resolution of lead poisoning symptoms and normalization of blood lead levels. Both courses of Succimer treatment were well tolerated by the patient, without any evident side effects. Seven months after the initial accident the patient was symptom-free, had regained weight, and had a normal pyrimidine 5'-nucleotidase level (table).

Conclusion.—Lead toxicity, although rare in adults, can lead to potentially fatal outcome if overlooked during differential diagnoses. In treating such patients, Succimer has the advantage of oral administration with far less toxicity than other commonly used agents. The importance of resecting retained lead pellets to reduce the risk of continued toxicity is also demonstrated.

▶ I included this interesting case report because it is important for hematologists to always expect the unexpected, and lead intoxication has certainly been documented to occur in unexpected ways. In Baltimore, with its past history of ship building, it is still possible to encounter cases of saturnine gout in individuals who worked with lead paint. Some years ago, there was also a report of lead intoxication due to exposure in a shooting gallery (1). Lead poisoning due to retained bullets has been well documented previously, but that did not initially benefit the patient described here. I suspect that earlier scrutiny of a blood smear would have defined the problem, but, unfortunately, that practice has been abandoned in many hospitals except when hematologists are involved. In this regard, let me call to your attention a nice review of lead intoxication in adults published in *Medicine* (2). An important diagnostic point raised by the case described by Aly et al. is that whereas in most cases of chronic lead poisoning, anemia is mild and basophilic stippling absent, with acute lead intoxication, hemolysis, basophilic stippling, and severe anemia are common and are usually associated with abdominal pain.—J.L. Spivak, M.D.

References

1. Fischbein A, et al: *JAMA* 241:1141, 1979.
2. Cullen MR, et al: *Medicine* 62:221, 1983.

Specific Defect in *N*-Acetylglucosamine Incorporation in the Biosynthesis of the Glycosylphosphatidylinositol Anchor in Cloned Cell Lines From Patients With Paroxysmal Nocturnal Hemoglobinuria

Hillmen P, Bessler M, Mason PJ, Watkins WM, Luzzatto L (Hammersmith Hosp, London)

Proc Natl Acad Sci U S A 90:5272–5276, 1993   116-95-1-10

Background.—Membrane-bound proteins are attached to the cell membrane in 1 of 2 ways: either with a membrane-spanning hydrophobic amino acid domain or by covalent linkage to a glycosylphosphatidylinositol (GPI) structure, as shown in Figure 1–5. Paroxysmal nocturnal hemoglobinuria (PNH) is caused by abnormal cells cloned from a mutation in a multipotent hemopoietic stem cell. These abnormal cells lack all of the GPI-linked proteins. Studies have shown differential reductions of these proteins in PNH types II and III red cells, which explains their differing complement sensitivity. The GPI-linked protein deficiency may be caused by a biochemical defect in GPI synthesis.

Methods.—The PNH cell lines derived from 9 different patients were analyzed by flow cytometry and labeled with mannose, *myo*-inositol, and uridine diphospho-N-acetyl[³H]glucosamine (UDP-[³H]GlcNAc).

Results.—The PNH cell lines did not produce the complete anchor precursor or the normal mannose-containing GPI biosynthetic intermediates, suggesting that the defect occurs earlier in the pathway. The PNH cells did normally incorporate *myo*-[³H]inositol, showing that they could produce Man-GlcN-phosphatidylinositol, an early intermediate in GPI synthesis. None of the PNH cells incorporated GlcNAc normally. When normal and PNH cells were mixed, GlcNAc was incorporated normally,

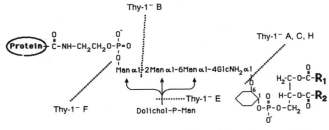

Fig 1–5.—Anchor structure of GPI. Sites of biosynthetic defects characterized in various Thy1⁻ mouse mutant cell lines are shown by *dotted lines.* R₁ and R₂ represent fatty acyl groups. (Courtesy of Hillmen P, Bessler M, Mason PJ, et al: *Proc Natl Acad Sci U S A* 90:5272–5276, 1993.)

indicating that PNH cells do not inhibit GlcNAc incorporation and that other GPI-anchor biosynthetic enzymes in PNH cells function normally.

Discussion.—In all 9 patients, including patients with PNH types II or III, the defective step occurs at the same point in the GPI biosynthetic pathway. The defect was localized at the first step of GlcNAc incorporation, which confirms a probable deficiency of UDP-GlcNAc:phosphatidylinositol-α-1, 6-N-acetylglucosaminyltransferase. This results in a blockage of the development from UDP-GlcNAc to Man-GlcN-phosphatidylinositol.

Abnormalities of PIG-A Transcripts in Granulocytes From Patients With Paroxysmal Nocturnal Hemoglobinuria

Miyata T, Yamada N, Iida Y, Nishimura J, Takeda J, Kitani T, Kinoshita T
(Osaka Univ, Japan; Nagoya Univ, Japan)
N Engl J Med 330:249–255, 1994
116-95-1–11

Background.—Paroxysmal nocturnal hemoglobinuria (PNH) is an acquired blood cell disorder caused by the deficient synthesis, by hematopoietic cells deriving from an abnormal stem cell, of the glycosyl-phosphatidylinositol molecules that serve to anchor proteins to the cell membrane. A previous study of 2 patients with PNH demonstrated that the disease was caused by the gene *PIG-A* (phosphatidylinositol glycan class A), a component of glycosyl-phosphatidylinositol synthesis.

Objective and Methods.—An attempt was made to characterize the somatically acquired abnormalities of *PIG-A* by examining granulocytes from 15 patients with PNH. The cellular contents of CD55 and CD59 were determined by fluorescence-activated flow cytometry. Gene transcripts were reverse-transcribed, amplified by the PCR technique, and cloned into plasmids. The structure of the cloned complementary DNA was analyzed by nucleotide sequencing, and it was tested for its ability to restore the abnormal phenotype of a gene-deficient cell line after transfection.

Findings.—Of the 15 patients, 3 had varying patterns of abnormal-sized *PIG-A* transcripts, and 1 had a very low level of transcript (table). In each of the 11 patients with normal-sized transcripts, the transfection assay showed that some of the transcripts were nonfunctional. The proportion of nonfunctional gene transcripts correlated with that of affected granulocytes. Sequencing demonstrated somatic mutations in 2 instances.

Conclusion.—It appears that *PIG-A* is responsible for somatic mutation, causing most, if not all, cases of PNH.

▶ Paroxysmal nocturnal hemoglobinuria is a rare disorder that gets publicity well out of proportion to its frequency, owing to the multifaceted nature of its clinical manifestations. Additionally, each passing year brings more insight

Results of *PIG-A* Messenger RNA Analyses in Patients With PNH

PATIENT No.	FLOW CYTOMETRY		REVERSE TRANSCRIPTION AND PCR*	TRANSFECTION
	ERYTHROCYTES	GRANULOCYTES		
	% deficient cells			no. of nonfunctional clones/ no. tested (%)
Patients with PNH				
1	98	95	100	100	Abnormal size	5/5 (100)
2	75	44	90	90	Abnormal size	5/5 (100)
3	68	73	96	97	Normal size	18/20 (90)
4	85	59	50	50	Normal size	11/22 (50)
5	63	67	77	65	Normal size	10/20 (50)
6	46	26	73	72	Normal size	12/17 (71)
7	98	85	63	60	Normal size	11/18 (61)
8	53	42	39	37	Normal size	8/19 (42)
9	97	93	95	95	Normal size	20/20 (100)
10	15	25	8	12	Normal size	8/21 (38)
11	50	38	83	83	Normal size	15/20 (75)
12	79	90	94	94	Normal size	19/20 (95)
13	75	75	89	87	Normal size	18/20 (90)
14†	37	46	44	43	Abnormal size	5/5 (100)
15	63	75	95	99	Very few transcripts	—
16	29	46	96	98	Abnormal size ‡	5/5 (100)§
Normal subjects				
N1	0	0	0	0	Normal size	3/15 (20)
N2	0	0	0	0	Normal size	2/10 (20)

* Entries in this column refer to the size or quantity of the polymerase chain reaction (PCR) products.
† Data for this patient were obtained from bone marrow samples.
‡ The affected B-lymphoblastoid cell line, rather than granulocytes, was used in this analysis.
(Courtesy of Miyata T, Yamada N, Iida Y, et al: N Engl J Med 330:249–255, 1994.)

into its pathophysiology, and this year is no exception. In Abstract 116-95-1-10, Dr. Hillmen and colleagues pinpoint the biochemical defect for the loss of GPI-linked membrane proteins to an abnormality in N-acetyl-glucosamine incorporation in nascent GPI molecules. Abstract 116-95-1-11 defines the gene *PIG-A*, which is involved in the early stages of GPI synthesis as the site of the genetic defects responsible for impaired N-acetylglucosamine incorporation. Interestingly, the genetic abnormality within *PIG-A* responsible for impaired GPI synthesis is heterogenous. Whether the *PIG-A* gene is involved in the defective stem cell proliferation that characterizes PNH remains to be determined.—J.L. Spivak, M.D.

Sickle Cell Disease

A Randomized Study of Outpatient Treatment With Ceftriaxone for Selected Febrile Children With Sickle Cell Disease

Wilimas JA, Flynn PM, Harris S, Day SW, Smith R, Chesney PJ, Rodman JH, Eguiguren JM, Fairclough DL, Wang WC (St Jude Children's Research Hosp,

Memphis, Tenn; LeBonheur Children's Med Ctr, Memphis, Tenn; Univ of Tennessee, Memphis)
N Engl J Med 329:472–476, 1993   116-95-1–12

Background. —Because children with sickle cell disease are susceptible to pneumococcal sepsis, they are usually hospitalized for antibiotic treatment when a fever develops. In selected cases, outpatient treatment may be a less expensive, safe alternative.

Methods. —Children aged 6 months to 12 years with sickle hemoglobinopathies and temperatures above 38.5°C were randomly assigned to inpatient or outpatient groups after emergency room evaluation. Children at greater risk for sepsis or with sickle cell disease complications were excluded and treated as inpatients. All children initially received ceftriaxone, 50 mg per kg of body weight, intravenously. Children in the outpatient group returned for a second dose of ceftriaxone 24 hours later. Inpatients were treated directly by their physicians.

Findings. —None of the 86 children in either group had sepsis, compared with 6 of the 70 children excluded from randomization because of increased risk. In the outpatient group, consisting of 44 patients, 11 subsequent hospitalizations were needed within 2 weeks of treatment. Only 1 child in the inpatient group needed rehospitalization. Outpatient treatment saved a mean $1,195 per febrile episode. Children randomized to the inpatient group had a median hospital stay of 3 days, compared with a median of 4 days for the high-risk inpatients. The reasons for children being assigned to the primary higher-risk group are shown in the table.

Reasons for Assignment to the Primary
Higher-Risk Group

Exclusion Criterion	No. (%) of Episodes
Seriously ill appearance	1 (1)
Severe pain	11 (13)
Temperature >40°C	29 (34)
Hemoglobin level, white-cell count, platelet count*	12 (14)
Pulmonary infiltrate	20 (23)
Poor fluid intake, decreased urine output	8 (9)
Previous sepsis	5 (6)

* A hemoglobin level below 5 g/dL; WBC count below 5,000/mm^3 or above 30,000/mm^3; or a platelet count below 100,000/mm^3.
(Courtesy of Wilimas JA, Flynn PM, Harris S, et al: *N Engl J Med* 329:472–476, 1993.)

Conclusion.—Using conservative eligibility criteria, at least half of the febrile episodes among children with sickle cell disease can be safely treated on an outpatient basis. This approach is not only more cost-effective but is well received by parents.

▶ The general thrust of medical economics is going to encourage more of this type of approach because we simply cannot afford to behave otherwise. In this particular instance, however, the benefits were not merely economic but also accrued to the patients involved. Dr. Serjeant has a thoughtful editorial in the same issue (1) that provides an excellent perspective on the delivery of outpatient care for sickle cell anemia patients.—J.L. Spivak, M.D.

Reference

1. Serjeant GR: N *Engl J Med* 329:501, 1993.

Human Parvovirus Infection in Homozygous Sickle Cell Disease

Serjeant GR, Serjeant BE, Thomas PW, Anderson MJ, Patou G, Pattison JR (Univ of the West Indies, Kingston, Jamaica; Univ College and Middlesex School of Medicine, London)
Lancet 341:1237–1240, 1993 116-95-1–13

Background.—Increased erythropoiesis maintains hemoglobin in patients with sickle cell disease. With aplastic crisis comes destruction of erythrocyte precursors, resulting in hemoglobin decline. The characteristics of aplastic crisis suggest an infectious cause. Human parvovirus infection B19 and aplastic crisis in patients with homozygous sickle cell

B19 Infections in SS and AA Genotypes

	No in study	No infected	% infected by 5 years	% infected by 10 years	% infected by 15 years	Comparison of survival curves*
Genotype						
AA	239	73	5·3	25·3	37·2	p=0·30
SS	107	33	5·9	31·1	40·0	
Sex within AA genotype						
Male	115	33	5·0	24·3	34·8	p=0·35
Female	124	40	5·5	26·2	39·5	
Sex within SS genotype						
Male	49	14	4·8	26·5	34·2	p=0·22
Female	58	19	7·0	35·6	45·8	

* Significance assessed with Lee-Desu statistic.
(Courtesy of Serjeant GR, Serjeant BE, Thomas PW, et al: *Lancet* 341:1237–1240, 1993.)

disease have been found at the same time during epidemics. Analysis of B19 and aplasia epidemiology may be useful for the management of sickle cell disease.

Methods.—Of 100,000 consecutive normal deliveries, 308 children with a sickle cell genotype were matched with 239 controls with normal hemoglobin. They were followed from birth with annual serum samples to determine the incidence of both B19 infection and aplastic crisis (defined as a daily decline in hemoglobin of more than 3 g/dL and either no peripheral blood reticulocytes or a daily increase indicating recovery).

Results.—Infection with B19 occurred equally in both sickle cell and normal hemoglobin genotypes (table). Infection with B19 was associated with all cases of aplastic crisis, although 20% of infected patients did not experience aplasia. Serologic IgG responses to B19 infection were similar in both genotypes; 45% of patients with sickle cell genotype maintained high IgG concentrations longer than 5 years, but no patients had more than 1 aplastic crisis, suggesting lifelong immunity. Hematologic effects of B19 did not differ between groups. An unexplained lack of hematologic effects occurred in 13 patients showing B19 seroconversion.

Discussion.—Aplasia generally lasts 7–10 days. However, in patients with sickle cell disease, this length exceeds the mean red cell survival, which leads to profound anemia requiring transfusion. Infection with B19 correlates with aplastic crisis in a number of hematologic diseases, but the relation is unclear. These findings did not reveal B19 influence on hemoglobin F or α-thalassemia, which are known to determine erythrocyte survival. However, the long immunity after B19 infection suggests that development of a B19 vaccine could be an important preventive treatment for patients with sickle cell disease.

▶ This useful study documents the epidemiology of parvovirus B19 infection in both patients with sickle cell disease and a cohort of controls with normal hemoglobin. Infection with B19 was consistently epidemic, and anemia was not a predisposing factor. Interestingly, a small number of infected patients with sickle cell disease did not manifest hematologic changes whereas some infected patients failed to seroconvert. Infection appeared to confer long-term immunity, even in those without evidence of seroconversion. Given the latter fact and the 40% to 60% incidence of B19 acquisition during childhood, a B19 vaccine would be useful. Because B19 infections tend to be epidemic, discovery of infection in a patient with sickle cell disease should lead to immediate evaluation of at-risk siblings. In this regard, I am reminded of the report years ago of glue sniffing–induced aplasia in a patient with sickle cell disease whose siblings remarkably shared the same consequence. This was obviously an example of unrecognized B19 infection.—J.L. Spivak, M.D.

Thalassemia

Brief Report: Treatment With Azacitidine of Patients With End-Stage β-Thalassemia

Lowrey CH, Nienhuis AW (Dartmouth-Hitchcock Med Ctr, Lebanon, NH; Natl Heart, Lung, and Blood Inst, Bethesda, Md)
N Engl J Med 329:845–848, 1993   116-95-1–14

Background.—Treatment of severe β-thalassemia relies on regular erythrocyte transfusions, which can produce serious adverse effects. The use of the nucleoside analog azacitidine to stimulate transcription of the fetal globin genes may be an alternative to regular transfusions. The effect of this treatment in 3 patients with end-stage β-thalassemia, in whom continued transfusion was no longer beneficial, was reported.

Case 1.—Man, 50, had β-thalassemia intermedia and a hemoglobin level of 6.2 g/dL without transfusion. Severe iron overload had developed several years earlier. His condition worsened despite daily deferoxamine, and he had congestive heart failure. After the first cycle of azacitidine, 2 mg/kg/day for 4 days, the

Hematologic Responses of 3 Patients With β-Thalassemia to Azacitidine

VARIABLE	PATIENT 1	PATIENT 2	PATIENT 3
Age (yr)	50	30	32
Hemoglobin (g/dl)			
No transfusion	6.2±0.27	3.4±0.17	3.2±0.24
Azacitidine			
Peak	10.6±0.60†	6.3±0.70†	6.3, 6.3
Trough	9.6±0.75†	5.6±0.82†	4.7, 4.7
Fetal hemoglobin (%)			
No transfusion	29	ND	72
Azacitidine	49, 52	100	ND
Mean corpuscular volume (μm³)			
No transfusion	69±10	79±7.1	103±2.3
Azacitidine	82±3.2†	96±6.3†	85±0.5†
Mean corpuscular hemoglobin (pg)			
No transfusion	19.0±1.1	23.2±3.8	20.4±1.6
Azacitidine	25.0±1.5†	29.6±3.0†	24.9±2.2‡
Mean corpuscular hemoglobin concentration (g/dl)			
No transfusion	27.7±2.3	29.0±2.2	19.9±1.8
Azacitidine	30.7±1.2†	30.8±2.0	29.2±2.8†

Abbreviation: ND, not determined.
* Measurements were made in the absence of transfusions and after treatment with azacitidine.
Plus-minus values are means ± SD. Only 2 hemoglobin measurements were made in patient 3 during therapy. Pretreatment fetal hemoglobin levels were not determined in patient 2 because she had been receiving regular transfusions before therapy was begun.
† P < .001.
‡ P = .01.
(Courtesy of Lowrey CH, Nienhuis AW: *N Engl J Med* 329:845–848, 1993.)

patient no longer needed transfusions. After tolerating 6 cycles of monthly treatment, the patient began more intensive treatment. Recurrent neutropenia necessitated a reduction in treatment frequency. After nearly 2 years of azacitidine therapy, the patient has a nearly normal ejection fraction at rest and a normal exercise response. Azacitidine was discontinued once the goals of substantial iron unloading and improved cardiac function were achieved.

Case 2.—Woman, 30, had β-thalassemia major and had received transfusions since age 7 years. Before azacitidine was initiated, she needed 20 units of erythrocytes to maintain her hemoglobin level above 5 g/dL. After azacitidine therapy, she no longer needed transfusions.

Case 3.—Man, 32, with β-thalassemia intermedia, was not receiving transfusions because of religious beliefs. His hemoglobin level had been 7–8 g/dL until age 20 years, when it started to decrease gradually. By day 5 of his first cycle of azacitidine treatment, the patient's reticulocytes increased. After 2 treatment cycles, his hemoglobin level increased from 3 to 6.3 g/dL.

Conclusion.—Azacitidine is a new treatment option for patients with thalassemia. The clinical regimen used produced long-term benefits in 2 patients (table). The pharmacologic manipulation of gene expression is a useful treatment approach.

▶ Dr. Lucarelli was honored this year at the American Society of Hematology meeting for his work on bone marrow transplantation in thalassemia (1, 2). Of course, not all such patients are eligible for bone marrow transplantation, and in this article, Lowrey and Nienhuis describe an alternative for iron-overloaded or alloimmunized patients. Obviously, both immediate and potential long-term risks are associated with this form of therapy. Given recent data that serum EPO levels in thalassemia intermedia are frequently less than 500 mU/mL even in untransfused patients (3), the patients described might have benefited additionally by receiving recombinant EPO as well as the azacitidine.—J.L. Spivak, M.D.

References

1. Lucarelli G, et al: *Blood* 80:1603, 1992.
2. Lucarelli G, et al: *N Engl J Med* 329:840, 1993.
3. Dore F, et al: *Ann Hematol* 67:183, 1993.

Spinal Deformities in Deferoxamine-Treated Homozygous Beta-Thalassemia Major Patients

Hartkamp MJ, Babyn PS, Olivieri F (Rijks Universiteit Utrecht, The Netherlands; Hosp for Sick Children, Toronto)
Pediatr Radiol 23:525–528, 1993   116-95-1–15

Background.—Osteoporosis with compression fractures, as well as paraspinal masses of extramedullary hematopoiesis, may develop in inadequately treated patients with homozygous β-thalassemia (HBT). Other skeletal changes have been seen since the advent of chelation therapy with deferoxamine, an iron-chelating agent used in conjunction with transfusion therapy.

Patients and Treatment.—Spinal involvement was examined retrospectively in 22 patients with HBT who were being treated with deferoxamine. All chest and spine radiographs obtained during the 3 years after the start of nightly subcutaneous deferoxamine treatment were reviewed, as were radiographs obtained before deferoxamine treatment. The current dose is 50 mg/kg. All patients had received transfusions to maintain the pretransfusion hemoglobin at more than 100 g/L.

Observations.—Of the 22 patients, 9 experienced a significant decrease in height after beginning deferoxamine treatment. All of them had metaphyseal abnormalities as well as spinal changes. Of the 13 patients without growth failure, 7 also had spinal changes, but only 1 had a subtle metaphyseal abnormality. In affected patients, the vertebral bodies were osteoporotic and had marginal sclerosis. The upper thoracic vertebrae appeared flattened and lengthened on lateral views and tapered anteriorly, producing exaggerated wedging and moderate kyphosis. The thoracolumbar vertebrae were reduced in height and appeared biconvex. Six patients had narrowed intervertebral disk spaces, and 2 had asymptomatic disk calcification. Some earlier patients had received as much as 80 mg of deferoxamine per kg, and those with spinal abnormalities tended to have received higher doses.

Discussion.—The spinal abnormalities seen in patients with HBT who receive deferoxamine are ascribed to impaired development of the spinal growth plates. A high daily dose of deferoxamine and reduced iron stores in the body both may contribute to abnormal spinal development in this setting. The spine may be more vulnerable to the effects of deferoxamine than the growth plates and metaphyses of the wrist and knee. Degenerative changes might take place earlier in these patients.

▶ For our pediatric colleagues, here is another potential adverse event to be added to the list of toxic effects associated with deferoxamine therapy.—J.L. Spivak, M.D.

Red Cell Aplasia and Aplastic Anemias

Treatment of Diamond-Blackfan Anemia With Recombinant Human Interleukin-3

Gillio AP, Faulkner LB, Alter BP, Reilly L, Klafter R, Heller G, Young DC, Lipton JM, Moore MAS, O'Reilly RJ (Mem Sloan-Kettering Cancer Ctr, New York; Mount Sinai School of Medicine, New York; Sandoz Pharmaceuticals Corp, East Hanover, NJ)
Blood 82:744–751, 1993   116-95-1–16

Clinical Characteristics and Laboratory Parameters at Study Entry

PT	Age*	Sex	Hgb† (g/dL)	Retic‡ (%)	ARC§ (10⁹/L)	BME|| (%)	Corticosteroids		Other RX	RBC TX	Chelation
							Initial Response	Dose at Study Entry			
Responders											
2	13.9	F	8.0	0.7	20	8	+	7.5 mg QD	Splenectomy, Epo	–	–
5	16.8	F	7.9	0.2	8	6	+	None	None	+	+
13	20.0	M	9.0	0.1	6	6	+	None	CSA	+	+
16	16.2	M	8.1	0.6	21	33	+	20 mg QD	None	–	+
Nonresponders											
1	4.8	M	7.7	0.7	30	36	+	30 mg × 3D Q14D	Epo	–	–
3	7.3	M	8.0	0.8	34	20	+	20 mg QOD	None	–	–
4	20.6	M	12.1	1.0	43	15	+	None	None	–	+
6	14.5	F	10.0	0.3	16	4	+	None	CSA	+	–
7	21.5	F	12.4	0.4	20	3	+	None	Androgens, CSA	+	+

(continued)

Table (continued)

Patient	Age*	Sex	Hgb†	Corrected retic‡	Absolute retic§	NE‖		Prednisone	Treatment		
8	11.1	M	*13.4*	0.1	5	0	+	None	None	+	+
9	0.4	M	*11.8*	0.2	8	1	−	None	None	+	−
10	15.5	M	*9.8*	0.2	10	5	+	None	GG, Plasmapheresis	+	+
11	12.3	F	*12.1*	0.5	23	9	+	15 mg QOD	None	+	−
12	31.3	F	*10.2*	0.2	9	1	+	20 mg QD	None	+	−
14	3.5	M	*12.1*	0.0	0	0	−	None	GG	+	−
15	1.7	M	*12.6*	0.0	0	0	−	None	GG, Epo	+	−
17	9.6	F	*11.8*	0.0	0	0	−	None	None	+	+
18	12.3	M	*7.0*	0.0	0	4	+	None	CSA, Epo, GM-CSF	+	−

Abbreviations: CSA, cyclosporin A; GG, gammaglobulin.
* Years at study entry.
† Values italicized in transfused patients.
‡ Corrected reticulocyte count.
§ Absolute reticulocyte count (nl 50–100).
‖ Percentage of nucleated erythroid cells in bone marrow.
(Courtesy of Gillio AP, Faulkner LB, Alter BP, et al: *Blood* 82:744–751, 1993.)

Background.—Diamond-Blackfan anemia (DBA) is a rare inherited anemia with a multifactor expression, possibly reflecting multiple causes. Corticosteroids currently provide the most effective treatment. Remissions are usually steroid-dependent or transfusion-dependent, or both.

Although erythropoietic growth factors appear to be at expected levels in patients with DBA, treatment with recombinant human IL-3 (rhIL-3) may stimulate erythroid development.

Methods.—Eighteen patients with DBA in a single center (table) were treated with escalating doses of rhIL-3 derived from *Escherichia coli.* All had significantly low hemoglobin levels. Patients receiving steroids were maintained with the same drugs. The rhIL-3 doses were escalated until patients responded or reached the maximum levels.

Results.—In 4 of the 18 patients, there was a significant erythroid response (Fig 1–6). Two of them were steroid-independent and transfusion-dependent. One of these patients became transfusion-independent and was maintained with 10 mg of rhIL-3 per kg/day until day 342, when a deep venous thrombosis developed. The other patient had decreased transfusion requirements but dose-dependent reticulosis developed. On day 131, DVT, which may have been trauma-induced, developed. Treatment was discontinued in both patients, and both returned to baseline levels. All responders experienced increased bone marrow cellularity without altered cell ratios and elevated mean corpuscular vol-

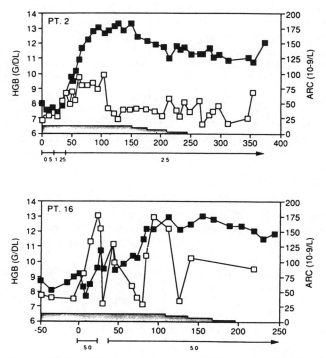

Fig 1–6.—Effect of rhIL-3 administration on hemoglobin (*filled squares*) and absolute reticulocyte count (*open squares*) in 2 steroid-dependent transfusion-independent DBA patients. The rhIL-3 dosing is depicted by the *horizontal arrows* and steroid taper by *dotted bars.* (Courtesy of Gillio AP, Faulkner LB, Alter BP, et al: *Blood* 82:744–751, 1993.)

ume and percentage of hemoglobin F, signs of DBA-characteristic stress erythropoiesis. White blood cell counts also increased significantly, caused by increased neutrophils and lymphocytes. The eosinophil count increased in a dose-dependent manner. In vitro growth of cloned cells was not predictive of in vivo erythroid response.

Discussion.—Treatment with rhIL-3 significantly stimulated erythroid development in about one fourth of patients. Other similar studies have produced different results. This may be explained either by the differences in the rhIL-3 administered (derivation or glycosylation, or both) or by differences in patient selection. The development of deep venous thrombosis may be related to hypereosinophilia. More research is required to determine the consequences of rhIL-3–induced eosinophilia.

▶ The Diamond-Blackfan syndrome, although rare, remains a vexing problem for physicians who manage these patients. Although it was once thought that W and Steel mice who lack either c-*kit* or stem cell factor, respectively, might be genetic models for this disorder, that contention has been disproved. Because IL-3 in vitro stimulates erythroid burst-forming unit proliferation in Diamond-Blackfan marrows, it was hoped that this cytokine might prove effective when administered in vivo in pharmacologic doses. In this study, 4 of 18 patients had a response to IL-3 that was not predictable based on their clinical status. Unfortunately, in 2, a thrombotic tendency led to cessation of therapy and was associated with hypereosinophilia. Whether there was a cause-and-effect relationship is unclear, but eosinophilia is a consistent effect of IL-3 and may well limit its long-term administration.—J.L. Spivak, M.D.

Erythrocyte P Antigen: Cellular Receptor for B19 Parvovirus
Brown KE, Anderson SM, Young NS (Natl Heart, Lung and Blood Inst, Bethesda, Md)
Science 262:114–116, 1993   116-95-1–17

Background.—The human parvovirus B19 causes fifth disease in normal persons, transient aplastic crisis in patients with hemolytic disorders, and chronic anemia secondary to persistent infection in immunocompromised patients. Infection during pregnancy can lead to hydrops and fetal loss or congenital infection. The virus is tropic for erythroid progenitors; it is possible that this tropism is mediated by a cellular receptor unique to these cells. Most parvoviruses can agglutinate red cells, and there is evidence that binding may be mediated by a glycolipid.

Objective.—The ability of membrane extracts of various cell types to block B19 binding was determined.

Results.—When red cells from 26 persons with different blood group P phenotypes were tested for their ability to agglutinate with parvovirus B19, only those lacking blood group P antigen failed to be agglutinated

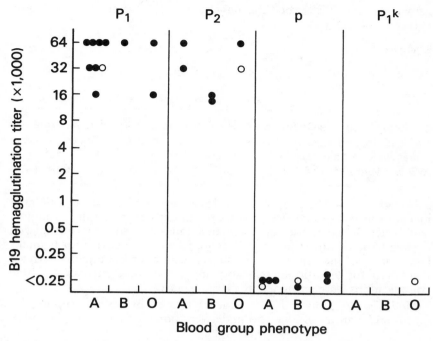

Fig 1-7.—Hemagglutination titers for B19 of human erythrocytes with different P phenotypes. Erythocytes were washed, suspended in saline (.5% v/v), and assayed with the use of recombinant B19 capsids (1 mg mL⁻¹). Rhesus-positive cells (*filled circles*); rhesus-negative cells (*open circles*). (Courtesy of Brown KE, Anderson SM, Young NS: *Science* 262:114-116, 1993.)

(Fig 1-7). Purified P antigen, or globoside, blocked binding of the virus to erythroid cells. It also eliminated the infectivity of B19 in a hematopoietic colony assay. Target cells preincubated with monoclonal antibody to globoside were protected against infection by B19.

Implications.—Blood-group P antigen is a receptor for parvovirus B19. The tissue distribution of P antigen helps explain the marked tropism of B19 for erythroid cells. Because the lipid nature of the red cell membrane can be chemically modified, introduction of a functional globoside receptor might be part of a gene therapy based on parvoviruses.

▶ This is an exciting observation in the saga that is parvovirus B19 from a laboratory that has led the way in parvovirus research. It appears that the blood group P antigen serves as the cellular receptor for parvovirus B19, which explains the exquisite tissue tropism of this virus. As a corollary, individuals who lack the P antigen phenotype are naturally resistant to parvovirus B19 infection (1). Although Dr. Young has some epidemiologic data suggesting an association between B19 infection and childhood paroxysmal cold hemoglobinuria, whether parvovirus B19 is involved in the pathogenesis of paroxysmal cold hemoglobinuria remains to be established.—J.L. Spivak, M.D.

Reference

1. Brown KE, et al: *N Engl J Med* 330:1192, 1994.

Malignant Tumors Occurring After Treatment of Aplastic Anemia

Socié G, for the European Bone Marrow Transplantation–Severe Aplastic Anaemia Working Party (Hôpital Saint Louis, Paris)
N Engl J Med 329:1152–1157, 1993   116-95-1–18

Background.—The proportion of long-term survivors of aplastic anemia is expected to increase, making treatment complications an important issue. Research has suggested that long-term survivors of aplastic anemia treated with immunosuppressive therapy are at risk for hematologic cancers. The incidence of solid cancers after bone marrow transplantation for aplastic anemia also appears to have increased. These complications were examined in a large cohort.

Methods.—A group of 860 patients treated by immunosuppressive means and a group of 748 who underwent bone marrow transplantation

Observed Cancers, by Treatment Group

Type of Cancer	Median Months from Treatment to Diagnosis (Range)	Immuno-suppressive Therapy	Bone Marrow Transplan-tation
Myelodysplastic syndrome†	52 (2 to 122)	28	0
Acute leukemia‡	47 (7 to 115)	15	2
Non-Hodgkin's lymphoma	33	1	0
Solid tumors§	52 (1 to 94)	7	7
Head and neck		1	5
Stomach		1	1
Liver		3	1
Breast		2	0

* There were 60 events in 51 patients.
† Three cases arose within 6 months of treatment in the immunosuppressive therapy group. According to French-British-American (FAB) classification, there were 7 cases each of refractory anemia and refractory anemia with an excess of blasts and 8 cases of chronic myelomonocytic leukemia.
‡ Nine cases occurred after myelodysplastic syndrome in the immunosuppressive therapy group. According to FAB classification, there were 2 cases each of M2 and M4 and 1 case of L2 acute leukemia in the immunosuppressive therapy group; 10 cases were unclassified.
§ Within 12 months of treatment, 2 cases arose in the immunosuppressive therapy group and 1 arose in the bone marrow transplantation group.
(Courtesy of Socié G: N Engl J Med 329:1152–1157, 1993.)

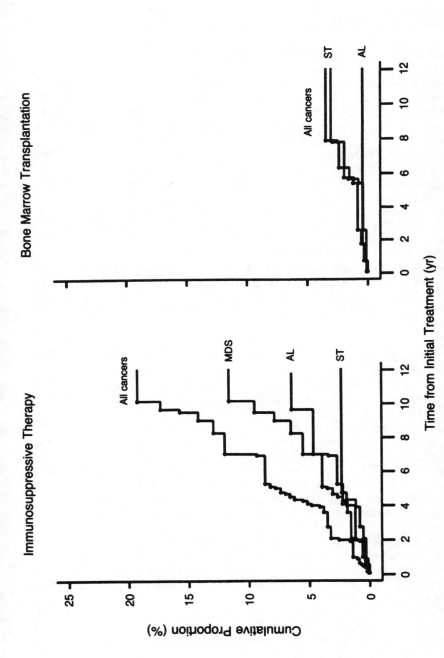

Fig 1-8.—*Abbreviations: MDS*, myelodysplastic syndrome; *AL*, acute leukemia; *ST*, malignant solid tumors. Cumulative incidence of observed cancer in 860 patients with aplastic anemia treated with immunosuppressive therapy and in 748 patients who underwent bone marrow transplantation. (Courtesy of Socié G: *N Engl J Med* 329:1152–1157, 1993.)

were included. Cancer risk was analyzed overall and by treatment and compared with the risk in the general population.

Findings.—The 42 malignant conditions among patients treated immunosuppressively included 19 cases of myelodysplastic syndrome, 15 of acute leukemia, 1 of non-Hodgkin's lymphoma, and 7 solid tumors. Among the patients who underwent bone marrow transplantation, the 9 cases of malignant disease included 2 cases of acute leukemia and 7 solid tumors (table). The overall risk was 5.5 compared with the general population. The immunosuppression and transplantation groups had cancer risks of 5.15 and 6.67, respectively. The 10-year cumulative incidence rate was 18.8% and 3.1% after immunosuppression and transplantation, respectively (Fig 1–8). Risk factors for myelodysplastic syndrome or acute leukemia after immunosuppression were the addition of androgens to the immunosuppressive regimen, older age, treatment in 1982 or later, splenectomy, and treatment with multiple courses of immunosuppression. Risk factors for solid tumors after marrow transplantation were age and the use of pretransplantation radiation therapy. Solid tumors occurred only in male patients.

Conclusion.—Aplastic anemia survivors have an increased risk of having malignant diseases. In this series, myelodysplastic syndrome and acute leukemia tended to follow immunosuppression. The incidences of solid tumors after immunosuppression and bone marrow transplantation were similar.

▶ This is an impressive study not only for the number of patients involved, but also for its conclusions. Where formerly we worried simply about how to keep aplastic anemia patients alive, now, owing to new therapies, success with respect to remission induction and longevity has led to different worries. It has been appreciated for some time that long-term survivors of aplastic anemia who received immunosuppressive therapy were at risk for myelodysplasia, paroxysmal nocturnal hemoglobinuria, and acute leukemia, whereas similar patients who received a marrow transplant were at risk for solid tumors. The current study, unfortunately, confirms these observations and adds solid tumors as a risk factor for the group receiving immunosuppressive therapy alone. Predisposing factors included age, androgen therapy, repeated courses of therapy and splenectomy, and, for the transplant group, irradiation and age. Certainly, avoidance of androgens that are not efficacious in severe aplastic anemia and splenectomy is easy. Unfortunately, those most likely to receive immunosuppressive therapy as opposed to a transplant are older individuals. They are also the group most likely to respond. The data raise again the issue of whether some cases of aplastic anemia actually represent a phase of acute leukemia. Clonal remissions of aplastic anemia have been reported, and immunosuppressive therapy has been observed anecdotally to alleviate the pancytopenia of myelodysplasia. We observed a partial remission of aplastic anemia associated with trisomy 8 and eosinophilic fasciitis after 2 courses of antithymocyte globulin and cyclosporine combined with long-term cyclosporine maintenance. If nothing else, these observations support the contention that aplastic anemia is a disorder with multiple causes. It is also worth emphasizing that in this study, not only was the cumulative 10-year incident rate of malignancies less than 20%, but survival before the onset of the malignancy was superior to no treatment at all. For an excellent review of clonality in aplastic anemia, see Dr. Young's article in *Blood* (3).—J.L. Spivak, M.D.

References

1. Tichelli A, et al: *Br J Haematol* 69:413, 1988.
2. de Planque MM, et al: *Br J Haematol* 70:55, 1988.
3. Young NS: *Blood* 79:1385, 1992.

Erythrocytosis and Polycythemia

Truncated Erythropoietin Receptor Causes Dominantly Inherited Benign Human Erythrocytosis

de la Chapelle A, Träskelin A-L, Juvonen E (Univ of Helsinki)
Proc Natl Acad Sci U S A 90:4495–4499, 1993   116-95-1–19

Background.—Erythroid precursor cell proliferation and differentiation are regulated through the EPO receptor (EPOR). A specific domain in the intracellular C-terminal region of the *EPOR* gene exerts negative control on erythropoiesis. Abnormalities in this domain could lead to erythrocytosis, inherited as a dominant trait linked to a polymorphic marker adjacent to the *EPOR* gene. A mutation in the C-terminal of the *EPOR* gene that cosegregates with the familial disease phenotype was described.

Phenotype.—Within a single family, 25 members with erythrocytosis and 72 unaffected members underwent clinical and laboratory examination. Laboratory findings revealed increased progenitor cell sensitivity to EPO as the pathogenic mechanism. Hemoglobin was very high: the mean male hemoglobin value was 204 g/L; the mean female value was 191 g/L. Bone marrow morphology was normal with signs of erythroid hyperplasia. Serum EPO was low or low-normal: 8.6 pmol/L for the proband and less than 8 pmol/L for 2 other individuals assayed.

Definition of Mutation.—Genomic sequences from GenBank were used to design primers to amplify the 3′ region of EPOR encompassing exons 7 and 8. This sequencing revealed a G-to-A mutation at position 6002 in an affected family member but only a G mutation in an unaffected family member. This mutation predicts a truncated EPOR molecule lacking the last 70 amino acids at the C-terminal end and destroys a restriction site for Nco I. All 29 affected family members, but none of the 21 unaffected individuals or 50 randomly chosen blood donors, were heterozygous for the mutation by the Nco I assay.

Conclusion.—The cosegregation of the mutation and phenotype in all cases and its absence in unaffected family members and healthy controls demonstrate that this defect in the *EPOR* gene causes the clinical phenotype of erythrocytosis.

▶ Three years ago, Juvonen and colleagues described an interesting kindred with erythrocytosis (1). A year ago, the same group (2) reported segregation of an *EPOR* gene polymorphism in affected family members, suggesting that the erythrocytosis in this family was due to a mutation in the *EPOR* gene. At that time, we predicted that the Juvonen group was sequencing the *EPOR* gene (3). That was not a difficult prediction, and the results are of great interest. It turns out that affected family members express a truncated EPOR resulting from a G-to-A mutation that creates a stop codon within the carboxyl-terminus of the molecule, leading to loss of the terminal 70 amino acids. It has been known for several years that the carboxyl-terminus region of the EPOR contains a negative regulatory domain (4, 5) and that cells expressing truncated EPORs lacking the terminal 40 amino acids were more sensitive to EPO than cells expressing the full-length receptor. Now, for the first time, not only has an EPOR defect been described for an abnormality of erythropoiesis (in this case erythrocytosis), but the particular receptor defect phenotypically recapitulated the behavior of the experimentally truncated receptor. This is an exciting observation and one that has led to renewed interest in seeking other EPOR defects associated with abnormalities in erythropoiesis.—J.L. Spivak, M.D.

References

1. Juvonen E, et al: *Blood* 78:3066, 1991.
2. de la Chapelle A, et al: *Lancet* 341:82, 1993.
3. 1994 YEAR BOOK OF HEMATOLOGY, p 48.
4. Yoshimura Y, et al: *Nature* 348:647, 1990.
5. D'Andrea A, et al: *Mol Cell Biol* 11:1980, 1991.

Interferon-α2b: A New Treatment for Polycythemia Vera
Silver RT (New York Hosp–Cornell Med Ctr, New York)
Ann Intern Med 119:1091–1092, 1993   116-95-1–20

Purpose.—Polycythemia vera, which features increased red cell mass and thrombohemorrhagic complications, has generally been treated by phlebotomy. Myelosuppressive agents are added to avoid the complications of early thrombosis or hemorrhage, but these drugs carry the risk of leukemia. Night sweats, pruritus, iron deficiency, progressive splenomegaly, and myelofibrosis make other treatments necessary. In a preliminary study, good results were reported with recombinant interferon (INF)-α2b in 5 patients with polycythemia vera. Extended follow-up and the addition of more patients were reported.

Patients.—Included were 11 patients treated during a period of 6 years. All had been treated previously by phlebotomy only, with a median of 4.5 procedures per year. Recombinant INF-α2b treatment began at a dose of 3 × 10⁶ units/m² 3 times a week subcutaneously. Four patients required supplemental phlebotomies during the first 6 months to maintain hematocrit at .45 or lower. Six had a 30% increase in dose or frequency to achieve the same purpose. The maintenance dose was reached by decreasing the maximum dose by 25% every 2 months to find the smallest dose that maintained hematocrit at .45 or lower.

Outcome.—The palpable spleen of 9 patients became nonpalpable in all but 2 in the first year of treatment. All patients had resolution of RBC microcytosis associated with iron deficiency as the hemoglobin level and RBC mass came into balance. The mean decrease in platelet count was 411 × 10⁹/L, and the maintenance dose was about 3 × 10⁶ units/m² 3–5 times a week. There were no thrombohemorrhagic events during a median follow-up of 36 months. Side effects, including asthenia, myalgia, and fever, occurred in all but 1 patient but decreased gradually.

Conclusion.—For patients with polycythemia vera, the recombinant INF-α2b treatment can control RBC values within 6–12 months of treatment. This promising new treatment avoids phlebotomy. However, polycythemia is a long-term disease, and additional follow-up is needed.

▶ This follow-up study extends the observation period for Dr. Silver's initial experience with the use of INF-α in the treatment of polycythemia vera (1). As such, it provides some interesting observations along with some misleading and erroneous comments about polycythemia vera that both the reviewers and editors of the *Annals of Internal Medicine* obviously share. The myths surrounding polycythemia vera have been discussed at length in this YEAR BOOK OF HEMATOLOGY before (2), but myths are frequently hard to dispel and nowhere more so than with polycythemia vera. Let me try again.

First, we are told by Dr. Silver that "treatment with phlebotomy only is associated with early, frequently fatal thrombosis or hemorrhage," and the work of the Polycythemia Vera Study Group (PVSG) is cited as the basis for this contention. In one regard, Dr. Silver is correct. If the original phlebotomy recommendations of the PVSG are followed, thrombosis can be anticipated (3). However, if men with polycythemia vera are phlebotomized to a hemoglobin of less than 15 gm%, and women to a hemoglobin of less than 12 gm%, thrombosis does *not* occur. A remarkable failing that I frequently encounter is that women with polycythemia vera are usually phlebotomized to a hemoglobin of 15 gm%, which might be appropriate for a man but certainly is not for a woman. Simple perusal of the PVSG's own data will reveal what they originally failed to appreciate: in patients with polycythemia vera, a hemoglobin or hematocrit in the upper range of normal can be misleading (4) because it is frequently associated with an elevated red cell mass. This is why PVSG patients initially had a 40% incidence of thrombosis.

Second, we are told that phlebotomy leads to iron deficiency, as if this is an undesired result instead of its objective. Phlebotomy is the initial treatment of choice in polycythemia vera because nothing else will reduce the red cell mass as quickly, thus eliminating the risk of thrombosis. Thereafter, once the red cell mass is normal, phlebotomy serves to keep it normal while inducing iron deficiency. A truly iron-deficient patient with polycythemia vera requires a phlebotomy no more than once every 2 to 3 months. In adults, iron deficiency in the absence of anemia might cause pica or thrombocytosis but does not impair aerobic function (5).

Third, there is no proof that platelet-derived growth factor is responsible for myelofibrosis in polycythemia vera, although it or a similar molecule could be involved in the autonomous hematopoiesis in polycythemia vera (6). With regard to Dr. Silver's patient population, it is instructive that of the 11 patients, 4 initially had hemoglobin levels above that which would be considered safe, only 4 had a substantial elevation in platelet number (not that platelet number per se requires therapy), and only 4 had substantial splenomegaly. Interestingly, in 1 patient there was not a significant correction in the hemoglobin level and in another the hemoglobin level actually rose. Most importantly, in all but 1 patient, splenomegaly was reduced. This is a significant observation because splenomegaly can be a distressing problem that is difficult to manage in polycythemia vera patients. Unfortunately, in this study, as in others involving similar patients, there is no control group so that the actual effectiveness of INF therapy cannot be assessed. As Dr. Silver correctly notes, polycythemia vera is a chronic disease, and because INF-α has many toxicities, it is difficult to make any recommendations about its long-term use in patients with polycythemia vera. From my perspective INF-α may be useful in reducing burdensome organomegaly, but as a substitute for phlebotomy or as a treatment for asymptomatic thrombocytosis, it has absolutely no role.—J.L. Spivak, M.D.

References

1. Silver RT: *Blood* 76:664, 1990.
2. 1988 YEAR BOOK OF HEMATOLOGY, pp 54–57.
3. Berk PD, et al: *N Engl J Med* 304:441, 1981.
4. Berlin NI: *Semin Hematol* 12:339, 1975.
5. Rector WG, et al: *Medicine* 61:382, 1982.
6. Eid J, et al: *Proc Natl Acad Sci U S A* 84:532, 1987.

Gaucher's Disease

Enzyme Therapy in Gaucher Disease Type 1: Dosage Efficacy and Adverse Effects in 33 Patients Treated for 6 to 24 Months

Pastores GM, Sibille AR, Grabowski GA (Mount Sinai School of Medicine, New York; Children's Hosp Med Ctr, Cincinnati, Ohio)
Blood 82:408–416, 1993   116-95-1-21

Background.—Gaucher's disease, an inborn error of glycosphingolipid metabolism, is the most common lysosomal storage disease. This highly

Characteristics and Outcomes of Patients With Gaucher's Disease Type 1 Treated With Alglucerase

Patient	Age (yr)	Age at Splenectomy (yr)	Genotype	Dose	Liver Volume				Spleen Volume			
					Initial	Phase 1	Phase 2	Overall	Initial	Phase 1	Phase 2	Overall
MB	11		N370S/84GG	60,60	2.74	37.2	2.3	38	49.3	54.6	23.6	65.2
GaR	12	2	?/?	60,60	4.52	6.5	1.2	7.7	0			
GrR	16	9	N370S/84GG	60,30	3.99	39	18.5	49.6	0			
YM	30	27	N370S/?	60,30	2.41	38.7	12.8	46.5	0			
HM	31		N370S/N370S	60,30,15	1.30	8.4	4.2	12.5	5.2	25	24.6	43.5
TM	36		N370S/L444P	60,30	1.70	21.6	4.5	24.7	14.4	45.8	17.9	55.6
LK	38	4	N370S/84GG	60,30	4.12	18.7	14.6	30.6	0			
EA	38	5	N370S/?	60,60	3.48	13.6	18.7	29.9	0			
MG	50	19	84GG/?	60,60	0.73		ND		0			
SoB	52	18	N370S/84GG	60	3.12	8.9	16.2	23.7	0			
EK*	63		N370S/N370S	60,60	ND	63.4	NL		ND	ND	19.8	41.3
SF	2		?/?	50	2.43	63.4		63.4	12.5	64.3		64.3
IT	5		N370S/L444P	50	1.94	21.9		21.9	13.8	23.2		23.2
JeL	9		N370S/IVS2+1	50,25	2.65	17.7	5.5	22.2	32.7	33.3	11.9	41.1
DD	12	9	?/?	50,50	1.85	16.9	16.2	30.2	0			
AG	21		N370S/84GG	50	2.72	19.1		19.1	13.8	24.6		24.6
AS	23	17	N370S/L444P	50	2.22	45.5		45.5	0			
JC	36		IVS2+1/?	50,50	1.13		NL	8.1	14.1	30.5	8.4	44.6
MM*	36	5	N370S/IVS2+1	50,50	ND		8.1		0			

(continued)

Table (continued)

	Age		Genotype	Dose								
JK	41	23	N370S/?	50	2.41	17.4	NL	17.4	0	27	27.3	46.7
BB	41		N370S/?	50,50,25	1.18	29	5.9	33.2	7.5	24.2	15.5	34.6
LR	41	14	N370S/84GG	50,25	2.62	21.9	4.1	24.9	0	18.4	56.5	65
DSm	48		N370S/?	50,50	3.09	28.3	27	47.6	33.1	20.1		20.1
StB*	52		N370S/84GG	50,50	1.91	10.1	NL	10.1	43.4	51.4	5.2	56.5
MR	59		N370S/84GG	50	1.68	34.3	NL	36.1	13.9	35.6	35.5	58.5
AM	18		S364T/L444P	40,20	1.83	19.3		37	27.2			
BP	46		N370S/N370S	40,20	1.92	9.4		9.4	12.7			
KL	47	15	N370S/?	40	1.36	17.4		30.8	0			
AK*	4		N370S/84GG	30,30	1.98	24.9	16	34.5	19	30	0.8	30.5
RS	15		N370S/?	30,60	2.38	14.5	12.4	25.5	61.9	8.9	52.6	79
CG	26		N370S/?	30,60	2.12		13.2		7.7	29.9	77.8	84.4
JoL	44	9	N370S/84GG	30	1.58	10.4		10.4	0			
DSk*	55	49	84GG/?	30	2.24	16.9		16.9	0			

Note: Doses are divided into 6-month intervals (e.g., 60,30 means 60 and 30 IU/kg per 2 weeks for 0–6 and 6–12 months, respectively). Initial liver and spleen volumes are expressed as fold increased over the predicted normal. Liver and spleen are 2.5% and .2% of body weight. For phases 1 and 2, the values present the percentage change during that phase. Overall values are normalized to body weight, so phase 1 plus phase 2 changes do not equal overall decreases.

* Antibody-positive patients.

(Courtesy of Pastores GM, Sibille AR, Grabowski GA: *Blood* 82:408–416, 1993.)

heterogenous disorder is inherited as an autosomal recessive trait. It is the most prevalent genetic disorder among Ashkenazi Jews. The outcomes of enzyme treatment in patients with type 1 Gaucher's disease were examined.

Methods.—Thirty-three patients were enrolled in the trial (table). In all patients' acid β-glucosidase activity was 5% to 15% of the mean normal activity. Intravenously administered alglucerase was given after dilution in .9% sodium chloride to a total volume of 100 mL through a blood transfusion filter for 1–2 hours after an initial 5-mL test dose.

Findings.—Within 3–12 months, hemoglobin levels and platelet counts increased by 0% to 178% in patients with anemia and 15% to 155% in patients with thrombocytopenia. In patients with splenomegaly or hepatomegaly, or both, liver and spleen volumes decreased 7% to 64% in 6 months and 8% to 84% by 12 months, respectively. Hematologic and visceral improvements occurred with 60–15 IU of treatment per kg every 2 weeks. These positive initial treatment responses persisted, with doses decreased by 50%. Three patients had no clinical improvement in pulmonary Gaucher's disease. The rate of patient improvement was unaffected by unrelated cirrhotic, cholestatic, or renal disease. Two of 5 patients having serum antibodies against alglucerase in the first 6–12 months had mild antibody reactions.

Conclusion.—Enzyme treatment at doses ranging from 30 to 60 IU/kg every 2 weeks induces similar regression of clinical Gaucher's disease manifestations. The treatment efficacy was not diminished after 50% to 75% reductions in dose or by the presence of antienzyme antibodies.

▶ Gaucher's disease is another uncommon disease that has achieved new prominence in the literature by virtue of the introduction of an effective therapy. The very expense of that therapy has additionally encouraged greater scrutiny of affected individuals, which has resulted in a better understanding of the natural history of the disorder (1, 2). Disease severity correlates with the particular genetic defect at the molecular level, and disease progression appears to stabilize with adulthood. These important observations emphasize the need to start enzyme replacement therapy in childhood, and dosage considerations might well be based on the particular genetic mutation involved. Currently, however, we are still coping with alleviating the complications that arose before an effective preparation of glucocerebrosidase was commercially available.

The study abstracted here is the largest therapeutic trial reported to date and documents not only the effectiveness of enzyme replacement but also that neither a reduction in dose nor splenomegaly compromised responsiveness. Importantly, antibody formation neither prevented nor impaired therapy. Because pulmonary involvement was not affected, the need for early therapy is evident. Whether the type of gene mutation will predict the intensity of enzyme replacement therapy remains to be determined.—J.L. Spivak, M.D.

References

1. 1994 YEAR BOOK OF HEMATOLOGY, pp 54–59.
2. Zimran A, et al: *Medicine* 71:337, 1992.

Call Mosby Document Express at **1 (800) 55-MOSBY** to obtain copies of the original source documents of articles featured or referenced in the YEAR BOOK series.

---

2 White Blood Cells

Introduction

This was a stutter-start year—one step back on cytokines, hold fast on gene therapy results, and—whoops—no common stromal hematopoietic stem cell. Now, what's really hot? Well, thrombopoietin seems to finally be here (not published yet). And is it IL-3? No. Is it IL-6? No. Well, it must be IL-11. Guess again—it's the ligand for the receptor encoded by the c-mpl proto-oncogene (c-Mpl)(1). A home run by Zymogenetics. More on this next year.

What else? Stem cells continue to mystify us: patent or no, we have a clue but only that. Medical economics and grant funding also continue to be big stories, but who wants to talk about them?

Inhibitors are probably here to stay, but we don't know which ones. Macrophage inflammatory protein-1α turned out to be the Dexter culture stem cell (CFU-S) inhibitor, and now its whole family of intercrine molecules appears to have similar actions. Transforming growth factor-β clearly inhibits early stem cells but may stimulate later progenitors. Then there are those fascinating small peptides, P-Glu-Glu-Asp-Cys-Lys (pentapeptide) and N-acetyl-Ser-Asp-Lys-Pro (the tetrapeptide, Seraspenide). The tetrapeptide first described by Frindel, Guigon, and colleagues (2) and the pentapeptide, initially described by Paukovits and Laerum (3), are inhibitors of early stem cell proliferation, presumably relatives of the old chalones, and were disparaged for years. The early data that they prevented CFU-S from cycling and could allow cytosine arabinoside treatment of leukemic mice with less toxicity and some cures were ignored for years. Guess what? The phenomenon seems real. The tetrapeptide appears to block entry of hematopoietic stem cells into S, whereas the pentapeptide removes cells from S. Both are now in phase 1 clinical trials as myeloprotective agents, and early results indicate that they are tolerated and may actually protect. Thus, the negative regulators continue to make news.

The biggest news, of course, is the Mpl-ligand, predicted by Dr. Vainchenker and colleagues (4) and cloned by Zymogenetics (Kaushansky and Porter [5]). The other putative thrombopoietins, IL-11, IL-6, and IL-3, have relatively meager effects on platelet levels, whereas Mpl-ligand gives "wall-to-wall megakaryocytes" and platelet counts in mice in the range of 5 to 6 million. This really appears to be the long-sought-after thrombopoietin. These results remain to be published.

45

I have addressed the issues of G-CSF and GM-CSF in past YEAR BOOKS OF HEMATOLOGY and will not reiterate the past (but still valid) arguments on why their use in cancer has not been established and why they should still be viewed as interesting experimental agents in the cancer chemotherapy setting. It is distressing to observe the total impact of skillful marketing on the clinical practice of supposedly intelligent hematologic-oncologic specialists. Amgen, with G-CSF, and even Immunex and associates, with an essentially noncompetitive product (GM-CSF), are registering brisk sales based on aggressive marketing without a valid clinical or scientific base. Amgen is marketing directly to patients and supplying many perks to clinician users at various meetings, especially those held in Europe. Worst of all, the American Society of Clinical Oncology has been generating a standard-of-care document. Inside information indicates that this document will be based not only on clinical and scientific data, but also on current clinical usage and practical political considerations. This is very depressing and indicates that the document will most likely be worthwhile only to the biotech marketing community. Other groups are beginning to draw up standard-of-care documents for the cytokines, which hopefully will be balanced and useful. Rumors, of course, could be wrong, and the American Society of Clinical Oncology document may in fact be helpful: however, I am not optimistic on this point.

Currently, there is reasonable information that G-CSF is a useful agent for chronic neutropenic states. There are no such data for the use of G-CSF or GM-CSF in cancer. In a review of published data since 1990, there are 29 studies covering therapeutic uses of GM-CSF and 30 covering uses of G-CSF that seem at least marginally interpretable. In these studies there is no evidence for increased survival or cure in patients with cancer who are treated with these agents. A palliative role is presumed by many, but we await data showing that simple chemotherapy dose reduction would not have the same results on survival rate and toxicity. Many of the recent studies are focused on the ability to escalate the dose of chemotherapy. This is, of course, based on the presumption that dose escalation in the particular tumors tested will lead to an increased therapeutic benefit. That presumption has not been established for most tumors, and there remain no data for long-term survival benefit in this setting. The critical information needed is whether dose escalation with G-CSF gives increased cure or survival rates as compared with lower-level therapy without G-CSF. Most of the studies do not seem to be addressing this point.

Stem cells remain a major focus of interest with regard to their basic biology, their use in transplantion, and their commercial potential. Patents have been issued on 1 specific stem cell as previously discussed, and, more recently, fights have broken out over who owns cord blood stem cells. This latter area is moving rapidly; cord blood transplants appear to work reasonably well in pediatric and younger patients and are just being explored now in adult patients. This discard product provides a potentially very interesting source of stem cells for transplant, and stem cells from cord blood may be more proliferative and less immunogenic. There should be a good deal of data in the next several years on their use in various transplant settings. The gold standard for stem cell assays in general has been repopulation in irradiated hosts, usually a mouse. This is essentially an amplification system, which not infrequently gives an oligoclonal readout. Data discussed from my group in Abstract 116-95-2-14 indicate that marrow can be transplanted in nonmyeloablated hosts and that in this setting, post–5-fluorouracil marrow is quite defective. This is dramatically different from results obtained in irradiated hosts and suggests the possibility that intrinsically different cells or the same cell in different functional states are monitored when engrafted in normal vs. irradiated animals. Characterization of stem cells in both settings is ongoing.

Last year we highlighted the article by Huang and Terstappen, "Formation of haematopoietic microenvironment and haematopoietic stem cells from single human bone marrow stem cells" (6). These investigators isolated cells from human fetal bone marrow with tremendous proliferative potential. The separations were elegant and the work impressive. However, it turns out that some of the antibodies for defining stromal vs. hemopoietic cells were not as specific as was previously thought, and, thus, this work had to be retracted. The elements from these individual cells appear to be essentially stromal. When this work was initially presented, a number of members of the audience were moaning about how close they were to defining the same cell. This remains an intriguing challenge, and my prediction is that at some point, a cell with this potential will in fact be identified.

Gene therapy remains a highly visible clinical-research interface. The initial studies on adenosine deaminase transfer have received a great deal of attention, and, clearly, adenosine deaminase has been transferred by repetitive injection of gene-transducted lymphocytes. Clinical benefit in this setting is less clear. Important marrow-marking experiments from Dr. Brenner of the St. Jude group (7) have shown the ability to transfer genes in the humans via hematopoietic stem cells and have further shown that tumor relapse in both acute myelogenous leukemia and neuroblastoma comes at least in part from the transplanted bone marrow. The Recombinant DNA Advisory Committee in Washington has loosened its restrictions considerably, and a relatively large number of gene therapy protocols have now been approved and are in various stages of clinical application. Murine studies have shown relatively high long-term gene transfer and expression rates under certain circumstances, but data with larger animals (primates and humans) have been relatively disappointing. There is continuing work on retroviral and adeno-associated viral vectors, with the major emphasis being to improve long-term expression of genes after in vivo transplantation.

What else? Well, the ILs continue to expand. We now have IL-14 and IL-15, and our knowledge of receptors is rapidly increasing. An intriguing article (Abstract 116-95-2–8) reviewed here relates to the potential of soluble gp130 receptors to block the action of IL-6.

Peter J. Quesenberry, M.D.

References

1. Lok S, et al: *Nature* 369:565, 1994.
2. Frindel E, Guigon M: *Exp Hematol* 5:74, 1977.
3. Laerum OD, Paukovits WR: *Pharmacol Ther* 44:335, 1989.
4. Methia N, et al: *Nature* 369:571, 1994.
5. Kaushansky K, et al: *Nature* 369:568, 1994.
6. 1994 YEAR BOOK OF HEMATOLOGY, pp 64-65.
7. Brenner MK, et al: *Lancet* 342:1134, 1993.

Cytokine Basic

Basic Fibroblast Growth Factor Promotes the Proliferation of Human Megakaryocyte Progenitor Cells

Bruno E, Cooper RJ, Wilson EL, Gabrilove JL, Hoffman R (Indiana Univ, Indianapolis; New York Univ; Mem Sloan-Kettering Cancer Inst, New York)
Blood 82:430–435, 1993   116-95-2–1

Background.—Basic fibroblast growth factor (bFGF) has been found both intracellularly and extracellularly. It is an important hematopoietic modulator that synergizes with other hematopoietic growth factors. The possibility that bFGF may operate either through an autocrine or paracrine regulatory loop was examined.

Methods.—Three bone marrow samples were obtained—low-density bone marrow (LDBM), the bone marrow subpopulation CD34+DR+, enriched for the CFU megakaryocyte, and the bone marrow subpopulation CD34+DR+, enriched for the more primitive burst-forming unit (BFU) megakaryocyte. Each was assayed with bFGF alone and in combination with IL-3, GM-CSF, and the antisera-neutralizing IL-3, GM-CSF, and IL-6. Their ability to produce colonies derived from CFU megakaryocyte or BFU megakaryocyte was measured.

Results.—Basic fibroblast growth factor stimulated CFU-megakaryocyte–derived colony formation in a dose-dependent manner. However, this effect was neutralized by either anti–IL-3 or anti–GM-CSF sera. When bFGF was added alone to either bone marrow subpopulation culture, it had no effect on formation of either CFU-megakaryocyte– or BFU-megakaryocyte–derived colonies and did not further potentiate the megakaryocyte colony-stimulating activity of IL-3. However, bFGF did significantly increase the numbers of megakaryocytes in both CFU-megakaryocyte– and BFU-megakaryocyte–derived colonies. These data suggest that bFGF might operate by inducing the release of cytokines with megakaryocyte colony-stimulating activity from accessory cells.

Discussion.—Basic fibroblast growth factor seems to regulate mega-karyocyte development in 2 ways: 1) it acts directly to stimulate prolifer-ation of both BFU-megakaryocyte and CFU-megakaryocyte, possibly by altering cellular mitosis in the individual CFU-megakaryocyte; and 2) it may also act indirectly by inducing bone marrow accessory cells to re-lease or synthesize megakaryocyte-stimulating cytokines, or both.

▶ Basic fibroblast growth factor appears to be a critical factor acting at a relatively early stem cell level. It interacts with other factors and may act both by autocrine and paracrine loops or by direct action. Further studies will have to determine its exact place in the hierarchy of hematopoietic cyto-kines.—P.J. Quesenberry, M.D.

Mechanism of Differential Inhibition of Factor-Dependent Cell Prolif-eration by Transforming Growth Factor-β1: Selective Uncoupling of FMS From MYC
Chen AR, Rohrschneider LR (Fred Hutchinson Cancer Research Ctr, Seattle)
Blood 81:2539–2546, 1993   116-95-2-2

Background.—Transforming growth factor (TGF)-β1 selectively inhib-its hematopoietic cell growth and differentiation. Research has suggested that TGF-β1 causes factor-selective inhibition of CSF, having inhibitory effects on GM-CSF receptor expression but no effect on macrophage-CSF (M-CSF) receptors.

Methods.—The MAC-11 cells were isolated from FDC-P1 cells of a murine factor–dependent bipotential hematopoietic cell line that ex-presses receptors for IL-3, GM-CSF, and M-CSF. These MAC-11 cells were cultured with either M-CSF, GM-CSF, or IL-3 and various concen-trations of TGF-β1 to measure proliferation or inhibition, or both. To identify the inhibitory mechanism, several factors were assessed, includ-ing cell cycle (maturity) and the M-CSF receptor (FMS) expression. The FMS expression was analyzed closely, focusing on its kinase activity, its internalization, and FMS-induced c-*myc* expression.

Results.—The TGF-β1 differentially inhibited proliferation depending on the CSF environment. However, although the greatest inhibitory re-sponse occurred with M-CSF, these cells also showed the greatest in-crease in FMS expression, an apparently paradoxical response. The FMS activity and internalization were not affected by TGF-β1. Expression of the early response genes c-*fos*, c-*jun*, and c-*myc* were induced by either M-CSF or GM-CSF; only M-CSF–induced c-*myc* was inhibited by TGF-β1. Cell cycle analysis showed altered cell cycle progression.

Discussion.—The TGF-β1 affects the early events in signal transduc-tion by inhibiting expression of FMS-induced c-*myc*. The differential re-sponse may explain the selective effects of TGF-β1. Cell cycle analysis revealed arrested cell development, supporting the view that normal cell cycle progression requires MYC. More research is required to test these results by rescuing cell proliferation with overexpression of c-*myc* and to determine the mechanism that regulates c-*myc* RNA levels.

▶ Transforming growth factor-β is a pleiotropic cytokine that has prominent inhibitory effects on relatively early hematopoietic progenitor stem cells. This contribution indicates that it may arrest cell cycle progression by blocking FMS induction of c-*myc*. This is the first step in studies that need to be carried out to fully elucidate the mechanism of action of a number of the potential myeloprotective inhibitors currently under evaluation, including as macrophage inflammatory protein-1α, the tetrapeptide of Frindel and Guigon, and pentapeptide, described by Paukovits and Laerum.—P.J. Quesenberry, M.D.

Human Interleukin-10 Can Directly Inhibit T-Cell Growth

Taga K, Mostowski H, Tosato G (Food and Drug Administration, Bethesda, Md)
Blood 81:2964–2971, 1993   116-95-2-3

Background.—Previous research has demonstrated the ability of human IL-10 to suppress multifactorial secretion in monocytes and to reduce growth of T cells; IL-10 inhibition of T-cell growth was believed to be indirect and to require monocyte presence. An anti-CD3 monoclonal antibody (MoAb) was used to stimulate human T-cell growth in the absence of monocytes, and the ability of IL-10 to inhibit T-cell growth was tested.

Methods.—Obtained from peripheral blood, T cells were purified to remove monocyte populations. Proliferation of T cells was then induced by OKT3, an anti-CD3 MoAb. Another purified T-cell sample was stimulated by the addition of monocyte-enriched populations in a wide range of concentrations. Interleukin-10 was added to both growth-stimulated samples. A neutralizing MoAb to human IL-10 was used to isolate the effects of IL-10. The inhibitory effects of IL-10 on a tetanus toxoid-specific (TM11) T-cell clone and T-cell secretion of IL-2 were studied with and without monocytes.

Results.—Proliferation of T cells was significantly inhibited by IL-10 in the absence of monocytes. In samples to which monocyte-enriched populations were added, initial T-cell proliferation increased, but IL-10 inhibitory effects did not decrease with a wide range of monocyte concentrations. The addition of anti–human IL-10 MoAb 19F1 reversed the inhibition of T-cell proliferation, thus isolating IL-10 as the direct inhibitory cause. Also, IL-10 inhibited proliferation of TM11 cells and inhibited IL-2 secretion by purified T cells, both with and without monocyte addition, at similarly significant levels.

Discussion.—Human IL-10 directly inhibits T-cell growth. Former research found that activated T cells in the presence of Epstein-Barr virus–immortalized cells and murine B cells could not be directly inhibited by IL-10. However, these findings suggest that these cells may produce

IL-10 inhibitors. Further research should examine the biochemical effects of T-cell activation pathways and the possible involvement of co-stimulatory signals between T cells.

▶ This is another example showing that the action of cytokines represents a moving target. Interleukin-10 was thought to have an indirect action on T cells, and this article appears to establish that in fact it acts directly under the appropriate assay conditions. Interleukin-10 inhibits interferon-γ production by activated TH1 cells, promotes survival and expression of class 2 major histocompatibility complex antigens in murine splenic B cells, and, in the presence of IL-3 or IL-4, stimulates mass cell proliferation. Finocyte and T cell proliferation are stimulated in the presence of IL-2 and IL-4. Human IL-10 has also been reported to inhibit IL-1α, IL-1β, IL-6, IL-8, tumor necrosis factor-α, GM-CSF, and G-CSF production by monocytes. It seems as though IL-10 may, in fact, be a major component of many dampening negative regulator systems.—P.J. Quesenberry, M.D.

Macrophage Colony-Stimulating Factor Regulates Both Activities of Neutral and Acidic Cholesteryl Ester Hydrolases in Human Monocyte-Derived Macrophages
Inaba T, Shimano H, Gotoda T, Harada K, Shimada M, Kawamura M, Yazaki Y, Yamada N (Univ of Tokyo)
J Clin Invest 92:750–757, 1993   116-95-2–4

Background.—Cholesterol metabolism is regulated both in vitro and in vivo by macrophage CSF (M-CSF). The effects of M-CSF on enzyme activities of acidic cholesterol ester hydrolase, neutral cholesterol ester hydrolase, and acyl-coenzyme A:cholesterol acyltransferase (ACAT) were examined. All investigated activities are involved in cellular cholesterol metabolism in macrophages.

Findings.—During the differentiation of monocytes to macrophages, all enzyme activities were induced and further enhanced by M-CSF. The introduction of M-CSF, 100 ng/mL, resulted in a 3.2-fold, fourfold, and 2.3-fold enhancement of acidic and neutral cholesterol ester hydrolase and ACAT activities, respectively, in the presence of acetyl low-density lipoprotein. These enzyme activities were influenced by acetyl low-density lipoprotein. An increase in ACAT and acidic cholesterol ester hydrolase activities and a decrease in neutral cholesterol ester hydrolase activity were noted. These findings suggest that these enzymes are regulated by intracellular cholesterol enrichment. The ratios of acidic cholesterol ester hydrolase to ACAT activity and neutral cholesterol ester hydrolase to ACAT activity were increased by M-CSF.

Conclusion.—The M-CSF seems to enhance net hydrolysis of cholesterol ester by stimulating the 2 cholesterol ester hydrolases to a greater degree than ACAT, and M-CSF may reduce the rate of atherogenesis.

▶ To the delight of the biotech marketers, CSF-1 and GM-CSF have been shown to reduce serum cholesterol levels. This article addresses the potential mechanisms of these actions. Although there are very strong correlations of cholesterol levels with atherogenesis, the information that altering these levels impacts in a positive way on the disease is marginal at best. Therefore, the supposition that M-CSF may reduce the rate of atherogenesis is quite premature.—P.J. Quesenberry, M.D.

Human Interferon-Inducible Protein 10: Expression and Purification of Recombinant Protein Demonstrate Inhibition of Early Human Hematopoietic Progenitors

Sarris AH, Broxmeyer HE, Wirthmueller U, Karasavvas N, Cooper S, Lu L, Krueger J, Ravetch JV (Mem Sloan-Kettering Cancer Ctr, New York; Indiana Univ, Indianapolis; Rockefeller Univ, New York; et al)
J Exp Med 178:1127–1132, 1993   116-95-2–5

Objective.—Human interferon-inducible protein 10 (IP-10) is an intercrine cytokine or chemokine. It is secreted by interferon-γ–stimulated T cells, monocytes, endothelial cells, and keratinocytes. Initial experiments were conducted to define the biological proteins of IP-10 via cloning and overexpression in baculovirus and in bacterial protein expression systems.

Findings.—Infected insect cells secreted a 9.9-kD protein. On sodium dodecyl sulfate–polyacrylamide gel electrophoresis, this protein comigrated with keratinocyte IP-10 and f(22-98), a bacterial recombinant fragment with all residues of IP-10 except for the signal sequence. The 9.9-kD protein, IP-10, and f(22–98) all reacted with antibodies recognizing IP-10 residues 10-98 (αIP-10) and 77-98 (α22). Thus, IP-10 was secreted by keratinocytes and insect cells after removal of the signal sequence but without proteolysis of the COOH-terminal end.

In early human bone marrow cells requiring r-steel factor (rSLF) and GM-CSF or rSLF and recombinant EPO, colony formation was suppressed by purified recombinant IP-10. This dose-dependent inhibition was complete at concentrations of 50 ng/mL or greater. It was prevented by preincubation of recombinant IP-10 with αIP-10 but not with α22. Inhibition was also noted with highly purified CD34+ cells, indicating that rIP-10 had a direct effect on the progenitors. Combined with other chemokines at inactive concentrations, recombinant IP-10 inhibited colony formation in a synergistic fashion. Colony formation was unaffected by recombinant IP-10 in the absence of any growth factors or in the presence of recombinant EPO or recombinant GM-CSF but in the absence of rSLF.

Conclusion.—The inhibition of early human hematopoietic progenitors by IP-10 was documented. These effects may play a role in normal marrow function and might be harnessed clinically to protect progenitor cells from cytotoxic chemotherapy.

▶ The IP-10 is a member of the intercrine family, which evidences chemotaxis activity with monocytes, neutrophils, T cells, basophils, and fibroblasts. Members of this family also appear to have inhibitory activity on bone marrow progenitors. The α-subfamily includes GRO-α, β-thromboglobulin macrophage inflammatory protein (MIP)-2α, MIP-2β, IL-8, neutrophil-activating peptide-2, and IL-10, whereas the β-family includes MIP-1α, MIP-1β, macrophage-chemotactic and activating factor, and RANTES. The MIP-1α, MIP-2α, PF4, IL-8, and macrophage-chemotactic and activating factor all seem to have inhibitory activity on marrow progenitors similar to that seen with IL-10. Action of IL-10 on CD34 cells seems to be direct, and IL-10 appears to synergize with the above intercrine molecules in inhibiting colony formation. This, along with the other intercrine molecules, offers the potential of myeloprotection in a chemotherapy setting.—P.J. Quesenberry, M.D.

Interleukin 3 Stimulates Proliferation and Triggers Endothelial–Leukocyte Adhesion Molecule 1 Gene Activation of Human Endothelial Cells
Brizzi MF, Garbarino G, Rossi PR, Pagliardi GL, Arduino C, Avanzi GC, Pegoraro L (Università di Torino, Italy)
J Clin Invest 91:2887–2892, 1993   116-95-2-6

Background.—The proliferation and functional activation of endothelial cells in an inflamed tissue site are regulated by humoral factors released by cells that infiltrate the perivascular space, for example, T lymphocytes and monocytes. The effects of IL-3, an activated T-lymphocyte–derived cytokine, on cultured human umbilical vein endothelial cells (HUVECs) were investigated.

Methods and Findings.—Proliferative activity was assessed both by estimation of the fraction of cells in the S phase and by direct cell count. Interleukin-3, 25 ng/mL, increased DNA synthesis and cell proliferation more than threefold above baseline control conditions. Binding studies with radioiodinated ligand showed that HUVECs constitutively expressed a small number of IL-3 binding sites. Molecular analysis demonstrated transcripts for both α- and β-subunits of the IL-3 receptor. The expression of the endothelial–leukocyte adhesion molecule 1 (ELAM-1) transcript and leukocyte adhesion were used to assess the functional activation of endothelial cells. The ELAM-1 gene transcript was evident 4 hours after the addition of IL-3 and began to decline after 12 hours. In addition, IL-3–induced ELAM-1 transcription was followed by increased neutrophil and CD4+ T-cell adhesion to HUVEC.

Conclusion.—Interleukin-3 stimulates proliferation of HUVEC, ELAM-1 gene activation, and neutrophil and CD4+ cell adhesion. Locally released IL-3 may support the coexistence of neovascularization and leukocyte recruitment in chronically inflamed sites.

▶ This extends the actions of IL-3 to endothelial cells. A general theme in the cytokine field is the pleiotropy of action of most cytokines. Cytokines are produced by most cell types, and a large number of cell types appear to be able to respond differentially to different cytokines. Part of the regulatory network also seems to be modulation of adhesion molecules. These molecules appear to act in the trafficking of different cell populations and probably also in the functional activation and, in certain circumstances, the regulation of proliferation and differentiation.—P.J. Quesenberry, M.D.

Transcription of Genes Encoding Granulocyte-Macrophage Colony-Stimulating Factor, Interleukin 3, and Interleukin 6 Receptors and Lack of Proliferative Response to Exogenous Cytokines in Non-hematopoietic Human Malignant Cell Lines
Guillaume T, Sekhavat M, Rubinstein DB, Hamdan O, Symann ML (Catholic Univ of Louvain, Brussels, Belgium; Boston Univ)
Cancer Res 53:3139–3144, 1993   116-95-2-7

Background.—It has been suggested that human tumor cell lines can respond in vitro to hematopoietic growth factors. The transcription of the α- and β-subunits of the GM-CSF receptor, the α- and β-subunits of the IL-3 receptor, and the single subunit of the IL-6 receptor and its associated gp130 transduction protein were studied in malignant cell lines.

Methods and Findings.—Polymerase chain reaction amplification of reverse-transcribed cellular messenger RNA was performed in 34 malignant cell lines derived from various histologic cell types. The messenger RNA for a single subunit polypeptide was detected in 23% of the cell lines. In 20%, both α- and β-subunits of either the GM-CSF receptor or the IL-3 receptor were found in a number of histologic cell types. In 38% of the cell lines, transcription of the gene encoding the IL-6 receptor was found. All cell lines transcribed the gp130 transduction protein, which is consistent with earlier findings of the ubiquity of that polypeptide. Then GM-CSF, IL-3, or IL-6 was added in therapeutic concentrations to assess the in vitro effect of exogenously added growth factors on those malignant cell lines transcribing complete cytokine receptor. Cellular proliferation was measured by incorporating [³H]thymidine. There was no stimulation at 3 or 6 days of culture. Cytokine production by these cell lines was studied at the transcription level and by assay of the peptide product. None transcribed messenger RNA for GM-CSF or IL-3. Five of 6 expressed IL-6 messenger RNA. Two of these latter cell lines produced IL-6 as determined by bioassay. None produced GM-CSF or IL-3 by enzyme-linked immunosorbent assay.

Conclusion.—In the case of GM-CSF and IL-3, the failure to proliferate after addition of cytokine is apparently not the result of the previous existence of endogenous production. However, at least a subset of malignant cell lines may involve a closed IL-6 autocrine loop that saturates cell surface sites. The ability to transcribe the genes encoding the cytokine receptor appears to be inadequate by itself to make cells cytokine-responsive. Malignant cells may lack the cellular machinery for cytokine-induced proliferation. The therapeutic administration of GM-CSF, IL-3, or IL-6 may therefore involve no additional risk of tumor regrowth in vivo.

▶ This is a nice study, but the conclusion that "therapeutic administration of either GM-CSF, IL-3, or IL-6 may involve no additional risk of tumor regrowth in vivo" may not be warranted. These results are based on tritiated thymidine incorporation at 3 or 6 days of culture. This can be misleading, and it would have been preferable if actual cell counts at different intervals and daily thymidine incorporation results had been presented. It appears that about 1 of 4 articles in this area provide negative results whereas the others show receptor expression and proliferation of various cell lines. I think, overall, the weight of evidence still suggests that tumor stimulation in vivo may be a problem, at least in some subsets of patients. An intriguing presentation at the recent European Hematology Association meetings actually suggested direct stimulation of solid tumor growth in patients during the administration of GM-CSF. Although this obviously needs confirmation, the issue remains of real concern, and it is my opinion that a subset of patients, which probably varies in percentage among different tumors, has tumor growth stimulated by the various cytokines. It is a challenge to the oncology community to adequately assess these patients and to provide appropriate tailored therapy rather than the current shot-gun approaches with cytokines. It is worth noting that as yet there have been no valid scientific results indicating a true patient benefit in cancer patients treated with either G-CSF or GM-CSF.—P.J. Quesenberry, M.D.

Soluble Forms of the Interleukin-6 Signal-Transducing Receptor Component gp130 in Human Serum Possessing a Potential to Inhibit Signals Through Membrane-Anchored gp130

Narazaki M, Yasukawa K, Saito T, Ohsugi Y, Fukui H, Koishihara Y, Yancopoulos GD, Taga T, Kishimoto T (Osaka Univ, Japan; Tosoh Corp, Kanagawa, Japan; Chugai Pharmaceutical Co, Ltd, Shizuoka, Japan; et al)
Blood 82:1120–1126, 1993   116-95-2–8

Background.—Interleukin-6 is a pleiotropic cytokine that has growth-promoting and growth-inhibiting effects on a wide range of cell types. In addition, it sometimes promotes cellular differentiation. Interleukin-6 exerts its multiple actions through a specific receptor system consisting of 2 membrane proteins, a ligand-binding receptor (IL-6R), and gp130. The IL-6 signal is transduced through membrane-anchored gp130, which is associated with IL-6R in the presence of IL-6. Soluble forms of gp130 (sgp130) having molecular weights of 90 and 110 Kd have been identified in human serum.

Objective.—The potential effects of sgp130 on various cytokines including oncostatin M, leukemia inhibitory factor, and ciliary neurotrophic factor were examined. A murine pro–B-cell line–derived transfectant, BAF-130, which expresses human gp130, was used to study the function of serum sgp130.

Findings.—Serum sgp130 was associated with soluble IL-6R in the presence of recombinant IL-6. Studies using the sandwich enzyme-linked immunosorbent assay showed that sera from healthy humans contained a mean of 390 ng of sgp130 per mL. Human serum supplemented with recombinant IL-6 induced DNA synthesis in BAF-130 cells, but serum deprived of soluble IL-6R did not. Induced DNA synthesis increased when the serum was deprived of sgp130. The synthesis of DNA induced by oncostatin M on the ciliary neurotrophic factor/recombinant-soluble ciliary neurotrophic factor receptor complex was significantly inhibited by recombinant sgp130. Its effect on the DNA synthesis induced by leukemia-inhibiting factor or the IL-6/soluble IL-6R complex was less marked.

Interpretation.—Naturally produced sgp130 and soluble IL-6R both are seen in human serum. The latter, in conjunction with IL-6, can act on cells that do not ordinarily respond to IL-6. Serum sgp130 may negatively regulate the IL-6 signal and may inhibit various cytokines in vivo.

▶ These intriguing data indicate an extracellular cytokine/cytokine receptor signaling pathway. Soluble IL-6R and IL-6 presumably interacting with membrane gp130 on cells may mediate biological effects on cells that do not express the IL-6R. This could be a cause of a number of pathophysiologic phenomena associated with infection or inflammation. Soluble gp130 may be the inhibitory arm of this regulatory network and conceivably could be effective in ameliorating certain signs and symptoms associated with elevated IL-6 levels (e.g., Castelman's disease, atrial myxoma, and infection).—P.J. Quesenberry, M.D.

Expression and Regulation of Human Neutrophil-Derived Macrophage Inflammatory Protein 1α
Kasama T, Strieter RM, Standiford TJ, Burdick MD, Kunkel SL (Univ of Michigan, Ann Arbor)
J Exp Med 178:63–72, 1993   116-95-2-9

Objective.—The acute inflammatory response is characterized by polymorphonuclear leukocyte (PMN) sequestration. As the inflammatory response evolves, PMNs are commonly replaced by mononuclear cells, usually as the lesion moves toward repair or resolution or progresses toward chronic inflammation. It was postulated that 1 possible mechanism for this shift is that PMNs are a rich source of monocyte chemotactic factors. An investigation was conducted to test this hypothesis.

Observations.—The PMNs treated with lipopolysaccharide showed a dose-dependent induction of monocyte chemotactic activity. This activity was significantly decreased in the presence of neutralizing anti–human macrophage inflammatory protein-1α (MIP-1α) antibodies. The antibody MIP-1α was expressed by stimulated PMNs on immunolocalization studies. Further studies to characterize MIP-1α steady-state messenger RNA and antigen expression showed a dose- and time-dependent production by lipopolysaccharide-treated PMNs. Although GM-CSF did not induce MIP-1α expression, PMNs stimulated in the presence of both GM-CSF and lipopolysaccharide showed enhanced and prolonged expression for both MIP-1α messenger RNA and antigen. Isolated MIP-1α had a longer messenger RNA half-life than that stimulated in the presence of lipopolysaccharide alone.

Conclusion. —It appears that PMNs are capable of producing MIP-1α in the presence of lipopolysaccharide; production is further influenced by GM-CSF, a portent activator of PMNs. Polymorphonuclear leukocyte–derived MIP-1α production, along with expression of appropriate adhesion molecules at the inflammation site, may be a key event contributing to the shift from PMNs to monocytes during the evolution of the inflammatory response.

▶ Here it is again, now in the guise of a chemoattractant as opposed to a stem cell inhibitor. We, of course, characterize all biological phenomena within the context of our own tunnel vision. We characterize molecular entities based on a favorite assay and then are disappointed when a "knockout experiment" does not confirm our preconceptions. For example, the src oncogene group was devastated by the meager impact of a src "knockout" (knockout meaning get rid of the gene in a transgenic mouse and see the effect). The leukemia inhibitory factor people were initially equally puzzled until they found that although the phenotype of the leukemia inhibitory factor knockout mouse was virtually normal, the blastocytes in this animal failed to implant. Thus, there is "no effect" on the individual, but the species is destroyed. Another example is the GM-CSF knockout on an op-op background: a mouse with no GM-CSF or CSF-1. It is hematologically normal, but guess what? It has a pulmonary disease closely resembling alveolar proteinosis. Thus, with a refreshing vigor, the hematologist investigators become pulmonologists.—P.J. Quesenberry, M.D.

Transforming Growth Factor β: Is It a Downregulator of Stem Cell Inhibition by Macrophage Inflammatory Protein 1α?
Maltman J, Pragnell IB, Graham GJ (Beatson Inst for Cancer Research, Glasgow, Scotland)
J Exp Med 178:925–932, 1993 116-95-2-10

Background. —Recent studies have shown that transforming growth factor-β1 (TGF-β1) and macrophage inflammatory protein-1α (MIP-1α) are potent hematopoietic stem cell proliferation inhibitors that appear to function in a similar way. An in vitro study was conducted to clarify the relationship between the 2 and to define their possible separate roles in the hematopoietic system.

Observations.—Both TGF-β and MIP-1α inhibited the CFU-A/CFU-S stem cell population with similar potency. In bone marrow–derived macrophages, from which MIP-1α is presumed to originate, TGF-β was a potent inhibitor of MIP-1α gene expression. This nonspecific inhibition of gene expression was also reflected in a reduction of MIP-1α protein production. In further experiments, TGF-β reversibly down-regulated MIP-1α receptor levels on a murine stem cell line as much as 70% after 24 hours. Increasing the concentration or length of exposure to TGF-β did not alter the observed level of downregulation. On Scatchard analysis, the down-regulation of MIP-1α receptors was unassociated with any change in the affinity of the remaining receptors.

Conclusion.—Transforming growth factor-β may have the potential to interfere with the stem cell inhibitory role of MIP-1α. Without active TGF-β in vivo, MIP-1α is probably no more than a weak contributor to overall stem cell inhibition. In the presence of active TGF-β and in the absence of upregulators of MIP-1α transcription, very little MIP-1α is probably produced in vivo.

▶ The inhibitors of hematopoietic stem cells are edging into their own. The ability to selectively and reversibly block proliferation of stem cells can be used as a myeloprotectant during cytoxic therapy directed against proliferating cancer cells. Inhibitors such as TGF-β may have both stimulatory and inhibitory action dependent on the stage of differentiation of a particular stem cell. Thus, an end result of in vivo action would be difficult to predict.

My mentor, the late Frederick Stohlman, cautioned me during my fellowship not to study inhibitors: It was hard enough to get things to grow in vitro! At that time he was right. Culture systems with mixed-cell populations, uncharacterized stimulators (conditioned media), and serum supplements provided dangerous hunting ground for inhibitors—lurking in the bushes was unpredictable artifact. Now, with purified cells and regulators and serum-free systems, inhibitors can be, and have been, validly characterized. The next big clinical hit was in this area of investigation.—P.J. Quesenberry, M.D.

Cytokine Clinical

Lymphoproliferative Disorder of Granular Lymphocytes Associated With Severe Neutropenia: Response to Granulocyte Colony-Stimulating Factor

Cooper DL, Henderson-Bakas M, Berliner N (Yale-New Haven Hosp, Conn)
Cancer 72:1607–1611, 1993   116-95-2–11

Purpose.—The term lymphoproliferative disorder of granular lymphocytes (LPGLs) refers to an indolent disorder, often associated with neutropenia, in which most patients are stable without any treatment. However, there has been little progress in the management of patients who do require treatment or in understanding the possible mechanisms of the associated, sometimes severe, cytopenias. A patient with LPGL who responded to treatment with G-CSF was described.

Case Report.—Woman, 76, had LPGL, severe neutropenia, and life-threatening pneumonia. Her WBC count was 4,900/μL with 70% lymphocytes and 1% neutrophils; all neutrophil counts were less than 20/μL. The patient's chest radiographic findings worsened despite antibiotic treatment, and her granulocyte count remained less than 10/μL. She was treated with G-CSF, 300 μg/day subcutaneously, on her twelfth hospital day. The neutrophil count increased to 4,200/μL within 5 doses, and to more than 10,000/μL within 7 doses. The lymphocyte count increased slightly, and the granulocyte count rapidly decreased to less than 100/μL. The infection resolved and did not recur.

Discussion.—This case and others like it from the literature suggest that LPGL with severe neutropenia may respond to treatment with G-CSF or GM-CSF. These CSFs are relatively nontoxic and have a rapid onset of action. They should be considered as initial therapy for such patients. The neutropenia may result from some defect of myeloid maturation rather than from accelerated granulocyte removal.

▶ The large granular lymphocytosis leukemias are a special subset of chronic neutropenia. The use of G-CSF in chronic neutropenias, based largely on work with cyclical neutropenia, chronic idiopathic, neutropenic, and Kaustman's syndrome, appears to be of clear clinical benefit. Although this is essentially an anecdotal paper, giving G-CSF in this setting is a reasonable intervention given the chronic nature of the problem. This is quite different from the setting of acute drug-induced neutropenia, in which there is virtually no rationale for the use of G-CSF. It is important to keep in mind that the large granular lymphocytosis leukemias, some of which at least are clonal T-cell diseases, may respond to corticosteroids or may spontaneously remit.—P.J. Quesenberry, M.D.

Development and Application of a Sensitive Radioimmunoassay for Human Granulocyte-Macrophage Colony-Stimulating Factor Able to Measure Normal Concentrations in Blood
Mortensen BT, Schifter S, Pedersen LB, Jensen AN, Hovgaard D, Nissen NI (Rigshospitalet, Copenhagen)
Exp Hematol 21:1366–1370, 1993   116-95-2–12

Background.—Measurement of the different hematopoietic growth factors and their fluctuations in states of health and disease is essential to a deeper understanding of them. Previously described techniques have been unable to measure GM-CSF in human serum under normal conditions. A sensitive radioimmunoassay for human GM-CSF was developed based on rabbit antibodies.

Description.—The radioimmunoassay was based on antibodies from rabbits immunized with glycosylated recombinant human GM-CSF (rhGM-CSF). These antibodies were specific for human GM-CSF, with no cross-reaction with other human hematopoietic growth factors or mouse GM-CSF. They do react with nonglycosylated rhGM-CSF, meaning that the assay can detect *Escherichia coli* –derived rhGM-CSF as well. In tests, the range of measurement of the new radioimmunoassay was approximately 10–200 pg/mL. The mean GM-CSF content of normal blood was 18.5 pg/mL, with a range of 3–24 pg/mL. Treatment of normal human serum with anti–GM-CSF monoclonal antibodies removed the growth factor, suggesting that the GM-CSF measured was real, not just the product of nonspecific reactivity with the polyclonal rabbit antibodies.

Conclusion.—This new radioimmunoassay is sensitive enough to detect small amounts of GM-CSF in normal human serum or plasma. This assay will permit more precise investigation of the nature and physiology of human GM-CSF in health and disease. Sensitive tests for the other hematopoietic growth factors and their receptors are needed as well.

▶ The idea that GM-CSF was a "noncirculating" factor only acting locally never did sit well. This study indicates the presence of detectable levels of GM-CSF in the serum and clarifies this area of cytokine physiology. It is difficult to know whether to characterize these as "low" levels. Data from our labs and others indicate that, in certain circumstances, the biological activity of various hematopoietic cytokines may be evident at levels several logs below those detectable in standard assays. This is especially true under serum-free conditions. Thus, these "low" levels may in fact be physiologically very significant, and I think it is appropriate now to consider GM-CSF as another of the circulating humoral marrow growth factors.—P.J. Quesenberry, M.D.

Liver Damage in Patients With Colony-Stimulating Factor-Producing Tumors

Suzuki A, Takahashi T, Okuno Y, Seko S, Fukuda Y, Nakamura K, Fukumoto M, Konaka Y, Imura H (Kyoto Univ, Japan; Kitano Hosp, Osaka, Japan)
Am J Med 94:125–132, 1993   116-95-2–13

Background.—Some malignant tumors produce CSFs that result in marked leukocytosis. Patients with such tumors also may be febrile and have a high serum level of C-reactive protein (CRP). Some have had abnormal liver function and progressive jaundice.

Clinical Observations.—Six patients with malignant tumors who had a WBC count of more than 15,000/μL were studied to determine whether liver damage in these cases is specifically related to the presence of a CSF-producing tumor. The tumors included carcinomas of the lung, stomach, and pancreas; a T-cell lymphoma; and a malignant fibrous histiocytoma. Five tumors produced G-CSF and 1 produced a GM-CSF. All the patients had spikes of fever exceeding 38°C. Neutrophilic leukocytosis persisted throughout the course of disease. The serum level of CRP was markedly elevated in nearly all patients. All patients had high levels of biliary enzymes but normal or only mildly increased levels of glutamic oxaloacetic transaminase and glutamic pyruvic transaminase. Three patients had a progressive increase in serum bilirubin with direct bilirubin predominating. No patient had hepatic coma. None of the autopsies showed evidence of major bacterial or fungal infection, but 2 patients had tumor metastases to bone. Changes in the liver included focal centrilobular necrosis associated with neutrophilic infiltration, fibrotic changes, and intrahepatic cholestasis.

Experimental Study.—Two tumor cell lines that produce G-CSF and IL-1 and IL-6, KHC287 and CHU-2, were transplanted into nude mice. With the exception of cholestasis, the same pathologic changes were seen in the liver of these animals as in the patients with CSF-producing tumors.

Conclusion.—This paraneoplastic syndrome of leukocytosis and liver damage presumably is caused by the tumoral production of multiple cytokines. The liver damage may result in jaundice, and caution is required in using drugs that could make the damage worse.

▶ This may be a fairly common occurrence in cancer patients given the difficulty in sorting out causation for signs and symptoms in those who are receiving some combination of chemotherapy, radiation therapy, antiemetics, and narcotics and are susceptible to various infections, etc. It would be easy to ascribe liver function abnormalities to other causes. Clinical trials with G-CSF and GM-CSF have not documented this complication, but it would be easy to miss, especially in a subset of patients. Count on hearing much more of multicytokine liver damage syndrome and seeing it in patients given therapeutic doses of cytokines.—P.J. Quesenberry, M.D.

Stem Cell and Transplantation

Long-Term Engraftment of Normal and Post–5-Fluorouracil Murine Marrow Into Normal Nonmyeloablated Mice
Stewart FM, Crittenden RB, Lowry PA, Pearson-White S, Quesenberry PJ (Univ of Virginia, Charlottesville)
Blood 81:2566–2571, 1993   1 16-95-2–14

Background.—Little is known about the effects of the intramedullary changes associated with myeloablation on marrow engraftment or long-term renewal. Also, virtually no information is available on engraftment and renewal of different marrow cell populations in normal noncytoablated hosts. The capacity of normal and post–5-fluorouracil murine marrow to engraft and persist in normal, nonirradiated host mice was investigated.

Methods and Findings.—Chromosomal banding and Southern blot analysis were used to identify transplanted male marrow cells. The long-term stability of the chimeric marrow was shown. The Balb/C, BDF1, or CBA-J female hosts received 40 × 10⁶ male cells of the same strain every day for 5 days. Repopulation patterns were observed. Parallel studies were done with tibia/femur equivalents of normal marrow or marrow from Balb/C mice pretreated with 150 mg of 5-fluorouracil per kg 6 days earlier. Chromosome banding methods demonstrated that 5% to 46% of marrow cells were male 3–9 months after transplantation with normal donor marrow. Southern blot analysis with the pY2 probe demonstrated continued engraftment 21–25 months after transplantation, with 15% to 42% male engrafted cells in the marrow. Normal donor male marrow engrafted significantly better than male marrow pretreated with 5-fluorouracil in noncytoablated females. Proportions of male engrafted cells in bone marrow ranged from 23% to 78% and .1% to 39% in recipients of normal marrow and recipients of 5-fluorouracil marrow, respectively. The mean engraftment for 6 mice receiving normal marrow was 38%, compared with 8% for 6 mice receiving post-5-fluorouracil marrow 1–3 months after transplantation. The mean engraftment was 46% and 16% for the normal and 5-fluorouracil groups, respectively, at 10–12 months. Engraftment patterns with normal and 5-fluorouracil marrow for spleen and thymus were similar.

Conclusion.—The successful long-term engraftment of normal male donor bone marrow into noncytoablated female mice challenges the assumption that niches must be created for marrow engraftment. Transplanted marrow apparently competes equally with host marrow for space.

▶ This article from our laboratory follows up on classic work by Brecher and colleagues (1) and Saxe and Boggs (2) showing that engraftment into non-myeloablated hosts is feasible. This present work extends those data, showing significant rates of engraftment up to 78% for female recipients of normal male marrow up to over 2 years post engraftment. Similar rates of engraftment were seen in thymus, spleen, and bone marrow. Perhaps most intriguingly, marrow harvested from animals 6 days after administration of 150 mg of 5-fluorouracil per kg was markedly deficient as compared with normal marrow in engraftment into nonmyeloablated mice. This contrasts with published data indicating that 6-day post–5-fluorouracil marrow competes equally well with normal marrow in irradiated hosts, suggesting that these 2 assays may monitor quite different stem cells or, alternatively, the same stem cell in a different functional state. More recent data indicate that the key to these high rates of engraftment may be scheduling and that the cycle status of the cell is critical, i.e., cycling cells appear to engraft quite poorly.—P.J. Quesenberry, M.D.

References

1. Brecher G, et al: *Proc Natl Acad Sci U S A* 79:5085, 1982.
2. Saxe DF, et al: *Exp Hematol* 12:277, 1984.

Declining Lymphocyte Counts Following Cytomegalovirus (CMV) Infection Are Associated With Fatal CMV Disease in Bone Marrow Transplant Patients

Fries BC, Khaira D, Pepe MS, Torok-Storb B (Fred Hutchinson Cancer Research Ctr, Seattle)

Exp Hematol 21:1387–1392, 1993   116-95-2-15

Introduction.—In previous reports of long-term cultures of bone marrow stromal cells, different cytomegalovirus (CMV) isolates infected different cell populations, with varying mechanisms and degrees of myelosuppression. In a pilot study of bone marrow transplant recipients, detection of CMV in lymphocytes was associated with decreased lymphocyte counts and death from CMV disease.

Methods.—This retrospective study examined the association between decreasing lymphocyte counts and CMV-related death in 332 CMV-infected bone marrow recipients. For the analysis, patients were divided into 3 groups: group I, consisting of 170 patients who survived CMV infection and were still alive at follow-up; group II, 103 patients who died of non–CMV-related causes; and group III, 59 patients who died of CMV disease. The lymphocyte counts of the 3 groups were observed during 24 days, beginning 10 days before the first CMV-positive culture.

Findings.—Group III had significantly lower lymphocyte counts throughout the period analyzed. Multivariate analysis found that the observed difference in lymphocyte counts did not result from any of the variety of factors that may affect lymphocytes in transplant patients, including acute graft-vs.-host disease, time since transplant, transplant type, and high-dose steroid treatment. In group III, the average lymphocyte count decreased by an average of 35% after day 0.

Conclusion.—Among bone marrow transplant recipients, decreasing lymphocyte counts may be a consequence of CMV infection associated with fatal CMV disease. Possible mechanisms of the decline include direct lymphocytic infection or defective immune response. The clinical outcome of CMV infection may be related to which specific cell types are infected.

▶ This is a simple but important clinical study. Decreased lymphocyte counts in CMV infections appear predictive of a lethal outcome. Happily, the prophylactic use of ganciclovir with the associated decreased incidence of CMV means that this observation may not become a predictor for therapeutic interventions. However, the clinician should keep aware of this correlation and the potential significance of a falling lymphocyte count in transplant patients with CMV infection.—P.J. Quesenberry, M.D.

Quantitation of Murine Hematopoietic Stem Cells In Vitro by Limiting Dilution Analysis of Cobblestone Area Formation on a Clonal Stromal Cell Line

Neben S, Anklesaria P, Greenberger J, Mauch P (Harvard Med School, Boston; Univ of Massachusetts, Worcester)
Exp Hematol 21:438–443, 1993   116-95-2–16

Background.—By limiting dilution analysis of cobblestone-area formation on stromal layers in micro–long-term bone marrow cultures, murine hematopoietic stem cells with different proliferative capacities can be assayed. Cobblestone-area–forming cell (CAFC), which is frequency determined on day 7, is correlated with mature stem cells measured as day 8 spleen CFUs (CFU-S). The CAFC frequency determined on day 28 is more closely associated with long-term marrow-repopulating ability. A modification of the CAFC assay was developed.

Methods and Findings.—In this modification, a clonal bone marrow stromal cell line, GB1/6, was substituted for fresh marrow-derived stromal layers. In vitro CAFC frequencies, in vivo CFU-S, and in vivo competitive repopulating ability using hematopoietic cell populations known to have different stem and progenitor cell content were compared. The GB1/6 cell monolayers supported the growth of overlaid fresh marrow with the same efficiency as fresh stromal layers. The GB1/6 cells were grown to confluence in as few as 2 days, compared with 2 weeks for fresh marrow. Good correlations were obtained between CAFC frequency at an early point in the assay and CFU-S frequency. The CAFC frequency at late time points and long-term in vivo repopulating ability were also well correlated.

Conclusion.—The modified CAFC assay is a more streamlined, less expensive alternative to previously described versions. The modified assay should be useful for predicting the stem cell content in various hematopoietic cell populations.

▶ This relates to the search for an in vitro stem cell assay. In the mouse, we have in vivo repopulating assays and thus can have some confidence that a true renewal stem cell is being assayed. This work suggests the critical nature of stromal cells for stem cell support and indicates that the CAFC may well monitor real stem cells. There are other in vitro assays that seem to monitor the same or a closely related stem cell. These are the multifactor responsive high proliferative potential colony-forming cell and the blast CFU. These assays are of particular importance because they may provide surrogate assays for marrow renewal cells in humans.—P.J. Quesenberry, M.D.

Bone Marrow Transplantation With Interleukin-1 Plus *kit*-Ligand Ex Vivo Expanded Bone Marrow Accelerates Hematopoietic Reconstitution in Mice Without the Loss of Stem Cell Lineage and Proliferative Potential
Muench MO, Firpo MT, Moore MAS (Mem Sloan-Kettering Cancer Ctr, New York)
Blood 81:3463–3473, 1993   116-95-2-17

Background.—Recombinant DNA technology has produced numerous cytokines used in regulating hematopoiesis. *Kit*-ligand (KL), or stem cell factor, is an important stimulator of murine mast cell growth but does not significantly stimulate myelopoiesis. However, combined with hematopoietic growth factors, it exhibits synergistic ability. The efficacy of 3 cytokine combinations (IL-1 + IL-3, IL-1 + KL, and IL-1 + IL-6 + KL) in expansion of murine bone marrow for bone marrow transplantation (BMT) was studied to measure the superiority of the IL-1 + KL expansion of d1 5-fluorouracil bone marrow in effecting swift and long-term recovery of lethally irradiated mice.

Methods.—Normal bone marrow or d1 5-fluorouracil bone marrow was expanded with and without cytokine combinations. Control mice receiving fresh BM transplants and mice receiving transplants expanded in varying amounts were studied to determine peripheral blood cell counts, numbers of high proliferative potential–colony-forming cells and low proliferative potential–colony-forming cells (to measure proliferative capacity), and host/donor source of splenic T cells in female mice (using Y chromosome–sensitive Southern blot analysis).

Results.—Expanded bone marrow significantly accelerated the recovery of peripheral blood cell counts, with neutrophils being the first cells to recover. Overall, bone marrow expanded with the IL-1 + KL combination effected the most rapid recovery of peripheral blood cells. Although deaths occurred at the lowest doses of expanded bone marrow, the long-term survival and cell reconstitution potential with bone marrow expanded with moderate doses of IL-1 + KL were strong and required dramatically decreased numbers of fresh bone marrow cells. Isolated splenic T cells in secondary female survivors reconstituted with male cells were clearly derived from expanded donor bone marrow cells. The numbers of high proliferative potential–colony-forming cells and low proliferative potential–colony forming cells in primary and secondary hosts receiving fresh bone marrow and expanded bone marrow were not significantly different, suggesting that long-term proliferative efficacy of stem cells is not affected by bone marrow expansion.

Discussion.—Bone marrow with expanded progenitors accelerates peripheral blood cell recovery. The decreased number of bone marrow cells required for long-term recovery suggests that survival is dependent not on the number of hematopoietic progenitors in the transplant, but rather on the number of committed progenitors that reconstitute peripheral blood cells after BMT. The data further show that stem cells are not responsible for this initial reconstitution. Bone marrow expansion may therefore have clinical significance in treating iatrogenic cytopenias and cancer.

▶ There has been a great deal of investigation into methods to expand hematopoietic stem cells, both to further our understanding of hematopoiesis and, more directly, to obtain potential methods for rapid repopulation in marrow or stem cell transplant settings. These data indicate that expanded stem cells can be quite effective for rapid marrow recovery but do not really address the long-term efficacy or potential of stem cells in this setting. There is clearly repopulation of the animals, perhaps showing that clinically this can be an effective approach; however, this does not address the number of stem cells carrying out the repopulation. Certainly, for gene therapy approaches, polyclonal hematopoiesis with the incorporated gene is probably the goal. The major question here is whether the long-term hematopoiesis is oligoclonal from a very small number of stem cells or polyclonal. My bet is that it is the former and that the irradiated mouse host represents, essentially, an amplification system. The model presented in Abstract 116-95-2–14 of engraftment into nonmyeloablated hosts probably represents a true competitive system without significant amplification, perhaps in part explaining the different results in these models.—P.J. Quesenberry, M.D.

Maintenance of Hematopoiesis in Serum-Free Bone Marrow Cultures Involves Sequential Recruitment of Quiescent Progenitors
Lansdorp PM, Dragowska W (British Columbia Cancer Agency, Vancouver, Canada; Univ of British Columbia, Vancouver, Canada)
Exp Hematol 21:1321–1327, 1993   116-95-2–18

Background.—CD34+CD71lo cells from adult human bone marrow maintain constant numbers in long-term suspension cultures supplemented with IL-6, IL-3, mast growth factor (MGF), and EPO. Several models have been proposed to explain this unexpected finding (Fig 2–1). Two experimental strategies were used to discriminate between the different models.

Methods.—In the first approach, sorted CD34+CD45RAloCD71lo cells were placed in serum-free culture supplemented with IL-6, IL-3, MGF, and EPO before and after labeling with fluorescent tracking dye PKH26. The PKH26 fluorescence of CD34+CD71lo and other culture cells was analyzed several times within 11 weeks. In the second approach, single CD+CD71lo cells were sorted into separate wells with serum-free medium supplemented with IL-6, IL-3, MGF, and EPO. Growing cells were analyzed by flow cytometry.

Results.—Although most CD34+CD71lo cells survived for as long as 6 weeks in the first experiment, the cell count diminished after 40 days. The PKH26 fluorescence was maintained in most CD34+ cells until day

1. Escape from G₀ pool **2. Self - renewal divisions** **3. Asymmetric divisions**

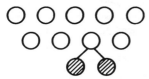 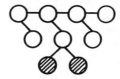 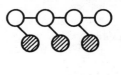

4. Combinations of above

Fig 2–1.—Models of hematopoietic stem cell maintenance in serum-free cultures that support extensive production of cells as well as maintenance of primitive hematopoietic (CD34$^+$CD71^{lo}) cells. *1*, survival in G$_0$. The cells are maintained in a quiescent state and the total cell production (> 10^6 cells per cell on day 30) is derived from a small fraction of input cells. *2*, self-renewal divisions. Some cells are capable of self-renewal, and maintenance of CD34$^+$CD71^{lo} cells is the net result of balanced self-renewal vs. loss of cells, for example, through differentiation or cell death. *3*, asymmetrical divisions. In this model, maintenance of cells is the result of asymmetrical cell divisions resulting in 2 different daughter cells, 1 of which has the CD34$^+$CD71^{lo} prototype. (Courtesy of Lansdorp PM, Dragowska W: *Exp Hematol* 21:1321–1327, 1993.)

40 but was lost in other culture cells by day 9. Overall, CD71 expression of CD34$^+$ cells decreased after day 40 in concert with a slight upregulation of CD34$^+$ expression in each experiment. The second experiment revealed substantial variability in cell survival and division: 10% of the input cells produced most of the new cells. Considerable heterogeneity was seen among progeny of clones containing more than 10^4 cells.

Conclusion.—Maintaining primitive CD34$^+$ cells in culture involves the survival of very-low-turnover CD34$^+$CD71^{lo} cells and very limited production of CD34$^+$ cells. Clonal heterogeneity, differences in CD34$^+$ and CD34$^-$ cell kinetics, and delayed proliferation of bone marrow–derived CD34$^+$CD45RA^{lo}CD71^{lo} cells in response to IL-6, IL-3, MGF, and EPO must be considered when experimental strategies for ex vivo expansion of primitive hematopoietic cells are developed.

▶ These intriguing in vitro data suggest that the key for long-term maintenance of early progenitor stem cells may be quiescence and that true expansion may be at the cost of losing these progenitors. A limiting problem with all in vitro expansion studies with human marrow remains the lack of an adequate in vivo engraftment model short of clinical transplantation.—P.J. Quesenberry, M.D.

CD4^{dull+} Hematopoietic Progenitor Cells in Murine Bone Marrow
Onishi M, Nagayoshi K, Kitamura K, Hirai H, Takaku F, Nakauchi H (Univ of Tokyo; Natl Med Ctr, Tokyo; Inst of Physical and Chemical Research (RIKEN), Tsukuba, Japan)
Blood 81:3217–3225, 1993   116-95-2–19

Background.—About 3% to 6% of murine bone marrow cells are positive for CD4, a glycoprotein that contributes to interactions between T cells and target cells through binding to the class II major histocompatibility complex molecule. Most CD4+ cells are CD4^{dull+}, but 2 distinct subpopulations are recognized: CD4 brightly positive Gr-1$^-$ cells and CD4+ Gr-1+ cells (CD4^{lo}Gr-1^{lo}). The former are thought to be mature T cells. The latter, composing about .6% of the bone marrow cells, express small amounts of B220 and Thy1 antigens.

Objective.—Studies were done in mice to determine whether CD4 is expressed on hematopoietic stem cells and has a role in hematopoiesis.

Findings.—Neither CFU-spleen nor CFU-culture were enriched in CD4^{lo}Gr-1^{lo} cells. However, when injected into lethally irradiated mice, these cells differentiated into T-cell, B-cell, and myelomonocyte lineages when cell assays were performed 26 weeks after transplantation. Donor-derived CD4^{lo} Gr-1^{lo} cells were seen in recipient bone marrow at least 16 weeks after transplantation.

Conclusion.—Murine CD4^{lo}Gr-1^{lo} cells are distinct from previously characterized hematopoietic stem cells. They are capable of renewing themselves, and they are able to differentiate into at least 3 hematopoietic lineages in the long term.

▶ This is a confirmation and extension of work showing that CD4 is present on murine pluripotent hematopoietic stem cells (1). This is of particular importance because of its impact on the issue of whether HIV infects early stem cells; most data on this point suggest that HIV does not infect early marrow stem cells.—P.J. Quesenberry, M.D.

Reference

1. Wineman JP, et al: *Blood* 80:1717, 1992.

Leukocytes

Mechanisms for Actin Reorganization in Chemotactic Factor-Activated Polymorphonuclear Leukocytes

Watts RG, Howard TH (Univ of Alabama, Birmingham)
Blood 81:2750–2757, 1993   116-95-2–20

Background.—Dynamic cytoskeletal reorganization in polymorphonuclear leukocytes is required for the motile processes necessary for normal functions. The cytoskeletal actin was thought to function in equilibrium between 2 forms, a monomeric form, globular actin (G-actin), and a polymeric form, filamentous actin (F-actin), by inducing, with soluble chemotactic factors or cellular activators, simple polymerization or depolymerization from 1 form to the other. However, recent findings have identified 2 distinct F-actin pools: a Triton-soluble and a Triton-insoluble pool. The tripartite equilibrium suggests that there may be additional mechanisms for actin reorganization.

Methods.—New actin filament formation in each pool was measured by quantification of NBDphallacidin binding and of cytoskeletal-associated actin by gel scanning. In addition, the quantity of actin in each actin pool was measured by moles at concurrent intervals during chemotactic factor–induced actin polymerization. To ensure physiologic relevance, and to prevent nonspecific actin reorganization, the experiments were also performed with a phalloidin buffer. To study kinetics, the effects of the addition of cytochalasin D, which inhibits end-to-end filament annealing but allows cross-linking, were observed.

Results.—After cytochalasin D activation, 60% of the F-actin increase occurred by new filament growth. The amount of actin increased exclusively in the Triton-insoluble F-actin pool and exceeded the amount accounted for by new filament growth. The actin increase in the Triton-insoluble F-actin pool exactly corresponded to the actin decrease in both the Triton-soluble F-actin pool and the G-actin pool. The phalloidin buffer did not prevent these effects. Cytochalasin D inhibited transfer of actin from the Triton-soluble F-actin pool and the G-actin pool by 75%.

Discussion.—Simple polymerization accounts for a minority of actin transformation. The data support a direct conversion from both G-actin and Triton-soluble F-actin exclusively to Triton-insoluble F-actin. The 75% cytochalasin D sensitivity suggests that end-to-end annealing is the primary process describing movement between the 2 F-actin pools but that some filament cross-linking may also occur.

▶ Neutrophil motility is a poorly understood process. Actin reorganization is clearly a major factor in the ability of these cells to move and function. These studies represent a nice step forward in our understanding of neutrophil motility.—P.J. Quesenberry, M.D.

β2-Integrin and L-Selectin Are Obligatory Receptors in Neutrophil Aggregation

Simon SI, Rochon YP, Lynam EB, Smith CW, Anderson DC, Sklar LA (Univ of New Mexico, Albuquerque; Los Alamos Natl Labs, NM; Baylor School of Medicine, Houston; et al)
Blood 82:1097–1106, 1993   116-95-2–21

Background.—Studies of neutrophil aggregation and adhesion to endothelium have shown that upregulation of β2-integrin is not necessary for initial adhesion, although it may be required for sustained adhesive function. Antibodies to L-selectin, the homing receptor on neutrophils, are as effective as anti-integrin antibodies in blocking formyl peptide-stimulated aggregation.

Objective and Methods.—Monoclonal antibodies against β2-integrin and L-selectin were used to examine adhesive receptor recognition in mixed populations of normal neutrophils and in cells from β2-integrin–

deficient patients. Fluorescence flow cytometry was used to characterize aggregates by size and color and to assess antibody binding. Formyl peptide–stimulated aggregate formation was measured in individual cell populations fluorescently labeled red or green.

Results.—Blocking either the β2-integrin or L-selectin adhesive epitope reduced 2-color aggregation by about half. Shedding L-selectin by preincubating cells with complexes of lipopolysaccharide and its plasma membrane–binding protein had the same effect. A study of neutrophils from patients genetically deficient in β2-integrin and clinically leukocyte adhesion–deficient showed that adhesion of leukocyte adhesion–deficient cells to normal neutrophils depended on the expression of L-selectin on leukocyte adhesion–deficient cells and the expression of β2-integrin on normal cells.

Conclusion.—Adhesion between 2 mixed populations of neutrophils requires, at a minimum, that 1 population expresses β2-integrin and that the other expresses L-selectin.

▶ This presentation highlights the key feature of ligand receptor binding, which is involved in all integrin-mediated interactions. Neutrophils express at least 3 adhesion proteins of the β2-integrin class: MAC-1, LFA-1, and L-selectin. Given the corresponding receptors for these ligands, the potential complexity of this system is apparent.—P.J. Quesenberry, M.D.

P-Selectin Mediates Spontaneous Leukocyte Rolling In Vivo
Doré M, Korthuis RJ, Granger DN, Entman ML, Smith CW (Baylor College of Medicine, Houston; Louisiana State Univ, Shreveport)
Blood 82:1308–1316, 1993   116-95-2–22

Background.—During an inflammatory reaction, rolling is the initial step leading to leukocyte extravasation from blood vessels. Previous in vitro studies suggest that P-selectin may be 1 of the ligands on endothelium involved in the occurrence of rolling. However, the molecular determinants that account for this transient attachment in vivo have not yet been defined. A blocking monoclonal antibody (MoAb) against canine P-selectin was developed and used in an investigation that used an intravital microscopy technique to examine the role of P-selectin in leukocyte rolling in vivo.

Methods and Findings.—P-selectin was immunoaffinity purified from canine platelets. It was then used to produce monoclonal antibodies. Enzyme-linked immunosorbent assay and flow cytometry revealed that MD6, 1 of the generated hybridomas, binded preferentially to stimulated platelets and completely prohibited binding of stimulated platelets to neutrophils. Examination of canine mesenteric venules visualized via intravital microscopy revealed that administration of MD6 led to a dramatic inhibition in the number of rolling leukocytes, at 18.96 compared with 156.4 leukocytes per minute (88.3% inhibition). Control antibody MD3, which recognizes a nonfunctional epitope of canine P-selectin, did not effect the number of rolling leukocytes or rolling velocity.

Conclusion.—P-selectin is directly involved in leukocyte rolling in vivo and may therefore be a key participant of the inflammatory response. The newly developed blocking MoAb against canine P-selectin should prove useful for future investigations of the functions of P-selectin in canine models of hemostasis and inflammatory diseases.

▶ Adhesion molecules carry out a number of biological roles, including migration of cells through tissue, fastening of cells to tissue sites, and, probably, the delivery of regulatory signals, at least to hematopoietic stem cells. P-selectin appears to be critical in leukocyte rolling, and a modulation of this integrin offers obvious opportunities for selectively inhibiting inflammatory responses in various pathologic states. The problem, of course, remains selectivity and therapeutic toxic ratios given the wide number of actions of these binding proteins.—P.J. Quesenberry, M.D.

Rapid IL-2-Induced Adherence of Human Natural Killer Cells: Expression of mRNA for Cytokines and IL-2 Receptors in Adherent NK Cells
Vitolo D, Vujanovic NL, Rabinowich H, Schlesinger M, Herberman RB, Whiteside TL (Univ of Pittsburgh, Pa; Hebrew Univ, Jerusalem)
J Immunol 151:1926–1937, 1993   116-95-2–23

Introduction.—A distinct subpopulation of human natural killer (NK) cells, characterized by an extremely rapid adherence response in the presence of 2–22 nM of IL-2, was recently isolated. These cells, termed adherent NK (A-NK) cells, may be more receptive to activation than other populations of NK cells. Expression of cytokine and IL-2 receptor genes was examined in these cells to determine whether A-NK cells are activated.

Methods.—Negative immunoselection with OKT3 monoclonal antibody was used to purify a population of normal human peripheral blood resting NK cells. These resting NK cells were then activated by exposure to 22 nM of IL-2 for 1, 3, 5, or 24 hours, and the A-NK and nonadherent NK cells were separated. In situ hybridization with labeled complementary DNA probes was used to examine expression of cytokine or IL-2 receptor messenger RNA.

Results.—In the population of receptor NK cells, few cells expressed IL-2 receptor p55 or cytokines IL-2, interferon-γ, tumor necrosing factor-α, and transforming growth factor-β. Much larger proportions of the receptor NK cells expressed IL-1-β (35%) and IL-6 (40%), indicating that these genes may be constitutively expressed in a significant proportion of circulating NK cells. In the A-NK cell population, a large proportion were positive for IL-2 receptor and cytokine expression. At 48 hours, there was also a high level of these proteins in culture superna-tants from A-NK cells, indicating that messenger RNA expression was followed by protein expression. In the nonadherent NK population, few cells expressed IL-2 receptor and cytokines, with the exception of in-creased expression of transforming growth factor-β.

Conclusion.—Exposure of normal peripheral human resting NK cells to 22 nM of IL-2 and selection for adherent cells can be used to purify a phenotypically and functionally distinct subset, A-NK cells. These adher-ent cells are also selectively activated for expression of IL-2 receptor and several cytokine genes. Therefore, A-NK cells appear to be a useful sub-set of cells for adoptive immunotherapy. These cells are currently being evaluated for therapeutic efficacy in animal tumor models.

▶ As I indicated in the comment for Abstract 116-95-2–24, we still are not really sure what a NK cell is, and we are now subsetting them. The problem, of course, with many cell populations is to determine when the subsetting is real vs. when one is simply looking at the same cell in a different functional state, especially in transit through the cell cycle. Hematopoietic cells show a wide range of responses to different cytokines and theoretically might be classified into multiple different subsets based on dose-response curves. We still need a better definition of NK cells.—P.J. Quesenberry, M.D.

Hematopoietic Cells and Radioresistant Host Elements Influence Nat-ural Killer Cell Differentiation
Sykes M, Harty MW, Karlhofer FM, Pearson DA, Szot G, Yokoyama W (Har-vard Med School, Boston; Mt Sinai Med Ctr, New York)
J Exp Med 178:223–229, 1993   116-95-2–24

Background.—Radioresistant host elements mediate the positive se-lection of developing thymocytes, whereas bone marrow-derived cells induce clonal deletion of T cells with receptors that are strongly auto-reactive. The elements governing the natural killer (NK) cell repertoire are not clearly understood. This repertoire, which is similar to the T-cell repertoire, differs among persons with different major histocompatibility complex (MHC) phenotypes. Murine bone marrow transplantation models were used to analyze the effects of donor and host MHC on a NK cell subset.

Methods and Findings.—To assess the effect of hematopoietic cell H-2^a expression on Ly-49 expression of H-2^b NK cells, mixed allogeneic chimeras were prepared by administering T-cell–depleted allogeneic and host-type marrow to lethally irradiated B10 mice or by administering B10.A marrow to B10 recipients conditioned by a nonmyeloablative regi-men. The expression of H-2^a on bone marrow–derived cells was suffi-cient to down-regulate Ly-49 expression on H-2^a as well as H-2^b NK cells, independent of the thymus. To assess the effect of H-2^a expressed on radioresistant host elements only, fully allogeneic chimeras were prepared by administering B10 bone marrow to lethally irradiated B10.A recipients. The B10 NK cells of these chimeras also showed down-regulation of Ly-49 expression.

Conclusion.—The differentiation of NK cells is determined by interactions with MHC molecules expressed on bone marrow–derived cells. To a lesser degree, MHC antigens expressed on radioresistant host elements also play a role.

▶ The NK cell still remains somewhat of a mystery. These important regulatory cells, as with most lymphohemopoietic elements, appear to be modulated by both hematopoietic cells and radioresistant stromal elements.—P.J. Quesenberry, M.D.

General

Clozapine-Induced Agranulocytosis: Incidence and Risk Factors in the United States

Alvir JMJ, Lieberman JA, Safferman AZ, Schwimmer JL, Schaaf JA (Hillside Hosp, Glen Oaks, NY; Sandoz Pharmaceuticals, East Hanover, NJ)
N Engl J Med 329:162–167, 1993   116-95-2–25

Background.—Clozapine offers substantial therapeutic advantages compared with standard antipsychotic drugs for patients with refractory schizophrenia. Although clozapine is not associated with acute extrapyramidal symptoms or tardive dyskinesia, it may cause potentially fatal agranulocytosis in as many as 2% of patients. Initially, clozapine was available only as part of a surveillance system that required a weekly white cell count before the patient could receive a supply of the drug.

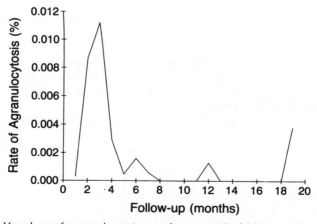

Fig 2–2.—Hazard rates for agranulocytosis, according to month of follow-up. (Courtesy of Alvir JMJ, Lieberman JA, Safferman AZ, et al: *N Engl J Med* 329:162–167, 1993.)

The incidence of and potential risk factors for clozapine-induced agranulocytosis in clozapine surveillance participants were examined.

Methods and Findings.—Clozaril Patient Management System (CPMS) records for 11,382 patients from February of 1990 to April of 1991 were reviewed. Forty-two women and 31 men had agranulocytosis. Twenty-three cases of agranulocytosis developed within 2 months after the start of clozapine therapy; 61 developed within 3 months, and 70 developed within 6 months; only 1 additional case developed within a year. Thus, the agranulocytosis hazard rate peaked in the third month (Fig 2–2). Patients who had agranulocytosis were considerably older than those who did not and had lower baseline white cell counts. Univariate survival analysis revealed correlations between risk of agranulocytosis and increasing age and female gender. Although the baseline white cell count was inversely related to the risk for agranulocytosis, the effect was not significant after adjustment for age and gender. Clozapine dose did not affect the risk for agranulocytosis.

Conclusion.—Although the hazard of agranulocytosis is substantial with clozapine treatment, monitoring the white cell count decreases the danger. The increasing risk associated with age and the reduced incidence after the first 6 months of treatment provide additional guidelines for future clozapine prescription and monitoring.

▶ This is an interesting summary of the risk of agranulocytosis with clozapine. It is my impression that the risk of death from agranulocytosis in drug-induced neutropenia is almost always overstated in the literature and that the risk of death in hospitalized patients under observation is really quite small. Two patients died in this series, although the data presented are inadequate to assess other potential clinical variables in these cases. It is worth emphasizing that there is no clinical or scientific base for the use of G-CSF in this setting, especially because G-CSF levels are virtually always quite high, although the number of patients with drug-induced agranulocytosis who are treated with G-CSF or GM-CSF continues to escalate.—P.J. Quesenberry, M.D.

A Recombinant Immunotoxin That Is Active on Prostate Cancer Cells and That Is Composed of the Fv Region of Monoclonal Antibody PR1 and a Truncated Form of *Pseudomonas* Exotoxin
Brinkmann U, Gallo M, Brinkmann E, Kunwar S, Pastan I (Natl Cancer Inst, Bethesda, Md)
Proc Natl Acad Sci U S A 90:547–551, 1993   116-95-2–26

Background.—Immunotoxins, IgG antibodies conjugated to plant or bacterial toxins, have been shown to exhibit potent cytotoxic effects on tumor cells. Truncated forms of the *Pseudomonas* exotoxin (PE) conjugated to antibody fragments (a variable light chain connected by a polypeptide linker to the variable heavy chain region) have also proven to be potent cytotoxic agents. Recently, a monoclonal antibody, PR1, that is reactive against both normal and cancerous prostate cells has been isolated. An investigation was conducted to determine the cytotoxicity of an immunotoxin derived from the variable light- and heavy-chain fragments of this antibody on prostate cancer cells.

Methods.—The DNA fragments encoding the PR1 variable light- and heavy-chain regions were obtained by reverse transcriptase. Polymerase chain reaction splicing was used to join the 2 fragments to a $(Gly_4\text{-}Ser)_3$ flexible spacer. This construct, PR1(Fv), was then fused to a truncated PE. The result was a fusion protein, PR1(Fv)-PE38KDEL, containing the single-chain variable light and heavy regions and the truncated PE cytotoxin. The fusion protein was induced by IPTG and isolated, solubilized, reduced, and refolded from *Escherichia coli* inclusion bodies.

Results.—N-terminal peptide sequencing and RNA sequencing confirmed that the fusion protein contained variable light- and heavy-chain regions. The PR1-reactive LNCaP cells were enriched from 1% to 3% to 40% PR1-reactive cells by fluorescence-activated cell sorter. Fusion protein bound specifically to these cells and displayed biphasic toxicity toward these cells. An ID_{50} of .8 ng/mL was found for 40% of these cells, whereas the remaining 60% had an ID_{50} of 250 ng/mL. In contrast, a PR1-negative cell line, OVCAR3, was unaffected.

Conclusion.—The immunotoxin PR1(Fv)-PE38KDEL binds specifically to cells containing the PR1 antigen. In addition, it is selectively toxic to LNCaP carcinoma cells that express the PR1 antigen on their surface. Because the PR1 antigen is strongly expressed in prostate carcinomas and normal prostate but only in several other normal tissues, PR1(Fv)-PE38KDEL should be considered for use in humans with prostate cancer.

▶ This is an interesting report on an immunotoxin active on prostate cancer. Immunotoxins continue to intrigue investigators, the key to their application being the specificity of the antibody. Aside from lymphoma idiotypes, we have yet to define true tumor-specific antigens, and this is an underlying flaw in the whole immunotoxin approach. However, relatively impressive results have been obtained with the use of pokeweed lectin/CD19 immunotoxin in lymphoma, and these approaches continue to be worth pursuing.—P.J. Quesenberry, M.D.

Stromal Cells From Human Long-Term Marrow Cultures Are Mesenchymal Cells That Differentiate Following a Vascular Smooth Muscle Differentiation Pathway

Galmiche MC, Koteliansky VE, Brière J, Hervé P, Charbord P (INSERM/CRTS, Besancon, France; Laboratoire de Physiopathologie du Developpement, Paris; Hopital Laennec, Paris)

Blood 82:66–76, 1993   116-95-2–27

Background.—In human long-term marrow cultures, connective tissue–forming stromal cells are an essential component of the adherent layer, in which granulomonocytic progenitors are produced after the second week. Most stromal cells in confluent cultures are stained by monoclonal antibodies against smooth muscle–specific actin isoforms. The time course of α-SM–positive stromal cells was evaluated.

Methods and Findings.—Other cytoskeletal proteins specific for smooth muscle cells were sought. The expression of α-SM in stromal cells was time dependent, with most adherent spindle-shaped, vimentin-positive stromal cells seen in the first 2 weeks being α-SM negative and most interdigitated stromal cells in weeks 3–7 containing stress fibers with backbones made of α-SM–positive microfilaments. Other proteins specific for smooth muscle were found in confluent cultures. These included metavinculin, h-caldesmon, smooth muscle myosin heavy chains, and calponin. In vitro studies of trephine bone marrow biopsy samples from adults with no hematologic abnormalities revealed α-SM–positive cells in diverse locations, including vascular smooth muscle cells in the media of arteries and arterioles, pericytes lining capillaries, myoid cells lining sinuses at the abluminal side of endothelial cells or in the hematopoietic logettes, and endosteal cells lining bone trabeculae. More or less mature granulocytic cells were in intimate contact with the thin cytoplasmic extensions of myoid cells, which may be the in vivo counterpart of the stromal cells with the vascular smooth muscle phenotype.

Conclusion.—Marrow mesenchymal cells, whose differentiation in culture results in immature vascular smooth muscle–like stromal cells, seem to give rise to myoid or barrier cells in vivo. The number and location of these cells appear to vary with hematopoietic cell need.

▶ This is further confirmation that vascular smooth muscle cells may be an important component of bone marrow stromal cells. Wiess and Geduldig (1) reported on barrier cells forming syncytial sheets and appearing to increase under conditions of increased hematopoiesis. Galmiche et al. suggest that these barrier cells may be related to vascular smooth muscle–like stromal cells.—P.J. Quesenberry, M.D.

Reference

1. Weiss L, Geduldig U: *Blood* 78:975, 1991.

HIV

Identification of a Novel Human Immunodeficiency Virus Strain Cytopathic to Megakaryocytic Cells

Kunzi MS, Groopman JE (Harvard Med School, Boston)
Blood 81:3336–3342, 1993
116-95-2–28

Background.—Studies and clinical evidence suggest that impaired megakaryocytopoiesis, caused by HIV interaction with megakaryocytes, may contribute to the development of thrombocytopenia. Thrombocytopenia is common with HIV infection. The HIV genome has been found in bone marrow karyocytes, and azidothymidine (AZT) treatment rapidly increases platelet count; both facts support the hypothesis.

Methods.—Three HIV viruses were isolated and cultured: HIV-WW from an asymptomatic HIV-seropositive patient with severe thrombocytopenia, HIV-1 JR-CSF from the CSF of a patient with AIDS dementia, and HIV-RJ9435 from an asymptomatic HIV-seropositive patient with severe neutropenia. Two megakaryocytic cell lines, CMK and DAMI, T-lymphocytic H9 cells, and monocytic U937 cells were challenged with each HIV isolate. The CMK and DAMI cells were then challenged with 2 inoculates derived from HIV-WW strains inactivated by filtration and heat to test specificity. To investigate the role of viral replication, CMK and DAMI cells were challenged by HIV-WW in the presence of AZT. The involvement of viral envelope glycoprotein binding in megakaryocytic cytotoxicity was tested with preinoculation of anti-Leu3A, a CD4-specific antibody.

Results.—Of the 3 HIV isolates, only HIV-WW (obtained from the patient with thrombocytopenia) induced megakaryocytic cytopathy; HIV-WW was not cytotoxic to either T lymphocytes or monocytes. The inactivated inoculates restored CMK and DAMI viability. The presence of AZT or anti-Leu3A did not control the cytopathic effects of HIV-WW.

Discussion.—The HIV-WW has cytopathic properties specific for megakaryocytic cells. Neither viral replication nor envelope glycoprotein binding was a determinant in HIV-WW cytotoxicity to megakaryocytes. The data suggest that the various HIV strains have multiple tropic, cytopathic, and replication characteristics and effects. In light of recent studies implicating CD4 binding as a critical determinant of cytotoxicity, these data suggest that several envelope domains may be required for viral inoculation. Further analysis of the genotypic structure of HIV envelope glycoprotein is required.

▶ This contribution provides further insight into potential mechanisms underlying thrombocytopenia in patients with AIDS. Perhaps of even more importance is the suggestion that different HIV isolates may have different tropisms, which explains varying clinical syndromes and predilections for infecting specific cell types. This may have very practical consequences in conventional or gene therapy approaches for AIDS.—P.J. Quesenberry, M.D.

HIV Infection Is Active and Progressive in Lymphoid Tissue During the Clinically Latent Stage of Disease
Pantaleo G, Graziosi C, Demarest JF, Butini L, Montroni M, Fox CH, Orenstein JM, Kotler DP, Fauci AS (Natl Inst of Allergy and Infectious Diseases, Bethesda, Md; Univ of Ancona, Italy; Yale Univ, New Haven, Conn; et al)
Nature 362:355–358, 1993   116-95-2-29

Background.—A burst of viremia, symptomatic or not, is usually seen after primary infection with HIV. This burst is typically followed by a prolonged period of clinical latency. Little if any viremia is detected during this latency period. In addition, the numbers of infected cells in the blood are very low, and viral expression in these cells is difficult to demonstrate.

Methods and Findings.—Viral burden and levels of virus replication were analyzed simultaneously in the blood and lymphoid organs of the same patients at varying stages of HIV disease (Fig 2–3). In the early stage, there was a dichotomy between the levels of viral burden and viral replication in peripheral blood vs. lymphoid organs.

Conclusion.—Human immunodeficiency virus disease is active in lymphoid tissue during the latency period, even when minimal viral activity is found in blood. This finding may have important implications in designing treatment strategies.

▶ This is a very important article on the intrinsic nature of infection with HIV. The concept of a latent period seems invalid. These data and others indicate that there is progressive loss of lymphoid architecture and stromal elements during the whole course of the infection, eventuating in the profound immunodeficiency and fatal syndrome of AIDS. Localization of HIV in lymph nodes, with trapping first in follicular dendritic cells, and then in germinal centers followed by disruption of the germinal centers and the death of the follicular dendritic cells, clearly indicates the progressive nature of the disease. This strongly suggests that any effective therapy should be initiated immediately. Unfortunately, it is not clear that the current antiviral therapies are effective or that their early use impacts positively on the disease. There is little question that more effective treatments are necessary and that a number of gene therapy strategies are appropriate for attempting to reverse the consequences of HIV therapy. The creation of HIV-resistant stem cells is one specific targeted goal. Such gene therapy approaches will probably have to be carried out early in the course of an infection rather than late, given the results reported in this paper. It seems likely that progressive destruction of microenvironmental elements may preclude effective immunoreconstitution at later points in the disease.—P.J. Quesenberry, M.D.

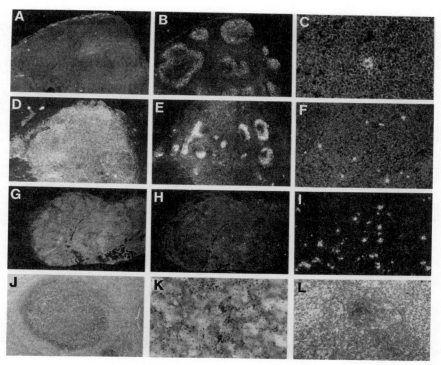

Fig 2-3.—In situ hybridization of lymph node sections from HIV-infected patients in different stages of disease. Autoradiograms were stained with hematoxylin-eosin and examined with dark-field microscopy. In double-labeling experiments (immunohistochemistry and in situ hybridization), slides were first subjected to staining with anti-CD21 antibody. Anti-CD21 antibody (clone 1F8) that specifically stains FDC in formaldehyde-fixed tissues was purchased from Dako Corporation, Carpinteria, Calif. **A–C,** early-stage disease. **A,** dark-field image of lymph node section not digested with protease. **B,** after protease digestion. Location of HIV RNA is indicated by the *silver grains,* which appear as *white dots.* An intense, granular, diffuse signal is predominantly restricted to the area of the germinal centers. **C,** dark-field image without protease digestion. Localization of HIV RNA signal over an individual cell in the paracortical area. **D–F,** patient with intermediate-stage disease. **D,** dark-field image without protease digestion. **E,** after protease digestion. Intense and diffuse signal is present over some germinal centers, whereas in the same section the signal is significantly decreased in other germinal centers. **F,** HIV RNA signal over individual cells in the paracortical area. **G–I,** patient with late-stage disease. **G,** dark-field image without protease digestion. Lymph node architecture is completely disrupted, and germinal centers are virtually absent. **H,** after protease digestion. A moderate increase in in situ hybridization signal is seen. **I,** higher magnification of a protease-digested section showing distribution of silver grains over several isolated cells expressing HIV RNA in copious amounts. **J,** bright-field image of a protease-digested lymph node section subjected to immunohistochemistry plus in situ hybridization showing the staining (New Fuchsin Red) of the FDC network with anti-CD21 antibody. **K,** localization of HIV RNA (with silver grains, which appear as *black dots*) coincides with the staining of the FDC network. **L,** presumed already involuted germinal center with a remnant of FDC network. Data are representative of the qualitative changes as well as the degree of changes among the different stages of disease seen in the 7 of 12 patients who had lymph node in situ hybridization done. These data were consistent with those from an additional 30 patients undergoing similar study. (Courtesy of Pantaleo G, Graziosi C, Demarest JF, et al: *Nature* 362:355–358, 1993.)

The Osteoclast: A Hematopoietically Derived Cell Unfamiliar to Hematologists

G. DAVID ROODMAN, M.D., PH.D.

Professor, Department of Medicine, Division of Hematology, University of Texas Health Science Center and the Audie L. Murphy VA Hospital, San Antonio, Texas

Introduction

The osteoclast is a hematopoietically derived cell that is the primary cell responsible for bone resorption. However, it is unfamiliar to most hematologists. The purpose of this review is to acquaint hematologists with the functional and morphologic characteristics of osteoclasts and to summarize some of the more recent data on the characterization of hematopoietic precursors for the osteoclast.

The osteoclast is a highly specialized multinucleated cell whose primary function is to participate in the control of calcium homeostasis. It is an extremely large cell, ranging in size from 50 up to 100 μm in diameter, and may contain as many as 100 nuclei per cell in pathologic conditions such as Paget's disease. Normal osteoclasts contain between 10 and 20 nuclei per cell and are located on endosteal bone surfaces within the haversian system and on periosteal surfaces beneath the periosteum. Osteoclasts are extremely rare cells in the bone marrow with only 1 to 2 being present per cubic micrometer of bone. Osteoclasts are found most frequently at sites of active bone resorption, such as metaphyses of growing bones, and in areas of active bone resorption, such as those seen in patients with hypercalcemia of malignancy. Recent evidence has suggested that a variety of cytokines produced in the marrow microenvironment regulate both osteoclast formation and osteoclastic bone resorption. The identity and characterization of these osteotropic factors have been areas of intensive research over the last 10 years and have led to some very important conclusions about the role of cytokines in osteoclastopoiesis. Until the last decade or so, little information has been available on understanding the ontogeny of the osteoclast or factors regulating its activity. This is primarily because the osteoclast is relatively inaccessible in its calcified matrix and is extremely fragile when isolated from bone. In subsequent sections of this review, current studies will be reviewed in an attempt to identify the origin of the osteoclast, to which hematopoietic cell lineage it belongs, and what factors control its formation and activity in normal and pathologic conditions.

Morphology of the Osteoclast

As noted, osteoclasts are extremely large cells. The nuclei are usually centrally located, and each nucleus contains 1 or 2 nucleoli (1). The cytoplasm is variable in appearance and can range from pale to basophilic in color. Osteoclasts are almost always found adjacent to bone and are very rarely seen away from bone surfaces. On electron microscopy, the osteoclasts that are actively resorbing bone display a ruffled border, comprising a series of fine finger-like cytoplasmic processes of the plasma membrane adjacent to bone (2, 3). These processes extend from the cell surface and terminate at the bone surface. This ruffled border acts as an extracellular vacuole in which extracellular demineralization and partial digestion of the bone matrix occur, most probably by release of proteolytic enzymes and hydrogen ions that cross the ruffled membrane. Studies by Gluck and others (4) have shown that a vacuolar proton pump is polarized to the ruffled border and actively excretes protons into the area adjacent to the ruffled border. Osteoclasts are extremely mobile cells with undulating membranes that show vigorous pinocytotic activity. Scanning electron micrographic studies have confirmed that these cells are multinucleated and vacuolated and that they contain prominent microvillae over the central portion of the cells. When these cells are incubated on a bone slice or other calcified matrices, a characteristic resorption pit is formed below the cell at the site of attachment of the ruffled border (5). Such resorption lacunae are never seen in the absence of activated osteoclasts and are not produced by macrophages or macrophage polykaryons (6). In addition to the ruffled border, the osteoclast has several unique characteristics that differentiate it from macrophage polykaryons. These include a clear zone, an organelle-free area in the cytoplasm adjacent to the plasma membrane that is closely opposed to the bone surface and is rich in actin filaments, centrally located nuclei, pleomorphic mitochondria, and prominent vesicles near the ruffled border.

Histochemical studies have shown that osteoclasts contain a variety of enzymes including high levels of tartrate-resistant acid phosphatase, carbonic anhydrase, and other acid hydrolases (7, 8). Resorbing osteoclasts also contain high levels of tricarboxylic acid–cycle enzymes, pentose phosphate shunt enzymes, and oxidative phosphorylation enzymes, which appear to be required for active bone resorption.

A variety of monoclonal antibodies have been developed that react with osteoclasts, including those that appear to be osteoclast specific. Osdoby and co-workers (9) were the first to report an osteoclast-specific monoclonal antibody. These antibodies were developed against chicken osteoclasts, and one of these, 121F, reacted only with osteoclasts and not with macrophage polykaryons. In addition, other antibodies from these preparations reacted both with osteoclasts and with macrophage giant cells and cultured monocytes. These studies showed that osteoclast-specific antigens existed but also that osteoclasts, macrophage giant cells, and cultured monocytes shared common antigen determinants not found on skin fibroblasts, liver, and a variety of other tissues. Horton (10) developed a panel of monoclonal antibodies against osteoclast-like giant cells isolated from human giant-cell tumors of bone. Giant cells from giant-cell tumors of bone have many unique characteristics of osteoclasts, including the capacity to form resorption lacunae on calcified matrices and expression of calcitonin receptors. One of these antibodies, 23c6, identified the osteoclast vitronectin receptor and preferentially reacted with osteoclasts as compared with macrophages and macrophage polykaryons. Figure 1 shows osteoclasts in a biopsy specimen of a giant-

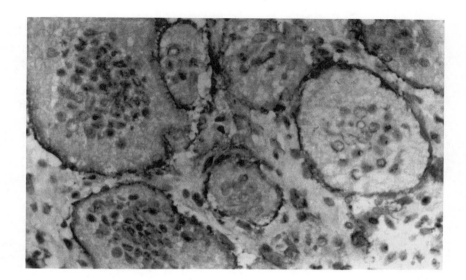

cell tumor of bone stained with an antibody that recognizes the osteo-clast vitronectin receptor. In addition, Horton and others have tested panels of monoclonal antibodies against granulocyte and monocyte anti-gens and hematopoietic cells and found that none of these antibodies cross-reacted with human osteoclasts. Athanasou and co-workers (11) have shown that osteoclasts express HLA, -B, and -C antigens but do not express HLA-DR and lack Fc receptors and C3B receptors. The only receptor that has been clearly demonstrated on the osteoclast surface has been the calcitonin receptor, which has been recently cloned by Gol-dring et al. (12). Thus, osteoclasts differ from other giant cells such as macrophage polykaryons because they have a ruffled border next to the bone surface, lack C3B and Fc receptors, form resorption lacunae on bone surfaces, and express calcitonin receptors.

Origin of the Osteoclast

The early studies of Walker (13, 14) clearly showed that the osteoclast is hematopoietic in origin. Using parabiotic unions of osteopetrotic mice with normal littermates, Walker demonstrated that osteopetrosis was cured in these animals and that a marrow cavity was formed. Similarly, Gothlin and Ericsson (15) showed that when 1 pair of parabiotic rats was lethally irradiated and the cells in a nonirradiated rat were labeled with thorotrast, osteoclasts that formed in the irradiated animal were de-rived from the nonirradiated animal. Studies using quail chick chimeras, in which quail bone rudiments were grafted onto a chick allantoic mem-brane, also showed that the osteoclasts were host-derived (16). More recently, studies of hematopoietic cells transplanted into lethally irradiated rodents and patients with osteopetrosis have confirmed that the osteoclast precursor is present in hematopoietic tissues. Walker (17) transplanted spleen and marrow cells into osteopetrotic mice and demonstrated that this resulted in removal of excess bone. Marks (18) has also shown that transplantation of spleen cells into osteopetrotic IA rats can cure this disease. Furthermore, bone marrow transplantation studies (19, 20) in patients with osteopetrosis have shown that some of the patients can be cured by bone marrow transplantation. The donor origin of the osteoclast was confirmed in these studies because female patients were transplanted with marrow from their HLA-matched male siblings. Karyotypic analysis of the osteoclasts in these patients revealed that the cells were male in origin. Transplantation of peripheral blood mononuclear cells that contain hematopoietic precursors into osteopetrotic rodents also cured osteopetrosis in these animals. Taken together, these studies support the hypothesis that the osteoclast precursor is a mononuclear cell in the marrow and that the osteoclast is hematopoietic in origin. However, the hematopoietic lineage of the osteoclast was not clearly defined by these studies and has been a topic of controversy.

Osteoclasts form by fusion of their mononuclear precursors. The mononuclear precursors have lost their capacity to proliferate at the time that they fuse. Studies by Kahn and Simmons (16) using quail-chick chimera show that some osteoclasts contain both quail and chick types of nuclei. Similarly, Feldman and co-workers (21) found no evidence for cell division when osteoclast numbers were increased in animals given parathyroid hormone. Furthermore, Young (22) showed that when marrow cells were exposed to ^{3}H-thymidine to label dividing cells, osteoclasts were formed by fusion of postmitotic mononuclear precursors, rather than endomitotic division. These data support the concept that multinuclear osteoclasts formed by fusion of mononuclear precursors that were hematopoietic in origin, rather than bone-derived, and that these precursors may pass through the circulation.

The identity of the osteoclast precursor remains in dispute. The first description of osteoclast precursors was by Ries and Gong (23). The cells were mononuclear, had ruffled borders, and contained tartrate-resistant acid phosphatase. The cells were in periosteal bone. It is unclear, however, if these cells represented mononuclear osteoclasts or osteoclast precursors. Baron and his co-workers (24) used a rat model to study osteoclast formation. In this model, the incisors were extracted, which resulted in a wave of bone resorption and new osteoclast formation. Using histologic techniques, they demonstrated that mononuclear cells that had a low nuclear-cytoplasmic ratio and an abundance of ribosomes invaded the site of the tooth extraction. The cells had polysomes with a characteristic rosette organization, multiple Golgi complexes, abundant mitochondria, and numerous cytoplasmic extensions. The cells initially contained nonspecific esterase. When the mononuclear precursors attached to the bone surface, the plasma membranes of the adherent precursor cells were closely associated with the calcified bone surface. Coated pits or coated patches were frequently demonstrated on the cytoplasmic processes that were surrounding the small, calcified spicules where the cells attached to bone. As these cells differentiated, they expressed tartrate-resistant acid phosphatase, eventually lost their nonspecific esterase activity, and only expressed tartrate-resistant acid phosphatase. These tartrate-resistant acid phosphatase–positive mononuclear cells then formed multinucleated osteoclasts. These data suggested that the precursor for the osteoclast was a cell in the monocytic lineage.

A number of other studies first performed in vivo and more recently in vitro have further supported the hypothesis that osteoclasts are derived from cells in the mononuclear phagocyte series. Fischman and Hay (25) showed that in regenerating newt limbs, osteoclasts were formed by fusion of leukocytes that were most probably monocytes histologically. Similarly, Jee and Nolan (26) showed that after surrounding macrophages had incorporated charcoal particles, the osteoclasts contained charcoal particles. Furthermore, Tinkler et al. (27) injected ^{3}H-thymidine–labeled peripheral blood monocytes into syngeneic hosts treated with 1,25-dihydroxy vitamin D_3 and showed that labeled nuclei were present in the osteoclasts that formed in response to this treatment. Similarly, Zambonin-Zallone et al. (28) found that some peripheral blood monocytes could fuse with purified chicken osteoclasts. Burger and co-workers (29) were one of the first groups to demonstrate formation of osteoclasts from marrow cells in vitro. They co-cultured murine fetal bone rudiments that lacked osteoclasts with marrow cells and a source of M-CSF in plasma clots and found that osteoclasts formed in these organ cultures. Using histologic techniques, these workers identified the precursor for these osteoclasts as a cell in the monocytic lineage. Consistent with the osteoclast being derived from a cell in the monocyte-macrophage lineage are the reports by Oursler and co-workers (9) who showed that a monoclonal antibody that identified macrophages and macrophage polykaryons also cross-reacted with osteoclasts. Athanasou et al. (11) have also shown that macrophage antigens are expressed in osteoclasts. More recently, Kurihara et al. (30) have shown, using human bone marrow cultures, that osteoclast-like multinucleated cells are formed from highly purified populations of GM-CFU–derived cells. In these studies, CD34+ nonadherent human marrow mononuclear cells were cultured in the presence of GM-CSF for 7 to 10 days, and then the colonies were isolated individually and pooled. The cells were then cultured in the presence of 1,25-$(OH)_2D_3$ to form osteoclast-like multinucleated cells. In addition, others (31) using murine systems have shown that fractions enriched for GM-CFU give rise to osteoclasts.

Taken together, these data suggest that the osteoclast precursors are derived from a cell in the monocyte-macrophage lineage. Mononuclear cells that contain both monocytic markers and osteoclast enzyme markers are present prior to formation of osteoclasts, and early precursors for cells in the monocyte-macrophage lineage (e.g., GM-CFU) can form os-

MODEL FOR OSTEOCLAST FORMATION

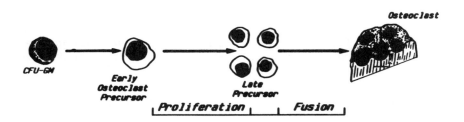

teoclast-like cells in vitro. Figure 2 shows our current model for human osteoclast formation.

However, others, such as Hattersley and Chambers (32), have suggested that the osteoclast precursors are not derived from the monocyte-macrophage lineage, but rather from more primitive cells, either the CFU-GEMM or even CFU blast. Consistent with their observations are the findings that macrophages are incapable of restoring osteoclast numbers in animals that have received total body irradiation, and that calcitonin decreases the cytoplasmic motility of osteoclasts but not mature monocyte macrophages. Furthermore, Horton and co-workers (33) have prepared monoclonal antibodies against human osteoclastoma cells that fail to react with the monocyte macrophages. Similarly, Nijweide et al. (34, 35) have shown that murine bone marrow cells enriched for hematopoietic stem cells can give rise to osteoclasts, and that cultures of fetal bone rudiments with pluripotent hematopoietic cell lines derived from mouse bone marrow cultures such as FDCP1 cells can form osteoclasts. These investigators have suggested that the osteoclast develops directly from a multipotent stem cell, rather than from a committed granulocyte-macrophage precursor. However, their data do not exclude the possibility that these early osteoclast precursors differentiate to GM-CFU prior to forming osteoclasts.

Further data that the osteoclast precursor is not derived from cells in the monocyte-macrophage lineage comes from the work of Hattersley and Chambers (32) who showed, using CFU-blast cultures, that if individual cells were allowed to differentiate, GM-CFU–derived cells formed only a small percentage of osteoclasts, but more primitive cells were able to form more osteoclasts. However, these workers were never able to identify a colony of pure osteoclast precursors by these techniques. Lee and her co-workers (36) have also proposed a model in which the osteoclast is not derived from GM-CFU. This model is based on in vitro studies using their newly described factor, CSF-O, which stimulates formation of colonies of tartrate-resistant acid phosphatase–positive mononuclear cells in semisolid marrow cultures. Using GM-CSF, rather than CSF-O, as a source of colony-stimulating activity in cultures of 5-fluorouracil–treated mouse marrow cells as a starting population, they failed to find any osteoclast-like cells formed. They were able to show after prolonged culture that tartrate-resistant, acid phosphatase–positive mononuclear cell colonies formed in these cultures. Again, their data do not negate the possibility that primitive cells may differentiate in the monocyte-macrophage lineage before branching to the osteoclast lineage. They have not done an experiment in which they treated GM-CFU–derived cells with CSF-O to determine whether they could form tartrate-resistant, acid phosphatase–positive colonies.

Suda and co-workers (37) have reported that co-culture of murine alveolar macrophages or peritoneal macrophages with a bone marrow stromal cell line or primary osteoblasts isolated from mouse calvaria in the presence of dexamethasone and $1,25\text{-}(OH)_2D_3$ formed osteoclast-like multinucleated cells. The cells expressed calcitonin receptors and formed resorption lacunae on calcified matrices. Overall, most studies support GM-CFU as the early osteoclast precursor, although there is still controversy about this point.

Methods for Studying Osteoclasts and Their Precursors

Progress in understanding the molecular events that occur during osteoclast differentiation and osteoclastic bone resorption has been difficult because, as noted, osteoclasts are few in number, are fragile when isolated from bone, and are difficult to isolate because they are embedded in a calcified matrix. To circumvent these problems, a variety of model systems have been developed to form osteoclast-like cells in vitro. These model systems have been used to identify osteoclast precursors and to characterize their surface phenotype and for studies of factors affecting osteoclast activity and formation.

Several techniques have been developed for isolating authentic osteoclasts from long bones. One of the most commonly used sources for osteoclasts has been the endosteal surface of chick long bones. In one approach, Osdoby et al. (38) prepared osteoclasts from embryonic chick tibia by removing the marrow and then releasing the osteoclasts using calcium and magnesium-free buffers. The cell suspension was then sieved through nylon mesh to trap the osteoclasts. The cells were then subjected to discontinuous density centrifugation to enrich the osteoclast fraction. Cell preparations by this method could yield up to 50% to 75% pure osteoclasts. These osteoclasts could then be cultured for 10 days and retain an osteoclast morphology, although only a small percentage of these cells could resorb bone. A similar approach has been used by Zambonin-Zallone and her co-workers (39) using hypocalcemic chicks. With their methods, large numbers of osteoclasts can be isolated, although the viability of these cells is still in question. Similarly, Chambers et al. (40) have isolated osteoclasts from rats or rabbits and used these osteoclasts to examine the effects of factors directly on osteoclasts. However, all these systems suffer from 2 shortcomings: most of these cells are not viable, and they are mixed-cell populations containing osteoblasts.

Recently, several groups have begun to use human giant-cell tumors of bone as a source of human osteoclasts. The giant cells from these tumors express an osteoclast phenotype. They are extremely large and highly multinucleated; contain high levels of tartrate-resistant acid phosphatase, a marker enzyme for osteoclasts; have calcitonin receptors; contract in response to calcitonin; and form resorption lacunae on calcified matrices. These cells most likely represent very highly activated osteoclasts. Using panning techniques and discontinuous Percoll gradients, Ohsaki et al. (41) were able to prepare cells that were 90% to 95% pure giant cells. They took advantage of the finding that they reacted strongly with the 23c6 monoclonal antibody developed by Horton, which cross-reacted with the osteoclast vitronectin receptor. Using immunomagnetic bead techniques, they could purify the 23c6-positive cell fraction and then further purify the multinucleated cells from mononuclear cells in this fraction on Percoll gradients. These types of studies have allowed testing to determine whether factors act directly on osteoclasts or must act via osteoblasts. Chambers (42) has popularized an assay of osteoclastic bone resorption in which isolated osteoclasts are deposited on bone slices, and the number of resorption pits and the area resorbed are quantified. Boyde and co-workers (43) argue that determining the volume of the pits is more important than measuring the area resorbed. In either case, factors are applied to the cells, and the number of resorption lacunae and the area of the calcified matrices resorbed are determined microscopically. However, such techniques can give only limited information on the effects of these factors on osteoclast differentiation and on the regulation of osteoclastic bone resorption, because no new osteoclasts form and the cell populations are not homogenous. Most of these studies have suggested that most factors act indirectly on osteoclasts via the osteoblast, but because of the impurity of the cell preparations and the difficulty in obtaining large numbers of viable osteoclasts, the interpretation of some of the results is extremely difficult.

As noted, Baron and co-workers (24) have developed an in vivo model for studying osteoclast formation in alveolar bone. Osteoclasts in alveolar bone are responsive to changes in the plasma concentration of parathyroid hormone or calcitonin and have enzymatic properties similar to those of osteoclasts in other parts of the skeleton. This system has been used to study formation of osteoclasts from mononuclear precursors when bone resorption is induced by extracting molars from adult rats. The absence of the antagonists' teeth leads to induction of bone remodeling along the periosteum of the mandible. The animals are then sacrificed every 24 hours and the mandibles processed for light microscopy, ultrastructural studies, and cytochemical studies to determine the sequence of osteoclast differentiation. However, these techniques are extremely cumbersome, and it is difficult to isolate cells from these preparations for further studies.

Bone organ culture systems have provided useful bioassays for studying factors controlling osteoclastic bone resorption and, in some cases, osteoclast formation. These organ culture systems have been useful in identifying new agents that stimulate, as well as inhibit, bone resorption. Among the most frequently used systems are the fetal rat or mouse calvarial assay or fetal rat long-bone system, in which pregnant rats or mice are injected with calcium-45, and the radius and ulnar or the calvaria are dissected from the fetuses or neonatal rodents. These bones are then floated on wire mesh or millipore filters over a chemically defined media, and various factors are then added to the media. After an appropriate time, the percentage of calcium-45 released from the bone relative to the total amount of calcium-45 in the bone fragment is determined. Light microscopic and ultrastructural studies can also be performed on these bone fragments, allowing some estimate of the number of osteoclasts present over time. However, because these organ cultures represent mixed-cell populations, determination of whether a factor(s) directly acts on osteoclasts or indirectly acts through marrow stromal cells or other cells within the bone organ culture is problematic. Furthermore, because most of these organ culture systems use fetal or neonatal tissues, these organ culture systems may not reflect the behavior of osteoclasts in adult animals.

Because, as noted, the osteoclast is hematopoietic in origin, a variety of bone marrow culture techniques have been developed in which osteoclast-like multinucleated cells form. The studies of Burger and her coworkers (29) who used fetal bone rudiments that were devoid of osteoclasts and cocultured them with marrow with a source of M-CSF were some of the initial marrow culture systems described. However, to determine the effects of a factor(s) in this system, histomorphometry had to be done, which was tedious, time-consuming, and labor intensive. Such culture systems could be used to ask the question whether a defined population of cells contains osteoclast precursors or not but were not as useful to determine the effects of various factors on osteoclast formation or identification of osteoclast precursors. Testa and co-workers (44) were the first to modify the classic Dexter long-term marrow culture systems to form osteoclast-like cells. In their original work, they used feline bone marrow and cultured it in α-minimum essential medium with horse serum in the absence of any osteotropic factors and found that multinucleated cells formed in these cultures. These cells were not well characterized but were called osteoclast-like because they were multinucleated.

Ibbotson and co-workers (45) extended these studies and demonstrated that a variety of factors could modulate formation of these osteoclast-like cells and that the precursor for these cells was a cell in the monocyte-macrophage lineage. Long-term marrow culture systems that form osteoclast-like cells have been expanded to include culture systems with mouse marrow, in which tartrate-resistant, acid phosphatase-positive multinucleated cells that resorb bone form in baboon cultures and human marrow cultures. In a typical human long-term marrow culture, nonadherent marrow mononuclear cells were cultured at 10^6 cells/ mL in the presence of 1,25-dihydroxy vitamin D_3 (10^{-8} M) for 3 weeks. Few, if any, multinucleated cells formed in the first week of culture, and most of the multinucleated cells formed during the second week of culture. Maximum numbers of osteoclast-like multinucleated cells formed in these cultures after 3 weeks. These cells persisted for approximately 4–5 weeks and then begin to detach and die. Multinucleated cells from these cultures fulfilled the functional criteria of osteoclasts. They were tartrate-resistant, acid phosphatase–positive, reacted with the 23c6 monoclonal antibody, expressed calcitonin receptors, contracted in response to calcitonin, and formed resorption lacunae on calcified matrices such as sperm whale dentine.

These human long-term marrow culture systems have been used to identify the mechanisms of action of a variety of factors on osteoclast formation. In the first week of the cultures, there is a growth phase in which the early precursors proliferate, and during the second and third week of culture, these cells differentiate and fuse to form multinucleated cells. Factors that stimulate proliferation of the precursors can be assessed by scoring the number of ^{3}H-thymidine–labeled nuclei incorporated into multinucleated cells in cultures treated for the first 24 hours with ^{3}H-thymidine. Factors that enhance fusion increase the number of nuclei per multinucleated cell. Using these culture systems, we have identified the mechanism of action of a variety of cytokines and osteotropic factors (Fig 3).

Recently, Udagawa et al. (46) have used mouse spleen cells as a source of osteoclast precursors. When these cells are cocultured with an appropriate bone marrow–derived stromal cell (MC3G-G2-4PA6 or ST2) or with primary mouse calvarial cells in the presence of dexamethasone and 1,25-dihydroxy vitamin D_3, multinucleated cells formed. Osteoclast-like cells formed in these cultures contained tartrate-resistant acid phosphatase and had enhanced cyclic adenosine monophosphate production in response to calcitonin. Calcitonin receptors were also demonstrated on the multinucleated cells formed in these cocultures by autoradiographic

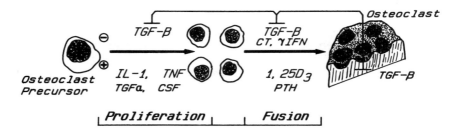

Model for Regulation of Osteoclast Formation

techniques with ^{125}I-labeled calcitonin, and numerous resorption lacunae were formed when spleen cells and ST2 cells were cocultured on sperm whale dentine in the presence of 1,25-$(OH)_2D_3$ and dexamethasone. Hattersley and Chambers (47) have recently reported the generation of osteoclast-like cells from murine hematopoietic multipotential cell lines in vitro. Using FDCPA4 cells cocultured with bone marrow stromal cells in the presence of 1,25-dihydroxy vitamin D_3, they demonstrated that these pluripotent hematopoietic cells could form multinucleated cells that expressed an osteoclast phenotype and formed resorption lacunae on calcified matrices. Nijweide and his co-workers (48) used FDCP-C2-GM cells, another multipotent hematopoietic murine cell line, and demonstrated that when these cells were co-cultured with fetal bone rudiments, osteoclast-like cells formed. Yoneda et al. (49) have also used HL-60 cells, a human promyelocytic cell line, to form osteoclast-like multinucleated cells. They cultured HL-60 cells in methylcellulose containing conditioned media from a squamous cell carcinoma tumor cell line that induced hypercalcemia in vivo. They then treated the cultures with 1,25-$(OH)_2D_3$ to form osteoclast-like multinucleated cells. However, the number of osteoclast-like cells formed from HL-60 cells was extremely low. Chambers et al. (50) recently reported that transgenic mice with a transgene composed of the SV40 large T antigen driven by a major histocompatibility complex promoter could be used to produce an osteoclast precursor cell line. They demonstrated that a cell line that formed osteoclast-like cells could be derived from these mice. Only a very low percentage of the cells formed osteoclasts, similar to their FDCP cell line experiments. They also isolated several marrow stromal cell lines from these mice that supported osteoclast differentiation from spleen cells or marrow cells.

Thus, cells derived from these transgenic mice do not appear to be committed to the osteoclast lineage but appear to be earlier precursors that have the potential to form small numbers of osteoclasts in vitro. None of the culture techniques described above form large numbers of osteoclasts required for biochemical or molecular biological studies, although Tamura and co-workers (51) have modified this culture system to form large numbers of osteoclast-like cells on collagen pads. However, as seen by the above discussions, development of an osteoclast cell line and an osteoclast precursor cell line would be a major advance.

In an attempt to try to develop an osteoclast cell line, we have cloned the promoter for tartrate-resistant acid phosphatase, a marker enzyme for the osteoclast, from a murine genomic library (52). We have characterized this promoter and demonstrated that the 5'-flanking sequence contains 2 promoters, as well as enhancer and repressor elements (53). We have fused this promoter to the complementary DNA for SV40 large T antigen and made transgenic mice to target the T antigen to the osteoclast (54). These transgenic mice develop osteopetrosis and have large numbers of transformed osteoclasts. The osteoclasts contain mitotic figures and transformed nuclei, and many of them are aneuploid. This is the first demonstration that T antigen can be targeted to the mature osteoclast by these techniques and suggests that there is a potential of isolating osteoclast or osteoclast precursor cell lines from these tartrate-resistant acid phosphostase–T-antigen mice.

Recently, we have also developed an in vivo model to examine the mechanism of action of osteotropic factors on various stages of osteoclast formation. In this model, mice are either injected with a factor or implanted with Chinese hamster ovary (CHO) cells, which have been transfected with the factor of interest and constitutively express the factor at high levels, to examine their effects on 3 specific stages of osteoclast formation: GM-CFU, the earliest identifiable osteoclast precursor, as assessed by colony assays; more committed osteoclast precursors, as assessed by osteoclast-like cell formation in long-term marrow cultures derived from these animals; and mature osteoclasts as determined by histomorphometry of calvariae from these animals. In preliminary studies (55), we have shown that IL-1, for example, increased the number of GM-CFU, the number of more committed osteoclast precursors, as well as the number of mature osteoclasts to resorb bone. In contrast, parathyroid hormone only increased the number of committed precursors and stimulated mature osteoclasts to resorb bone. This in vivo model system may further help to dissect the role of various cytokines in normal bone remodeling, as well as in states of increased bone turnover, such as osteoporosis.

In addition to the development of long-term marrow cultures and in vivo systems for studies of osteoclast formation, we have modified semisolid marrow culture techniques to identify the committed precursor for the human osteoclast-like cells formed in vitro (30). In this culture system, CD34+ marrow mononuclear cells are cultured in the presence of GM-CSF for 7 to 10 days, and then the cultures are overlayered with 1,25-dihydroxy vitamin D_3 for an additional 2 weeks. At the end of the second culture period, 4 types of colonies are found in the cultures: granulocytic, macrophage, colonies of mixed hematopoietic lineages, and cells that have unique polygonal morphology. One hundred percent of these polygonal cells react strongly with the 23c6 monoclonal antibody. The cells express calcitonin receptors, fuse to form only osteoclast-like multinucleated cells, and multinucleated cells formed from these polygonal cells form resorption lacunae on calcified matrices.

Using these types of systems, we have tested cytokines for the effects on both immature and committed mononuclear osteoclast precursors. We demonstrated that for example, parathyroid hormone is a mitogen for the immature osteoclast precursor but does not affect the committed osteoclast precursor. All of the multinucleated cells form from these committed precursors contract in response to calcitonin, express the osteoclastic vacuolar proton pump, and react strongly with the 23c6 monoclonal antibody. Thus, these cells appear to be committed precursors for the osteoclast. In addition to examining the cytokine responsivity of both immature and committed precursors for these osteoclast-like cells, these culture systems can be used to begin to examine the molecular events controlling osteoclast differentiation and commitment to the osteoclast lineage.

Takahashi and co-workers (56) have utilized these semisolid culture techniques to determine when during osteoclast differentiation commitment to the osteoclast lineage occurs. They did this by examining expression of calcitonin receptor messenger RNA in immature precursors after treatment with 1,25-dihydroxy vitamin D_3. They found that it required at least 7 days of treatment with 1,25-$(OH)_2D_3$ to induce commitment of immature precursors to the osteoclast lineage. Interestingly, they also found that calcitonin down-regulated expression of the messenger RNA for the calcitonin receptor in these highly purified osteoclast precursors and that removal of calcitonin resulted in reexpression of the messenger RNA for the calcitonin receptor. Thus, there are now a variety of in vitro and in vivo techniques for examining osteoclast formation and osteoclastic bone resorption. These techniques now permit studies to further characterize the molecular events that occur during osteoclast differentiation, as well as to identify novel factors that stimulate osteoclast formation.

Cytokines Involved in Osteoclast Formation and Activity

INTERLEUKIN-1

Interleukin-1 is one of the most extensively studied cytokines for its effects on bone. It is a very potent bone-resorbing agent when administered either in vivo or in vitro and can induce hypercalcemia because of its marked stimulatory effects on mature osteoclasts. In vivo studies have shown that IL-1 increases the number of GM-CFU, the probable early precursor for the osteoclast, as well as more committed osteoclast precursors, in addition to increasing the bone-resorbing activity of osteoclasts already present in bone (55). Osteoclasts formed from bone marrow cultures of IL-1–treated animals have a markedly enhanced bone-resorbing capacity per osteoclast compared with osteoclast formed from bone marrow cultures of animals treated with vehicle. Gowen and her co-workers (57) were the first to show that IL-1 stimulated osteoclastic bone resorption in organ culture, and Boyce and co-workers (58) have extensively studied IL-1's capacity to induce hypercalcemia and bone resorption in vivo. Interleukin-1 can induce hypercalcemia in animals when given continuously or intermittently over 3 to 4 days. In addition, IL-1 can stimulate osteoclast formation in vitro in long-term marrow cultures both from human and murine sources, and it has been suggested as the mediator for the effects of IL-6 in long-term human marrow cultures (59, 60). It is unclear whether IL-1 works directly or indirectly on osteoclasts. Using isolated osteoclast assays, Chambers and co-workers (61) have suggested that osteoblasts mediate the effects of IL-1. Interleukin-1 can increase IL-6 production by osteoblasts, and IL-6 can stimulate osteoclast formation in vitro and in vivo. Interleukin-1 may be involved in increased bone resorption seen in chronic inflammatory diseases including malignancies and osteoporosis. However, its role in osteoporosis has not been clearly defined. Pacifici and co-workers (62) have reported that monocytes from patients with osteoporosis produce high levels of IL-1 compared with nonosteoporotic age-matched controls and that IL-1 receptor antagonists blocked the increased bone loss seen in ovariectomized mice. Thus, IL-1 appears to be a major regulator of osteoclast activity in normal and pathologic states.

TUMOR NECROSIS FACTOR-α

Tumor necrosis factor (TNF)–like IL-1 is a powerful stimulator of osteoclastic bone resorption in vivo and can induce hypercalcemia. It has not been studied in as much detail as IL-1, but Johnson and co-workers (63) have shown in mice bearing CHO cells, which have been transfected with the human TNF-α gene and constitutively produced high levels of TNF, that these animals developed hypercalcemia and increased numbers of osteoclasts. Pfeilschifter and co-workers (59) have also demonstrated that TNF-α and -β can stimulate osteoclast formation in long-term human marrow cultures. Tumor necrosis factor-β, also known as lymphotoxin, can also stimulate osteoclastic bone resorption and induce hypercalcemia and has been implicated in the increased bone resorption associated with myeloma (64). Established myeloma cell lines produce TNF-β, and part of the bone-resorbing activity produced by these cells can be accounted for by TNF-β. However, these studies suggest that TNF-β may not be the sole mediator of bone resorption in patients with myeloma.

Tumor necrosis factor-α may also be responsible for the hypercalcemia seen in some patients with cancer. This has been clearly demonstrated in a number of human and animal tumors and is best documented in animals bearing the MH85 human squamous cell carcinoma tumor. Yoneda and co-workers (65) have shown that this tumor stimulates normal host immune cells to produce TNF-α and that antibodies to TNF-α blocked the hypercalcemia in these animals. It appears that the MH85 tumor cells produce a factor that induces TNF production by host macrophages. Thus, TNF-α may amplify the effects of other hypercalcemia agents in patients with malignancy.

INTERLEUKIN-6

Interleukin-6 is a pleotropic cytokine that can increase WBC counts and platelet counts in animals and primates and can stimulate osteoclastic bone resorption. The effects of IL-6 on bone have been controversial because different results have been found in murine and human systems. Interleukin-6, by itself, appears not to stimulate osteoclastic bone resorption in mice, except at levels greater than 20 ng/mL. However, IL-6 appears capable of stimulating osteoclast formation in these animals. Using CHO cells transfected with the murine IL-6 gene, Black and co-workers (66) have shown that animals bearing these tumor cells have hypercalcemia, leukocytosis, and thrombocytosis develop. More recently, our laboratory has shown that IL-6 stimulates GM-CFU production in mice bearing CHO–IL-6 cells but by itself does not induce marked hypercalcemia. However, IL-6 appears to be capable of acting synergistically with other osteotropic factors such as parathyroid hormone–related peptide and can induce extreme hypercalcemia in animals bearing both CHO tumors transfected with the IL-6 and the parathyroid hormone–related protein genes. Thus, IL-6 appears to be a cofactor that may play an important role in the hypercalcemia of malignancy.

We have shown that IL-6 may also be the mediator of the increased osteoclast formation in patients with Paget's disease of bone (67). Pagetic osteoclasts actively produce IL-6 messenger RNA, as well as express the IL-6 receptor. Similarly, giant cells from osteoclastomas produce large amounts of IL-6. Interleukin-6 acts as an autocrine factor regulating bone resorption by human osteoclasts. This has been shown by the work of Ohsaki et al. (41) and Reddy et al. (68) who used either neutralizing antibodies to IL-6 or antisense constructs to IL-6 to show that either of these agents could block bone resorption by highly purified populations of osteoclasts from giant-cell tumors of bone. Furthermore, Kurihara et al. (60) have shown that IL-6 is a potent stimulator of osteoclast cell formation in long-term human marrow cultures, and Tamura and co-workers (69) have suggested that IL-6 stimulates osteoclast formation in murine systems only in the presence of soluble IL-6 receptor. Interleukin-6 has also been implicated as a potential mediator for postmenopausal osteoporosis by Jilka and colleagues (70). These workers reported that murine bone cells express IL-6, and IL-6 production by these cells can be modulated by estrogens. They also reported that there was overproduction of IL-6 in mice after ovariectomy and that the rapid bone loss associated with estrogen withdrawal could be ablated by neutralizing antibodies to IL-6, as well as estrogens. Osteoblasts are an important source of IL-6, and IL-6 production by osteoblasts can be stimulated by parathyroid hormone, IL-1, TNF, and lipopolysaccharide. Interleukin-6 has also been implicated as a mediator of bone loss associated with myeloma. Thus, IL-6 appears to be an autocrine/paracrine factor that stimulates osteoclast formation and mediates human osteoclastic bone resorption. Its role in osteoporosis and normal osteoclast function is still controversial and remains to be clarified.

MACROPHAGE COLONY-STIMULATING FACTOR

Macrophage colony-stimulating factor exerts its effects through the M-CF receptor, which is the c-*fms* proto-oncogene. This receptor is expressed on cells in the osteoclast lineage. Macrophage colony-stimulating factor probably plays an important role in murine osteoclast formation, because a point mutation in the M-CSF gene in the op/op mouse results in osteopetrosis (71). These mice can be cured of their osteopetrosis by infusion of M-CSF. In vitro experiments have shown that M-CSF can induce osteoclast formation in murine long-term marrow cultures if the cultures are treated sequentially with M-CSF followed by

1,25-dihydroxy vitamin D_3. In addition, M-CSF is the factor produced by murine ST2 stromal cells and calvarial cells that stimulate spleen cells to form osteoclasts in coculture systems. It is unclear when M-CSF acts during osteoclast differentiation because other investigators (72) have reported that osteoclast formation is decreased by M-CSF. Macrophage colony-stimulating factor is also capable of stimulating osteoclast-like cell formation in long-term human marrow cultures (73) if the cultures are treated sequentially for the first week with M-CSF followed for the next 2 weeks by 1,25-dihydroxy vitamin D_3.

GRANULOCYTE-MACROPHAGE COLONY-STIMULATING FACTOR

Granulocyte-macrophage colony-stimulating factor has been reported to have both stimulatory inhibitory effects on osteoclasts and osteoclast differentiation. MacDonald and co-workers (73) have shown that treatment of long-term human marrow cultures with GM-CSF followed by 1,25-dihydroxy vitamin D_3 markedly increased osteoclast-like cell formation. Similarly, Kurihara et al. (30) have shown that GM-CSF stimulates proliferation of less differentiated precursors for osteoclast-like cells formed in these long-term human marrow cultures but does not affect their subsequent differentiation. Takahashi et al. (74) reported recently that GM-CSF can stimulate murine osteoclast formation when the cultures are treated sequentially with GM-CSF followed by 1,25-dihydroxy vitamin D_3. However, when bone marrow cultures are treated simultaneously with GM-CSF and 1,25-$(OH)_2D_3$, there is inhibition of osteoclast-like cell formation. Shuto and co-workers (75) have also shown that addition of GM-CSF in the absence of dexamethasone to murine marrow cultures treated with 1,25-$(OH)_2D_3$ inhibits osteoclast-like cell formation. Lorenzo and co-workers (76) reported that GM-CSF has little effect on osteoclasts in murine organ cultures, but it significantly decreased osteoclast formation in organ cultures treated with parathyroid hormone. Thus, the role of GM-CSF in osteoclast formation and differentiation is still controversial. It appears that GM-CSF stimulates early precursors for osteoclasts, but it may actually suppress the later differentiation of these cells toward the osteoclast lineage and subsequent osteoclastic bone resorption.

INTERLEUKIN-3

Interleukin-3 stimulates the growth of primitive hematopoietic progenitors. Kurihara and co-workers (30) have shown that IL-3 can stimulate the growth of precursors for osteoclast-like cells formed in human marrow cultures. Similarly, Hattersley and Chambers (77) reported that IL-3 can stimulate the growth of murine pluripotent stem cells, which, in turn, can differentiate into calcitonin receptor–positive cells that resorb bone. Barton and Mayer (78) demonstrated that IL-3 can also increase multinucleated cell formation in long-term murine marrow cultures and that these multinucleated cells appear to be osteoclasts. However, no one has been able to show that IL-3 stimulates mature osteoclasts to resorb bone.

Thus, the overall effects of hematopoietic growth factors, such as IL-3, are to stimulate the growth of osteoclast precursors and to induce the differentiation toward other lineages unless the cells are exposed to potent osteoclast differentiation agents such as 1,25-dihydroxy vitamin D_3. It appears that 1,25-dihydroxy vitamin D_3 cannot compete equally with hematopoietic growth factors for the differentiation of the common precursor for the osteoclast and the monocyte macrophage, because when IL-3 and 1,25-$(OH)_2D_3$ are added simultaneously to coculture systems that form osteoclasts, IL-3 inhibits osteoclast-like cell formation. In contrast, when IL-3 is added initially and then the cultures are subsequently treated with 1,25-$(OH)_2D_3$, IL-3 can stimulate the growth of murine hematopoietic precursors that give rise to osteoclasts.

TRANSFORMING GROWTH FACTOR-β

Transforming growth factor (TGF)-β, which is produced by a number of normal tissues including bone, inhibits osteoclast-like cell formation as well as the growth of hematopoietic progenitors such as GM-CFU and blast-forming unit–erythroid (79). It will stimulate osteoclastic bone resorption in neonatal mouse calvariae, but this is due to induction of prostaglandin synthesis by TGF-β. Prostaglandins are potent stimulators of bone resorption in this murine organ culture system. In systems where prostaglandins are not important, TGF-β is a potent inhibitor of osteoclast formation. Chenu and co-workers (79) showed that TGF-β inhibits human osteoclast-like cell formation in 2 ways: by blocking fusion proliferation of early precursors and shifting the precursors toward the granulocytic lineage. Bone is a rich source of latent TGF-β, and TGF-β may be released in an active form when osteoclasts resorb bone, thus serving to inhibit excessive bone resorption. In addition, TGF-β can stimulate the growth of osteoblasts and may serve as a coupling factor between the osteoclastic bone resorption and new bone formation by osteoblasts.

INTERFERONS

Interferons are produced by activated lymphocytes and macrophages and appear to inhibit osteoclastic bone resorption stimulated by a variety of cytokines (80). Interferons appear to inhibit the differentiation of precursors to osteoclast-like cells formed in long-term human marrow cultures (81) by inhibiting the fusion of these precursors, as well as blocking proliferation of the more immature precursors. Thus, in vitro studies suggest that interferons are extremely potent cytokines that inhibit both osteoclast formation and osteoclastic bone resorption. They may play an important role in controlling the excess bone resorption seen in patients with inflammatory conditions such as rheumatoid arthritis.

INTERLEUKIN-4

Interleukin-4 is produced in the marrow microenvironment and has been suggested as a potential regulator of osteoclast activity in vivo. Interleukin-4 can inhibit formation of osteoclast-like cells in vitro (82) and osteoclastic bone resorption in murine organ cultures (83). Thus, IL-4, like the interferons, appears to block both osteoclast formation and osteoclast activity.

Abnormal Osteoclast Precursors

Little information is available about abnormalities in osteoclast precursors that may exist in conditions of increased bone turnover such as osteoporosis. However, we have recently characterized the osteoclast precursor in Paget's disease of bone. Paget's disease of bone, the second most common metabolic bone disease, is characterized by an intense phase of bone resorption followed by excessive new bone formation. The bone that is formed is of poor quality. Increased numbers of extremely large osteoclasts are present in pagetic bone biopsy specimens, and there are increased numbers of nuclei per osteoclast. We have used long-term human marrow culture techniques to study osteoclast formation from bone marrow samples of patients with Paget's disease (84). We found that osteoclast-like cells are formed in these cultures more rapidly than in normals and that the precursors appear to be hyperresponsive to 1,25-dihydroxy vitamin D_3. Demulder and co-workers (85) have shown that the early pagetic precursor for the osteoclast is hyperresponsive to 1,25-D_3 and also hyperresponsive to cells in the marrow microenvironment. Furthermore, stromal cells present in pagetic marrow samples appear capable of stimulating the growth of normal osteoclast precursors as well. Thus, there appear to be 2 abnormalities in the pagetic marrow, 1 being increased sensitivity of the precursors to both the marrow microenvironment and to 1,25-dihydroxy vitamin D_3, and the other being an abnormality in the marrow stromal cells themselves. This is the first demonstration of an abnormality in an osteoclast precursor.

Ultrastructural studies of osteoclasts in pagetic bone biopsy specimens have shown that they contain nuclear inclusions that appear to be paramyxovirus nucleocapsids. Ultrastructural, immunocytochemical, and in situ hybridization studies have all suggested that measles virus, respiratory syncytial virus, or canine distemper virus may play a role in the pathogenesis of Paget's disease. Reddy and co-workers (86) have recently shown that osteoclast precursors from marrow samples from patients with Paget's disease contain measles virus nucleocapsid transcripts and suggest that these types of studies may be useful in isolating the virus present in pagetic osteoclasts. Thus, studies using bone marrow culture techniques of osteoclast precursors may help to unravel the pathogenesis of Paget's disease, a very common disease of bone.

Summary

The osteoclast is a hematopoietic-derived cell that is unfamiliar to most hematologists. It is the major mediator of bone resorption and plays an important role in both the hypercalcemia of malignancy and postmenopausal osteoporosis. The osteoclast is derived from early hematopoietic precursors, with the earliest identifiable precursor being the GM-CFU. Hematopoietic growth factors produced by the marrow microenvironment can affect osteoclast formation by stimulating proliferation of the immature precursors or fusion of more committed precursors for the osteoclasts, as well as enhancing osteoclastic bone resorption. Further studies will be required to confirm the differentiation pathway for the osteoclast, as well as to identify specific differentiation markers that may be unique to the osteoclasts. Model systems are now available both to examine osteoclast precursors and osteoclast formation and to identify the mechanisms of action of a variety of osteotropic factors in this process. Both in vitro and in vivo model systems have been developed, and recently a transgenic mouse has been produced in which the SV40 large T antigen has been targeted to the osteoclast. Osteoclast precursors can now be isolated and identified in relatively pure populations so that molecular and biochemical studies may be possible to understand factors regulating the genetic events that control osteoclast differentiation and activity. One would anticipate that in the near future, osteoclast precursor or osteoclastic cell lines may be available from these transgenic mice or from osteoclast precursors transfected with transforming genes to help further the understanding of osteoclast biology.

References

1. Roodman, GD: Osteoclast differentiation, in *Critical Reviews in Oral Biology and Medicine.* Boca Raton, Fla, CRC Press, 2(2):389–409, 1991.
2. Holtrop ME, King GJ: The ultrastructure of the osteoclast and its functional implications *Clin Orthop* 123:177, 1977.
3. Lucht U: Osteoclasts—ultrastructure and function, in Carr I, Daems WT (eds): *The Reticuloendothelial System. A Comprehensive Treatise,* Vol 1 (Morphology). New York, Plenum Press, 1980, p 705.
4. Blair HC, Teitelbaum SL, Ghiselli R, et al: Osteoclastic bone resorption by a polarized vacuolar proton pump. *Science* 245:855, 1989.
5. Chambers TJ, McSheehy PMJ, Thomson BM, et al: The effect of calcium-regulating hormones and prostaglandins on bone resorption by osteoclasts disaggregated from neonatal rabbit bones. *Endocrinology* 116:234, 1985.
6. Chambers TJ, Horton MA: Failure of cells of the mononuclear phagocyte series to resorb bone. *Calcif Tissue Intl* 36:556, 1984.
7. Lucht U: Acid phosphatase of osteoclasts demonstrated by electron microscopic histochemistry. *Histochemistry* 28:103, 1971.
8. Gay C, Mueller WJ: Carbonic anhydrase and osteoclasts: Localization by labeled inhibitor autoradiography. *Science* 183:432, 1974.
9. Oursler MJ, Bell LV, Clevinger B, et al: Identification of osteoclast specific monoclonal antibodies. *J Cell Biol* 100:1592, 1985.
10. Horton MA: Osteoclast-specific antigens, ISI Atlas of Science. *Immunology* 35, 1988.

11. Athanasou NA, Quinn J, McGee JO: Immunocytochemical analysis of the human osteoclast: Phenotype relationship to other marrow-derived cells. *Bone Miner* 3:317, 1988.
12. Goldring SR, Gorn AH, Yamin M, et al: Characterization of the structural and functional properties of cloned calcitonin receptor cDNAs. *Horm Metab Res* 25:477, 1993.
13. Walker DG: Congenital osteopetrosis in mice cured by parabiotic union with normal siblings. *Endocrinology* 91:916, 1972.
14. Walker DG: Osteopetrosis cured by temporary parabiosis. *Science* 180:875, 1973.
15. Gothlin G, Ericsson JLE: On the histogenesis of the cells in fracture callus. Electron microscopic and autoradiographic observations in parabiotic rats and studies on labeled monocytes. *Virchows Arch B Cell Pathol* 12:318, 1973.
16. Kahn AJ, Simmons DJ: Investigation of the cell lineage in bone using a chimera of chick and quail embryonic tissue. *Nature* 258:325, 1975.
17. Walker DG: Control of bone resorption by hematopoietic tissue. The induction and reversal of congenital osteopetrosis in mice through the use of bone marrow mononuclear phagocytes. *J Exp Med* 156:1604, 1975.
18. Marks SC Jr: Osteopetrosis in the IA rat cured by spleen cells from a normal littermate. *Am J Anat* 146:331, 1976.
19. Coccia PF, Krivit W, Cervenka J, et al: Successful bone marrow transplantation for infantile malignant osteopetrosis. *N Engl J Med* 302:701, 1980.
20. Sorell M, Kapoor N, Kirkpatrick D, et al: Marrow transplantation for juvenile osteopetrosis. *Am J Med* 70:1280, 1981.
21. Feldman RS, Krieger NS, Tashjian AH Jr: Effects of parathyroid hormone and calcitonin on osteoclast formation in vitro. *Endocrinology* 107:1137, 1980.
22. Young RW: Cell proliferation and specialization during endochondral osteogenesis in young rats. *J Cell Biol* 141:357, 1962.
23. Ries WL, Gong JK: A comparative study of osteoclasts: In situ versus smear specimens. *Anat Rec* 203:221, 1982.
24. Baron R, Neff L, Van PT, et al: Kinetic and cytochemical identification of osteoclast precursors and their differentiation into multinucleated osteoclasts. *Am J Pathol* 121:363, 1986.
25. Fischman DA, Hay ED: Origin of osteoclasts from mononuclear leukocytes in regenerating newt limbs. *Anat Res* 143:329, 1962.
26. Jee WS, Nolan PD: Origin of osteoclasts from fusion of phagocytes. *Nature* 200:225, 1963.
27. Tinkler SMB, Williams DM, Johnson NW: Osteoclast formation in response to intraperitoneal injection of 1, alpha hydroxycholecalciferol in mice. *J Anat* 133:91, 1981.
28. Zambonin-Zallone A, Tete A, Primavera MV: Monocytes from circulating blood fuse in vitro with purified osteoclasts in primary culture. *J Cell Sci* 66:335, 1984.
29. Burger EH, Vander Meer JWM, Gevel JS, et al: In vitro formation of osteoclasts from long-term cultures of bone marrow and splenic transplants. *J Exp Med* 192:651, 1982.
30. Kurihara N, Chenu C, Civin CI, et al: Identification of committed mononuclear precursors for osteoclast-like cells formed in long-term marrow cultures. *Endocrinology* 126:2733, 1990.
31. Schneider GB, Relfson M: A bone marrow fraction enriched for granulocyte-macrophage progenitors gives rise to osteoclasts in vitro. *Bone* 9:303, 1988.
32. Hattersley G, Chambers TJ: Generation of osteoclasts from hemopoietic cells and a multipotential cell line in vitro. *J Cell Physiol* 140:478, 1989.
33. Horton MA, Rimmer EF, Lewis D: Cell surface characterization of the human osteoclast: Phenotypic relationship to other bone marrow-derived cell types. *J Pathology* 144:281, 1984.
34. Scheven BAA, Visser JWM, Nijweide PE: In vitro osteoclast generation from different bone marrow fractions, including a highly enriched haematopoietic stem cell population. *Nature* 321:79, 1986.

35. Hagenaars CE, van der Kraan AAM, Kawilarang-de Haas EWM, et al: Osteoclast formation from cloned pluripotent hemopoietic stem cells. *Bone Miner* 6:179, 1989.

36. Lee MY, Eyre DR, Osborne WR: Isolation of a murine osteoclast colony-stimulating factor. *Proc Natl Acad Sci U S A* 88:8500, 1991.

37. Udagawa N, Takahashi N, Akatsu T, et al: The marrow-derived stromal cell line (ST2) induces differentiation of not only spleen cells but also mature monocyte-macrophages into osteoclast-like cells. *J Bone Miner Res* 5:563A, 1990.

38. Osdoby P, Martini MC, Caplan AI: Isolated osteoclasts and their presumed progenitor cells, the monocyte, in culture. *J Exp Zool* 224:331, 1982.

39. Zambonin-Zallone A, Tete A, Primavera MV: Isolated osteoclasts in primary culture: First observations on structure and survival in cultured media. *Anat Embryol* 165:405, 1982.

40. Chambers TJ, Thomson BM, Fuller K: Resorption of bone by isolated rabbit osteoclasts. *J Cell Sci* 66:383, 1984.

41. Ohsaki Y, Takahashi S, Scarcez T, et al: Evidence for an autocrine/paracrine role for IL-6 in bone resorption by giant cell tumors of bone. *Endocrinology* 131:2229, 1992.

42. Chambers TJ: The pathobiology of the osteoclast. *J Clin Pathol* 38:241, 1985.

43. Boyde A, Dillon CE, Jones SJ: Measurement of osteoclastic resorption pits with a tandem scanning microscope. *J Microscopy* 158:261, 1990.

44. Testa NG, Allen TD, Lajtha LG, et al: Generation of osteoclasts in vitro. *J Cell Sci* 44:127, 1981.

45. Ibbotson KJ, Roodman GD, McManus LM, et al: Identification and characterization of osteoclast-like cells and their progenitors in cultures of feline marrow mononuclear cells. *J Cell Biol* 94:471, 1984.

46. Udagawa N, Takahashi N, Akatsu T, et al: The bone marrow-derived stromal cell lines MC3T3-G2/PA6 and ST2 support osteoclast-like cell differentiation in cocultures with mouse spleen cells. *Endocrinology* 125:1805, 1989.

47. Hattersley G, Chambers TJ: Generation of osteoclasts from hemopoietic cells and a multipotential cell line in vitro. *J Cell Physiol* 140:478, 1989.

48. Hagenaars CE, van der Kraan AAM, Kawilarang-de Haas EWM, et al: Interleukin-3 dependent hemopoietic stem cell lines are capable of osteoclast formation in vitro. *J Bone Miner Res* 4:588A, 1989.

49. Yoneda T, Mundy GR, Roodman GD: Induction of differentiation of the human promyelocytic HL-60 cells into cells with the osteoclastic phenotype. *J Bone Miner Res* 4:559A, 1989.

50. Chambers TJ, Owens JM, Hattersley G, et al: Generation of osteoclast-inductive and osteoclastogenic cell lines from the H-2KbtsA58 transgenic mouse. *Proc Natl Acad Sci U S A* 90:5578, 1993.

51. Tamura T, Takahashi N, Akatsu T, et al: New resorption assay with mouse osteoclast-like multinucleated cells formed in vitro. *J Bone Miner Res* 8:953, 1993.

52. Reddy SV, Scarcez T, Windle JJ, et al: Cloning and characterization of the 5'-flanking region of the mouse tartrate-resistant acid phosphatase (TRAP) gene. *J Bone Miner Res* 8:1263, 1993.

53. Reddy SV, Hundley JE, Windle JJ, et al: Characterization of the mouse tartrate-resistant acid phosphatase (TRAP) gene promoter. *J Bone Miner Res* (submitted).

54. Brendan BF, Windle JJ, Reddy SV, et al: Targeting SV-40 T antigen to the osteoclast in transgenic mice causes osteopetrosis, transformation and apoptosis of osteoclasts. *ASBMR Meeting* Tampa, Fla, September 1993.

55. Uy HL, Dallas M, Calland JW, et al: Development of a simple in vivo model to determine the effects of factors on cells at different stages in the osteoclast lineage. *J Bone Miner Res* (submitted).

56. Takahashi S, Goldring S, Katz M, et al: Downregulation of calcitonin receptor mRNA expression by calcitonin during human osteoclast-like cell differentiation. *J Clin Invest* (submitted).

57. Gowen M, Meikle MC, Reynolds JJ: Stimulation of bone resorption in vitro by a non-prostanoid factor released by human monocytes in culture. *Biochem Biophys Acta* 762:471, 1983.

58. Boyce BF, Aufdemorte TB, Garrett IR, et al: Effects of interleukin-1 on bone turnover in normal mice. *Endocrinology* 125:1142, 1989.

59. Pfeilschifter J, Chenu C, Bird A, et al: Interleukin-1 and tumor necrosis factor stimulate the formation of human osteoclast-like cells in vitro. *J Bone Miner Res* 4:113, 1989.

60. Kurihara N, Bertolini D, Suda T, et al: IL-6 stimulates osteoclast-like multinucleated cell formation in long term human marrow cultures by inducing IL-1 release. *J Immunol* 144:4226, 1990.

61. Thomson BM, Saklatvala J, Chambers TJ: Osteoblasts mediate interleukin-1 stimulation of bone resorption by rat osteoclasts. *J Exp Med* 164:104, 1986.

62. Pacifici R, Rifas L, McCracken R, et al: Ovarian steroid treatment blocks a postmenopausal increase in blood monocyte interleukin-1 release. *Proc Natl Acad Sci U S A* 86:2398, 1989.

63. Johnson RA, Boyce BF, Mundy GR, et al: Tumors producing human TNF induce hypercalcemia and osteoclastic bone resorption in nude mice. *Endocrinology* 124:1424, 1989.

64. Garrett IR, Durie BGM, Nedwin GE: Production of the bone-resorbing cytokine lymphotoxin by cultured human myeloma cells. *N Engl J Med* 317:526, 1987.

65. Yoneda T, Alsina MA, Chavez JB, et al: Evidence that tumor necrosis factor plays a pathogenetic role in the paraneoplastic syndromes of cachexia, hypercalcemia, and leukocytosis in a human tumor in nude mice. *J Clin Invest* 87:977, 1991.

66. Black K, Garrett IR, Mundy GR: Chinese hamster ovarian cells transfected with the murine interleukin-6 gene cause hypercalcemia as well as cachexia, leukocytosis and thrombocytosis in tumor-bearing nude mice. *Endocrinology* 128:2657, 1991.

67. Roodman GD, Kurihara N, Ohsaki Y, et al: Interleukin-6: A potential autocrine/paracrine factor in Paget's disease of bone. *J Clin Invest* 89:46, 1991.

68. Reddy SV, Takahashi S, Dallas M, et al: Il-6 antisense deoxyoligonucleotides inhibit bone resorption by giant cells from human giant cell tumors of bone. *J Bone Miner Res* 9:753, 1994.

69. Tamura T, Udagawa N, Takahashi N, et al: Soluble interleukin-6 receptor triggers osteoclast formation by interleukin-6. *Proc Natl Acad Sci U S A* 90:11924, 1993.

70. Jilka RL, Hangoc G, Girasole G, et al: Increased osteoclast development after estrogen loss: Mediation by interleukin-6. *Science* 257:88, 1992.

71. Yoshida H, Hayashi S, Kunisada T, et al: The murine mutation osteopetrosis is in the coding region of the macrophage colony-stimulating factor gene. *Nature* 345:442, 1990.

72. Shinar DM, Sato M, Rodan GA: The effect of hemopoietic growth factors on the generation of osteoclast-like cells in mouse bone marrow cultures. *Endocrinology* 126:1728, 1990.

73. MacDonald BR, Mundy GR, Clark S, et al: Effects of human recombinant CSF-GM and highly purified CSF-1 on the formation of multinucleated cells with osteoclast characteristics in long-term bone marrow cultures. *J Bone Miner Res* 1:227, 1986.

74. Takahashi N, Udagawa N, Akatsu T, et al: The role of colony stimulating factors in osteoclast development: Osteoclast progenitors proliferate in response to macrophage colony stimulating factor. *J Immunol* (submitted).

75. Shuto T, Kukita T, Hirata M, et al: Dexamethasone stimulates osteoclast-like cell formation by inhibiting granulocyte-macrophage colony-stimulating factor production in mouse bone marrow cultures. *Endocrinology* 134:1121, 1994.

76. Lorenzo JA, Sousa SL, Fonseca JM, et al: Colony-stimulating factors regulate the development of multinucleated osteoclasts from recently replicated cells in vitro. *J Clin Invest* 80:160, 1987.
77. Hattersley G, Chambers TJ: Effects of interleukin-3 and of granulocyte-macrophage and macrophage colony stimulating factors on osteoclast differentiation from mouse hemopoietic tissue. *J Cell Physiol* 142:201, 1990.
78. Barton BE, Mayer R: Il-3 induces differentiation of bone marrow precursor cells to osteoclast-like cells. *J Immunol* 143:3211, 1989.
79. Chenu C, Pfeilschifter J, Mundy GR, et al: Transforming growth factor β inhibits formation of osteoclast-like cells in long-term human marrow cultures. *Proc Natl Acad Sci U S A* 85:5683, 1988.
80. Gowen J, Mundy GR: Actions of recombinant interleukin-1, interleukin-2, and interferon gamma on bone resorption in vitro. *J Immunol* 136:2478, 1986.
81. Takahashi N, Mundy GR, Roodman GD: Recombinant human gamma interferon inhibits formation of osteoclast-like cells by inhibiting fusion of their precursors. *J Immunol* 137:3544, 1986.
82. Shioi A, Teitelbaum SL, Ross FP, et al: Interleukin-4 inhibits murine osteoclast formation in vitro. *J Cell Biochem* 47:272, 1991.
83. Watanabe K, Tanaka Y, Morimoto I, et al: Interleukin-4 as a potent inhibitor of bone resorption. *Biochem Biophys Res Commun* 172:105, 1990.
84. Kukita A, Chenu C, McManus LM, et al: Atypical multinucleated cells form in long-term marrow cultures from patients with Paget's disease. *J Clin Invest* 85:1280, 1990.
85. Demulder A, Takahashi S, Singer FR, et al: Evidence for abnormalities in osteoclast precursors and the marrow microenvironment in Paget's disease. *Endocrinology* 133:1978, 1993.
86. Reddy SV, Singer FR, Roodman GD: Bone marrow mononuclear cells from patients with Paget's disease contain measles virus nucleocapsid mRNA that have mutations in a specific region of the sequence. *Proc Natl Acad Sci U S A* (submitted).

3 Coagulation Factors and Platelets

Introduction

The literature this year concerning blood platelets and coagulation factors is reasonably replete with modifications of various therapeutic regimens for the treatment of immune-mediated thrombocytopenia, thrombotic disease, and the prevention of recurrence of thrombosis. Several new therapeutic agents have been introduced in an attempt to improve on time-honored agents with defined efficacy.

Major among these new therapeutic agents is a glut of low-molecular-weight preparations of heparin. Only 1 of the approximately 15 preparations available worldwide has been approved by the Food and Drug Administration for use in the United States. Demonstration that the newer low-molecular-weight preparations are substantially more efficacious in the prevention and treatment of thrombotic disease has not been obvious. Because these agents do not bind to several different plasma proteins, endothelial cells, and platelets, the heparin molecules of the low-molecular-weight species are more bioavailable to interfere in an inhibitory mechanism with the serine proteases of the coagulation system. Because of this predictable bioavailability, there is no need for monitoring the degree of anticoagulation provided by the various low-molecular-weight-heparin preparations. Because these agents do not bind to platelets, it was expected there would be less bleeding compared with unfractionated heparin. This feature has been observed in a few preclinical animal models. Many clinical studies with an appreciable magnitude in the number of patients have been completed. Each of these studies generates copious quantities of instructive data. All of these studies almost without exception state in their final summary that low-molecular-weight heparin is at least as good as unfractionated heparin. In some studies, particularly in studies of patients receiving pelvic surgery, appreciably more bleeding has been documented than in control patients receiving standard unfractionated heparin. That these low-molecular-weight heparin preparations need to be administered once or twice every 24 hours via the subcutaneous route and do not require monitoring or a hospital environment are attractive features.

Considerable work continues in the study of platelet physiology and biochemistry of the platelet membrane. This work is primarily directed at prevention of platelet initiation of thrombus formation inducing reocclusion of coronary arteries that have been rendered patent by thrombolytic therapy. Although a large number of agents have been generated and a host of different strategies employed, the problem still exists without a satisfactory solution. Two important, frequently overlooked facts must be realized by investigators in this area. First, whenever platelets are sufficiently altered so that they do not interact with subendothelial collagen, do not interact with coagulation proteins, or do not cohere to each other, then hemorrhage is a definite result. Second, platelets can initiate thrombus formation, but extensive thrombus formation can occur in the absence of platelets, i.e., platelets are not required for thrombus formation to occur.

One of the most active areas in the world of coagulation continues to be study of the hypercoagulable state. This area has reached a sizzling point in the diagnostic arena with the identification of a new mechanism for spontaneous thrombus formation. This new mechanism for predisposition to thrombosis is "resistance to activated protein C" (1–6). In patients with this problem, activated protein C is unable to degrade and destroy factor V or activated factor V; therefore the normal inhibitory function of activated protein C is absent and thrombus formation ensues. The most recent study identified a mutation, an amino acid substitution in the factor V molecule, that prevents the normal activated protein C molecule from interacting with and thus degrading activated factor V (6). Some studies have already suggested that this will account for 30% of all thrombus formation seen in patients with venous thrombosis, arterial thrombosis, and pulmonary emboli. Details of these publications will be found in next year's edition of the YEAR BOOK OF HEMATOLOGY.

William R. Bell, M.D.

References

1. Dahlback B, et al: *Proc Natl Acad Sci U S A* 90:1004, 1993.
2. *Proc Natl Acad Sci U S A* 91:1396–1400, 1994.
3. Svensson PJ, Dahlback B: *N Engl J Med* 330:517, 1994.
4. Tuddenham EG: *Lancet* 342:1501, 1993.
5. Koster T, et al: *Lancet* 342:1503, 1993.
6. Sun X, et al: *Blood* 83:3120, 1994.

Platelet Physiology

Essential Thrombocythemia: A Relative Benign Long-Term Course
Meisel S, Shpilberg O, Ramot B, Ben-Bassat I (Chaim Sheba Med Ctr, Tel-Hashomer, Israel; Tel Aviv Univ, Israel)
Isr J Med Sci 29:190–194, 1993   116-95-3-1

Background.—Thrombocytosis is identified much more often now than in the past because of wide population screening. Some patients with thrombocytosis have essential thrombocythemia (ET), which is known to carry a significant risk for bleeding and thrombosis. However, the current impression is that most patients with ET have minor symptoms, with a very low incidence of life-threatening complications.

Patients and Findings.—Disease manifestations, treatment response, and follow-up course in 35 patients with ET at 1 center were reviewed. Patients ranged in age from 17 to 81 years. In 12 patients who were asymptomatic at the initial examination, the diagnosis was incidental. Twenty-three patients initially had thrombocytosis-associated symptoms, usually neurologic, microcirculatory, or thromboembolic. None of the patients had bleeding as an initial symptom. At diagnosis, the mean platelet count was 858×10^9/L. The mean maximal count during follow-up was 989×10^9/L. The overall median follow-up was 54 months. Of the 12 asymptomatic patients, 10 remained so during observation, and 10 patients seen with thrombocytosis-related symptoms became asymptomatic after a single treatment course. Thirty patients received busulfan or hydroxyurea treatment, or both. In most patients, the response to cytoreductive treatment was prompt and continuous.

Conclusion.—Although ET may be of grave consequence, its course with treatment generally appears to be more benign than previously believed. These observations suggest that a conservative, individual approach to ET treatment is warranted. Only patients who are symptomatic or at high risk for cardiovascular disease should be treated, preferably with intermittent hydroxyurea.

▶ This carefully prepared report of 35 patients with strikingly elevated platelet counts once again indicates the relative benign course of an elevated platelet count with this disease process. This, as other studies have pointed out, indicates that there is not a need for aggressive treatment and that in many instances, aggressive treatment is the incorrect maneuver in the management of these patients. For additional findings by other investigators, please consult the following references (1–5).—W.R. Bell, M.D.

References

1. Kessler CM, et al: *Br J Haematol* 50:157, 1982.
2. Mitus AJ, et al: *Am J Med* 88:371, 1990.
3. Buss DH, et al: *Am J Hematol* 20:365, 1985.
4. McIntyre KJ, et al: *Mayo Clin Proc* 66:149, 1991.
5. Colombi M, et al: *Cancer* 67:2926, 1991.

Effect of Extracorporeal Membrane Oxygenation on Platelets in Newborns

Robinson TM, Kickler TS, Walker LK, Ness P, Bell W (Johns Hopkins Hosp, Baltimore, Md)
Crit Care Med 21:1029–1034, 1993   116-95-3-2

Background.—Support with neonatal extracorporeal membrane oxygenation (ECMO) has been effective in saving the lives of infants who would otherwise have had little chance of surviving. It has been most

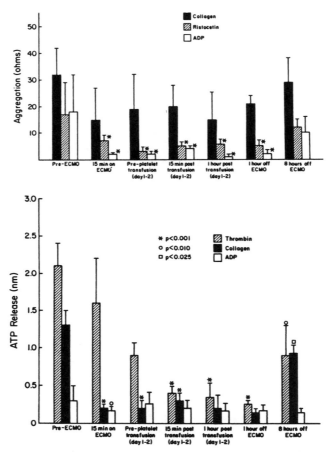

Fig 3–1.—Top, aggregation studies were done immediately before the start of ECMO and 15 minutes after the start of ECMO. The studies were repeated before the first platelet transfusion and 15–60 minutes after platelets were transfused. After stopping ECMO, the aggregation studies were done at 1 and 8 hours after ending the treatment. *Significant at $P < .05$. **Bottom,** amount of adenosine triphosphate (ATP) released was also measured after addition of collagen and adenosine 5′-diphosphate (ADP) agonists. Results in both graphs are expressed as standard error of the mean. (Courtesy of Robinson TM, Kickler TS, Walker LK, et al: *Crit Care Med* 21:1029–1034, 1993.)

beneficial in term infants with disorders involving severe impairment of blood oxygenation secondary to reversible pulmonary hypertension. However, there has been no systematic research on the effect of ECMO on platelet counts and function or on the recovery of transfused platelets in neonates. Qualitative platelet abnormalities, uncorrectable by platelet transfusions, may occur during ECMO.

Methods.—Ten infants aged younger than 1 week were prospectively studied in a neonatal intensive care unit. All had respiratory failure necessitating ECMO. Platelet counts were determined at certain intervals, and changes in platelet counts after transfusion were documented. Whole blood platelet aggregation studies were also done to assess the effect of ECMO on platelet function.

Findings.—Fifteen minutes after ECMO initiation, the platelet count was decreased by a mean 26% compared with baseline values. By the end of 1 hour, this mean had decreased an additional 16%. Fifteen minutes after platelet transfusions, the mean platelet count increased by 17%. Platelet counts declined to pretransfusion values 1 hour after platelet transfusion. Platelet aggregation studies 15 minutes after ECMO was begun indicated a 46% mean reduction in response to collagen from baseline and a significant decrease in the response to ristocetin and adenosine 5'-diphosphate. Significant decreases also occurred in platelet adenosine triphosphate release. Single-unit platelet transfusions did not correct platelet aggregation abnormalities. Eight hours after ECMO, the infants had a resolution of platelet aggregation abnormalities and normalization of platelet counts (Fig 3–1).

Conclusion.—Qualitative and quantitative platelet changes occur during ECMO in neonates. The survival rate of transfused platelets is reduced. Furthermore, the transfusion of platelets with normal function does not reverse the acquired platelet dysfunction while the infant is receiving ECMO treatment.

▶ This detailed study provides firm and quantified information on how much disturbance there is to platelets when ECMO is employed. When using this device, the physicians involved must realize that there will be a considerable disturbance and, to some extent, damage to the platelets that are passed through it.—W.R. Bell, M.D.

Abnormal Cytoskeletal Assembly in Platelets From Uremic Patients

Escolar G, Díaz-Ricart M, Cases A, Castillo R, Ordinas A, White JG (Hosp Clínic i Provincial, Barcelona; Univ of Minnesota, Minneapolis)
Am J Pathol 143:823–831, 1993   116-95-3–3

Introduction.—Little is known about the mechanisms of the bleeding tendency of patients with uremia. Some findings suggest that the platelets of patients with uremia may have some abnormality of cytoskeletal

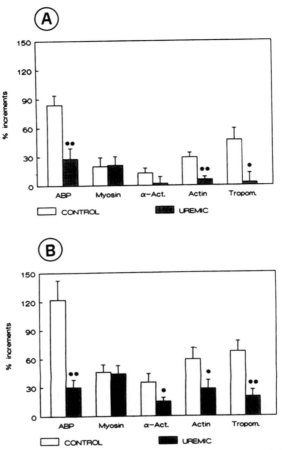

Fig 3–2.—*Bars* showing percentages of increase in the association of cytoskeletal proteins as calculated by scan densitometry of the electrophoretic gels. *Bars* display results (mean ± standard error) obtained in control (*white bars*) and uremic (*shaded bars*) cytoskeletons after .01 units (**A**) or .1 units of thrombin. (**B**) per mL. Values are expressed as percentages of increase vs. the amount of the same protein found in the cytoskeletons of nonactivated platelets. Triton-insoluble cytoskeletons analyzed were derived from the same individuals involved in spreading experiments. Amounts of actin-binding protein (ABP), α-actinin (α-*Act.*), actin, and tropomyosin (*Tropom.*) bound into uremic platelet cytoskeleton are significantly less than those incorporated by control cells, except for myosin. *Asterisks* denote statistical significance with respect to controls (*P < .05; **P < .01). (Courtesy of Escolar G, Díaz-Ricart M, Cases A, et al: *Am J Pathol* 143:823–831, 1993.)

function. The cytoskeletal assembly of uremic and normal platelets was compared.

Methods.—The response of normal and uremic platelets to surface activation at the ultrastructural level was observed. The changes occurring in the platelet cytoskeleton–associated proteins after stimulation with thrombin, .01 and .1 units/mL, were examined. Triton X-100 was used to extract the cytoskeletons, and, in addition, sodium dodecylsulfate–polyacrylamide gel electrophoresis was used to process them. Scan densitometry was used to look for cytoskeletal proteins.

Results.—Fewer uremic than control platelets fully spread on formvarcoated grids under static conditions. Resting uremic platelets demonstrated an impairment in cytoskeletal organization, more so after thrombin activation. On stimulation with thrombin, actin incorporation into the cytoskeletons of uremic platelets was significantly less than that in controls: 6% vs. 29% at the low dose and 28% vs. 59% at the high dose. The cytoskeletons of uremic platelets had decreased associations with actin-binding protein, α-actinin, and tropomyosin. However, myosin incorporation into the cytoskeletons of activated uremic platelets was no different (Fig 3–2).

Conclusion.—In uremia, the platelet cytoskeleton shows functional and biochemical changes that may play a role in impaired platelet function. Uremic platelets fail to spread fully after surface activation, and resting and thrombin-activated platelets both show impaired cytoskeletal organization. The clinical platelet dysfunction could result from abnormal cytoskeletal assembly in response to activation by surfaces or strong agonists in suspension.

▶ The bleeding tendency in uremic patients, although recognized for hundreds of years, has not been absolutely defined. There is no question that platelets are dysfunctional in uremic patients. Studies reported by these authors clearly demonstrate distinct differences between uremic and normal platelets. However, it remains to be absolutely demonstrated that these biochemical and functional alterations seen in the platelet cytoskeleton in uremic patients are truly responsible for the problem of hemorrhage. These studies need to be extended and confirmed by others. With this type of information, better directed therapy will be possible.—W.R. Bell, M.D.

Cocaine-Induced Platelet Defects
Jennings LK, White MM, Sauer CM, Mauer AM, Robertson JT (Univ of Tennessee, Memphis)
Stroke 24:1352–1359, 1993   116-95-3-4

Background.—Cocaine use has been associated with strokes and acute cardiac events, but its role in coagulation disorders has not been extensively investigated. Studies have demonstrated that local anesthetics inhibit platelet adhesion to foreign surfaces, platelet aggregation initiated by adenosine diphosphate (ADP) and thrombin, and platelet activation. Conflicting evidence from various in vitro models has shown that cocaine has either an inhibitory or proaggregatory effect on platelet function. The effect of cocaine and its carrier on the activation and aggregation of human platelets in vitro was examined.

Method.—Platelets from 4 medication-free donors were preincubated with increasing concentrations of cocaine or carrier and challenged with the agonists ADP or collagen in the aggregometer.

Results.—Cocaine inhibited the platelet aggregation response to challenge with ADP, collagen, or arachidonic acid. Cocaine had a direct effect on fibrinogen binding to the activated platelet and also dissociated preformed platelet aggregates. Cocaine's effect appears selective because there was no evidence of inhibition of agonist-mediated increases in cytosolic calcium or platelet shape change. Cocaine did disrupt the organization of the cytoskeleton of activated platelets, a secondary event critical to cell receptor clustering and clot retraction. Preincubation of platelets with cocaine produced alterations in platelet protein electrophoretic patterns.

Conclusion.—This in vitro data suggest that cocaine has an effect on mechanisms mediating both adhesive and cohesive properties of platelets. Cocaine may have a direct inhibitory effect on the ability of platelets to participate in thrombus formation. The contribution of this inhibitory effect on sudden death in cocaine abusers is still unclear.

▶ Although thrombocytopenia and platelet dysfunction have been recognized to be associated with excess cocaine ingestion for many years, the precise mechanism of interaction by cocaine with platelets remains unclear. Although the authors of this thoughtfully performed, detailed study have demonstrated a number of disturbing alterations to the platelet, one must question whether these are applicable to the addict with an excess of cocaine in his or her body. The cocaine used in this study was highly purified, which is in sharp contrast to what is used by the overwhelming majority of abusers. Almost certainly, some of the impurities found in "street preparations" are responsible for many of the abnormalities seen in cocaine addicts. However, purified cocaine is unquestionably capable of severely altering platelet metabolism and platelet function.—W.R. Bell, M.D.

Point Mutation in a Leucine-Rich Repeat of Platelet Glycoprotein Ibα Resulting in the Bernard-Soulier Syndrome
Ware J, Russell SR, Marchese P, Murata M, Mazzucato M, De Marco L, Ruggeri ZM (Scripps Research Inst, La Jolla, Calif; Centro Trasfusionale e Chimica Clinica, Pordenone, Italy)
J Clin Invest 92:1213–1220, 1993   116-95-3–5

Background.—Most cases of Bernard-Soulier syndrome stem from a genetic defect within 1 of the β-subunits of the glycoprotein (GP)-Ib-IX-V receptor. In a variant of Bernard-Soulier syndrome, designated type Bolzano, giant platelets incapable of binding vWF express a dysfunctional GP Ib-IX-V complex. The cause of the Bolzano variant of Bernard-Soulier syndrome was explored.

Methods.—Blood samples were obtained from an index patient with type Bolzano Bernard-Soulier syndrome, from family members, and from normal blood donors. Genetic studies were complemented by immunologic and functional analysis of expressed recombinant GP-Ibα fragments.

Results.—Two C-to-T mutations were found on 1 allele derived from the GP-Ibα gene of the proband: the codon for Thr[145] (ACG) was changed to Met (ATG); the codon for Ala[156] (GCT), to Val (GTT). The proband was homozygous for both mutations; his parents were heterozygous, with cosegregation of the Met[145] and Val[156] codons. The Thr[145] to Met mutation was found in 11% of the normal population, but the Ala[156] to Val mutation was not detected. The mutated GP-Ibα fragment was markedly less reactive to LJ-Ib1 and other conformation-dependent anti-GP Ib monoclonal antibodies. A similar abnormality was found only in the fragment with the single Ala[156] to Val mutation. This finding confirmed the Ala[156] to Val mutation as the cause of the altered antibody recognition and abnormal platelet GP Ib-IX-V complex.

Conclusion.—In this family, the molecular basis of the Bernard-Soulier syndrome was a single amino acid substitution within a leucine-rich repeat in the α-subunit of GP Ib. This finding suggests that structural integrity of a leucine-rich repeat is required for normal GP Ib-IX-V receptor function as well as normal platelet morphology.

▶ The results of these carefully done, detailed studies for the first time identify the molecular basis of the Bernard-Soulier syndrome. It is apparent from these studies that the integrity of a leucine-rich repeat is necessary for normal function of the GP Ib-IX-V receptor on the platelet membrane. When the amino acid alanine at address 156 (Ala[156]) is replaced by valine, this leucine-rich repeat is no longer functional and does not properly bind the von Willebrand protein. This finding should be verified in other families with the Bernard-Soulier disorder.—W.R. Bell, M.D.

Antiplatelet Agents

Aspirin Does Not Inhibit Adenosine Diphosphate-Induced Platelet α-Granule Release
Rinder CS, Student LA, Bonan JL, Rinder HM, Smith BR (Yale Univ, New Haven, Conn)
Blood 82:505–512, 1993   116-95-3–6

Background.—The role of arachidonic acid metabolites in homotypic platelet interactions is well characterized. The role of these metabolites in heterotypic interactions requiring α-granule secretion is less well understood. Platelet-surface expression of P-selectin was used as a marker of α-granule secretion to examine the effects of inhibiting platelet cyclooxygenase and lipoxygenase exchange on platelet α-granule secretion in response to adenosine diphosphate (ADP).

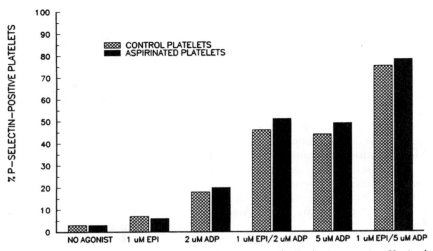

Fig 3–3.—Effect of aspirin on epinephrine and ADP synergy for P-selectin expression. Unstirred PRP was incubated with 500 μmol of acetylsalicylic acid per liter (*black bars*) or diluent (*hatched bars*) for 60 minutes, then stimulated with either a single agonist (epinephrine or ADP) or diluent for 15 minutes or for synergy experiments, with epinephrine for 10 minutes followed by ADP for 5 minutes. The percentage of P-selectin–positive platelets was then measured. Data for single experiment are representative of 4 so performed. (Courtesy of Rinder CS, Student LA, Bonan JL, et al: *Blood* 82:505–512, 1993.)

Methods.—Platelet-rich plasma (PRP), adjusted to 2.5 × 10⁸/mL, and platelet-free plasma were prepared from whole blood from normal volunteers who were receiving no medications. Standard platelet aggregometry was performed at 37°C. The percentage of platelets expressing P-selectin was determined using flow cytometry.

Results.—At doses sufficient to block dense granule secretion, aspirin did not inhibit α-granule secretion in response to ADP. Preincubation of PRP with 1 μmol of epinephrine per liter enhanced aggregation response to low-dose ADP. The addition of 1 μmol of epinephrine per liter to unstirred PRP did not significantly increase P-selectin expression compared with no agonist, indicating that homotypic contact is important for epinephrine-induced α-granule release (Fig 3–3). However, PRP preincubation with 1 μmol of epinephrine per liter followed by 2 or 5 μmol of ADP per liter produced a synergistic increase in P-selectin expression. Aspirin treatment did not affect the synergistic increase in P-selectin–positive platelets to epinephrine and ADP. Aspirin also did not affect the ability of P-selectin to mediate adhesion of activated platelets to monocytes and polymorphonuclear lymphocytes in whole blood.

Conclusion.—Leukocyte-platelet interactions mediated by P-selectin occur independently of arachidonic acid metabolites. As the regulation of this pathway is further elucidated, it may be possible to inhibit α-granule secretion selectively and to preserve platelet aggregation.

▶ This thorough investigation of the various alterations in platelet biochemistry induced by aspirin points out that aspirin is very selective and actually does not disturb all platelet functions. There are still several platelet functions remaining after aspirin has exerted its maximum inhibitory effect, and the platelets still can participate in a number of biochemical reactions, some of which may have hemostatic relevance.—W.R. Bell, M.D.

Transdermal Modification of Platelet Function: A Dermal Aspirin Preparation Selectively Inhibits Platelet Cyclooxygenase and Preserves Prostacyclin Biosynthesis

Keimowitz RM, Pulvermacher G, Mayo G, Fitzgerald DJ (Gundersen Clinic, La Crosse, Wis; Vanderbilt Univ, Nashville, Tenn)
Circulation 88:556–561, 1993   116-95-3–7

Background.—Prostaglandin-I_2 formation and gastrointestinal toxicity can occur in patients taking even low doses of aspirin. Even with controlled-release oral aspirin, which shows a high degree of platelet selectivity, the gut is still exposed to the drug. The possibility of using the skin as a route for continuous, low-dose aspirin administration and selective inhibition of platelet cyclo-oxygenase was investigated.

Methods.—Eighteen volunteers were divided into 3 groups: 1 received aspirin, 250 mg/day, a second, aspirin, 750 mg/day; and the third, placebo for 10 days. Aspirin was dissolved in isopropyl alcohol or ethanol and propylene glycol and applied to the forearm and upper arm. The 3 groups were compared for thromboxane-A_2 and prostaglandin-I_2 biosynthesis.

Results.—Both aspirin doses inhibited serum thromboxane-B_2 in a dose-dependent fashion. Five of 6 patients in the high-dose group responded, achieving mean serum thromboxane-B_2 reductions of 95%. There was a 68% decrease in urinary 2,3-dinor thromboxane-B_2, measured as an index of in vivo thromboxane-A_2 formation. This finding was consistent with the in vivo inhibition of platelet cyclo-oxygenase. Excretion of 2,3-dinor-6-keto prostaglandin-F_{1a}, measured as an indicator of prostaglandin-I_2 biosynthesis, decreased to 81% of baseline at 10 days. Before aspirin treatment, giving intravenous bradykinin resulted in a fivefold increase in prostaglandin-I_2 synthesis. This effect was negated by oral aspirin, 75 mg/day for 14 days, whereas dermal aspirin at the higher dose had no such effect. At the higher dose, aspirin reached its peak level of .24 μg/mL at 3 hours and salicylate peaked at .79 μg/mL within 6–12 hours.

Conclusion.—Transdermal aspirin can achieve selective inhibition of platelet cyclo-oxygenase in humans. Although further analysis is needed to determine whether transdermal aspirin reduces the risk of gastrointestinal side effects, this route of administration might be useful in patients with peptic ulcer disease or in those taking aspirin and oral anticoagulants in combination. Other antiplatelet agents might also be administered by the transdermal route.

▶ This very important report suggests that when aspirin is administered via the dermal route, it facilitates selective inhibition of platelet cyclo-oxygenase and does not disturb the synthesis of prostacyclin. However, it is important to point out that the prostacyclin is not totally spared of inhibition; there was approximately 20% inhibition of prostacyclin in contrast to 95% inhibition of thromboxane-A_2. The authors postulate that this is possible because of the exquisite sensitivity of cyclo-oxygenase to acetylation by aspirin. They suggest that the dermal tissues sufficiently deacetylate aspirin to protect the synthetic production of prostacyclin. One must ask whether this observation would hold up if this form of treatment was administered for longer than 10 days and whether the same effect could be achieved by administering exceedingly small doses of aspirin via the oral route.—W.R. Bell, M.D.

Prevention of One-Year Vein-Graft Occlusion After Aortocoronary-Bypass Surgery: A Comparison of Low-Dose Aspirin, Low-Dose Aspirin Plus Dipyridamole, and Oral Anticoagulants
van der Meer J, for the CABADAS Research Group of the Interuniversity Cardiology Institute of The Netherlands (Univ Hosp, Groningen, The Netherlands)
Lancet 342:257–264, 1993   116-95-3–8

Background.—Aspirin with or without dipyridamole can prevent aortocoronary vein graft occlusion. There is ongoing debate as to whether dipyridamole should be added and whether antiplatelet drugs are superior to oral anticoagulants. This prospective, randomized study compared the safety and efficacy of low-dose aspirin, aspirin plus dipyridamole, and oral anticoagulants in the prevention of vein graft occlusion in the first year after aortocoronary bypass surgery.

Methods.—A total of 948 patients at 7 hospitals were included. Aspirin, 50 mg/day, was started after surgery. Dipyridamole was administered at a dose of 5 mg/kg/24 hours intravenously for 28 hours, followed by 200 mg twice daily. Oral anticoagulants were administered to produce a prothrombin time of 2.8–4.8 international normalized ratio. Both were started before surgery. The oral anticoagulant arm of the study was open because of the necessity for dose adjustments. The 3 groups were compared for incidence of myocardial infarction, major bleeding, and death.

Results.—Occlusion of distal anastomoses occurred at a rate of 11% in the aspirin plus dipyridamole group, 15% in the aspirin-only group, and 13% in the oral anticoagulant group (table). Clinical events listed above occurred in 20.3% of the aspirin plus dipyridamole group, 13.9% of the aspirin-only group, and 16.9% of the oral anticoagulant group.

Frequency of Vein Graft Occlusion

Unit of analysis	Aspirin + placebo (A + P)	Aspirin + dipyridamole (A + D)	Oral anticoagulants (OA)	RR (95% CI)	
				A + D vs A + P	OA vs A + P
Distal anastomoses*	15 (757)	11 (764)	13 (797)	0·76 (0·54–1·05)	0·90 (0·65–1·25)
Grafts	20 (440)	15 (461)	19 (448)	0·76 (0·57–1·02)	0·95 (0·72–1·24)
Patients	27 (270)	26 (249)	27 (257)	0·97 (0·73–1·29)	0·99 (0·75–1·32)

Note: Data are percentage occluded (total number). A few patients were excluded from analysis because of a graft being defined as neither patent nor occluded.
* Comparison by ratio estimate analysis.
(Courtesy of van der Meer J, for the CABADAS Research Group of the Interuniversity Cardiology Institute of The Netherlands: *Lancet* 342:257–264, 1993.)

Conclusion.—Adding dipyridamole to low-dose aspirin does not appear to significantly improve aortocoronary vein graft patency and may even increase the rate of clinical events somewhat. Oral anticoagulants are no better than aspirin in preventing vein graft occlusion. Low-dose aspirin is preferable because of its efficacy, safety, practicality, and low cost.

▶ This critically important study is long overdue. The results clearly demonstrate that the efficacy of aspirin plus dipyridamole in many previously published reports is unquestionably due to the aspirin. The addition of dipyridamole to aspirin is actually associated with more adverse events than aspirin alone. This report clearly establishes that dipyridamole is not efficacious in the management of vascular occlusive diseases. Nearly identical information and data were reported in the past (1), and this report confirms the earlier observations.

Reference

1. FitzGerald GA: N Engl J Med 316:1247, 1987.

A Comparison of Aspirin With Placebo in Patients Treated With Warfarin After Heart-Valve Replacement

Turpie AGG, Gent M, Laupacis A, Latour Y, Gunstensen J, Basile F, Klimek M, Hirsh J (McMaster Univ, Hamilton, Ont, Canada; Univ of Western Ontario, London, Canada; Hôtel-Dieu Hosp, Montreal)
N Engl J Med 329:524–529, 1993
116-95-3-9

Causes of Death Among Patients Treated With High Doses of Heparin and Those Treated With Low Doses of Heparin

CAUSE OF DEATH	TREATMENT GROUP	
	HIGH-DOSE (N = 112)	LOW-DOSE (N = 109)
Cardiac arrest ≤48 hr	6	3
Cardiac arrest >48 hr	1	4
Myocardial rupture	2	3
Cardiogenic shock	2	2
Pulmonary embolism	0	1
Total	11	13

(Courtesy of Turpie AGG, Gent M, Laupacis A, et al: N Engl J Med 329:524–529, 1993.)

Background.—Thromboembolism remains a serious complication after heart valve replacement, despite the use of anticoagulants. The addition of an antiplatelet agent has been recommended as a means of further decreasing the risk of embolism. A trial was designed to assess the safety and efficacy of adding aspirin, 100 mg/day, to warfarin treatment in patients with mechanical heart valves or with tissue valves plus atrial fibrillation or a history of thromboembolism.

Methods.—The study was randomized, double-blind, and placebo-controlled. From February of 1987 to May of 1991, 557 patients at 3 Canadian hospitals had heart valve replacement. The criteria for inclusion were met by 370 patients; a group of 186 were assigned to enteric-coated, slow-release aspirin, and a group of 184 received placebo. Patients received anticoagulant therapy with warfarin as soon as they were able to take the medication orally. The initial dose was 10 mg/day, and patients were monitored to obtain an international normalized ratio of 3–4.5. Follow-up averaged 2.5 years.

Results.—Patients in the aspirin and placebo groups were comparable in age, sex distribution, preoperative rhythm, and site and type of valve. Major systemic embolism or death from vascular causes occurred in 6 aspirin-treated patients and in 24 placebo-treated patients. Twelve patients in the aspirin group and 28 in the placebo group experienced major systemic embolism or nonfatal intracranial hemorrhage or died of hemorrhage or vascular causes. Death from all causes occurred in 9 patients assigned to aspirin and in 22 patients assigned to placebo. Outcomes are annualized in the table. Bleeding was more common in the aspirin group (35% per year) than in the placebo group (22% per year). However, the difference in the rate of major hemorrhagic events was not statistically significant (8.5% for aspirin vs. 6.6% for placebo).

Conclusion.—The addition of aspirin to warfarin therapy decreased the mortality rate and the rate of major systemic embolism in patients with mechanical heart valves and in high-risk patients with prosthetic tissue valves. Even when an increase in bleeding was considered, the net beneficial effect of aspirin was substantial. Low doses of aspirin may prove valuable in other thromboembolic disorders.

▶ Results of this study strongly support the contention that for those patients with artificial cardiac valves who experience thrombotic problems when treated with warfarin therapy alone, the addition of aspirin, 100 mg/ day, may be beneficial. It is apparent from this study that not all patients with artificial cardiac valves should receive this combination because there is a higher frequency of bleeding when aspirin is added. Thus, appropriate selection of those patients experiencing trouble with warfarin alone must be carefully made before introducing the combination of warfarin plus aspirin.—W.R. Bell, M.D.

Thrombocytopenia

IMMUNE-MEDIATED THROMBOCYTOPENIA

Splenectomy Is Safe and Effective in Human Immunodeficiency Virus-Related Immune Thrombocytopenia

Oksenhendler E, Bierling P, Chevret S, Delfraissy J-F, Laurian Y, Clauvel J-P, Seligmann M (Hôpital St Louis, Paris; Hôpital Henri Mondor, Créteil, France; Hôpital Kremlin-Bicétre, France; et al)

Blood 82:29–32, 1993   116-95-3-10

Background.—Immune thrombocytopenic purpura (ITP) is a frequent early complication of HIV infection. Treatment is complicated by disappointing response rates, poor tolerance, and the risk of increased immune deficiency. Azidothymidine is the best first-line therapy, producing an increase in platelet counts in more than half of the treated patients. However, splenectomy is warranted in patients with persistent, severe, and symptomatic thrombocytopenia that does not respond to medical treatment. The influence of splenectomy on the rate of AIDS progression and of survival was evaluated.

Methods.—Sixty-eight patients who were part of a prospective cohort of 185 patients with HIV and severe ITP underwent splenectomy. Splenectomy was performed a median of 10 months after the diagnosis of ITP. A Cox's multiple regression model was used to assess the impact of splenectomy on AIDS-free survival. Splenectomy was incorporated as a time-dependent covariate.

Results.—In the patients who underwent splenectomy, the mean platelet count increased from $18 \times 10^9/L$ to $223 \times 10^9/L$, with a persistent increase in 58 patients. The mean CD4 cell count increased from $475 \times 10^6/L$ to $725 \times 10^6/L$ within a mean delay of 10 months, but the percentage of CD4 cells continued to decrease. In the whole cohort, the 5-year estimated rate for progression to AIDS was 23%, and the AIDS-free survival was 69% after a mean follow-up of 63 months. After adjustment on the CD4 cell count, there were no statistically significant differences between patients who underwent splenectomy and those who did not. Splenectomy did not influence the AIDS progression rate, survival, or AIDS-free survival.

Conclusion.—Splenectomy is a safe and effective treatment for severe, refractory ITP associated with HIV infection. However, after adjusting the CD4 count, it did not influence AIDS progression rate, survival, or AIDS-free survival at the 5-year follow-up.

▶ The results of this study suggest that splenectomy may be beneficial to patients who have severe refractory thrombocytopenia in association with AIDS. However, it seems critically important that one be somewhat selective in choosing patients for splenectomy. In the absence of the spleen, infection is much more difficult to control and eradicate. Immediately following splenectomy, abscess formation in the abdomen underneath the left diaphragm is fairly frequent even with the best of circumstances. Fatal fulminant sepsis is well known in patients who have had splenectomy. If everything else has been tried and the patient continues to be severely thrombocytopenic and is experiencing bleeding, splenectomy perhaps should be very selectively considered. See reference 1 for further reading.—W.R. Bell, M.D.

Reference

1. Alonso M, et al: *Br J Surg* 80:330, 1993.

Combination Chemotherapy in Refractory Immune Thrombocytopenic Purpura

Figueroa M, Gehlsen J, Hammond D, Ondreyco S, Piro L, Pomeroy T, Williams F, McMillan R (Scripps Research Inst, La Jolla, Calif)
N Engl J Med 328:1226–1229, 1993   116-95-3–11

Background.—Chronic idiopathic thrombocytopenic purpura is a destructive form of thrombocytopenia caused by an autoantibody. About 80% of patients remit after splenectomy or steroid therapy, but a substantial number of patients resist the usual treatments.

Patients.—Ten patients with refractory immune thrombocytopenia received combination chemotherapy. They had received an average of about 7 treatments previously, including steroids, splenectomy, vincristine, danazol, colchicine, cyclophosphamide, and azathioprine. Gammaglobulin and plasmapheresis had also been tried.

Treatment.—Three to 8 cycles of combination chemotherapy were administered. The most often used regimens consisted of cyclophosphamide and prednisone combined with vincristine and procarbazine, or with etoposide. One patient received vincristine alone in conjunction with cyclophosphamide and prednisone.

Results.—Six of the 10 patients responded completely to treatment, 4 of them for periods of 11 months to 10½ years. In 3 responders, autoantibodies were no longer demonstrated. Two patients had partial responses to treatment, and 2 had no response and died of intracerebral bleeding. Side effects were minimal. Only 2 patients were leukopenic, and there were no infections.

Conclusion.—Combination chemotherapy can benefit some patients whose chronic idiopathic thrombocytopenic purpura resists the usual treatments.

▶ The conclusions reached by the authors of this article must be very seriously questioned. This manuscript must be read very carefully because a uniform protocol was not employed in the patients studied. The authors clearly state in their Methods section that additional corticosteroids, intravenous γ-globulin, or platelet transfusions were given to patients at random during the course of this study. It is recommended that serious consideration be given before employing combination chemotherapy in the management of refractory immune thrombocytopenic purpura in view of the well-known risks of appreciable magnitude with the cytotoxic medications that constitute the therapeutic combination employed in this study.—W.R. Bell, M.D.

Dapsone for Autoimmune Thrombocytopenic Purpura
Godeau B, Oksenhendler E, Bierling P (Hôpital Henri Mondor, Créteil, France; Hôpital Saint Louis, Paris)
Am J Hematol 44:70–72, 1993   116-95-3–12

Background.—The common platelet disorder autoimmune thrombocytopenic purpura (AITP) resulting from the presence of platelet autoantibody can develop on its own or as a complication of HIV infection or other diseases. Corticosteroids yield lasting, complete remissions in only 20% of patients, and steroid-refractory AITP represents a management challenge. Experience with dapsone treatment in 27 patients with refractory AITP was assessed.

Patients.—Six patients were infected with HIV; the other 21 were free of HIV. All were treated with dapsone, 100 mg/day, orally. The median duration of disease was 13 months, and the median platelet count was $16 \times 10^9/L$. All patients but 1 had been previously treated; 4 had undergone splenectomy. A complete response was defined as a platelet count greater than $150 \times 10^9/L$.

Outcome.—Four patients had a complete response, and 9 had a partial response. The median platelet count in the 13 responders improved from 25 to $109 \times 10^9/L$. Four responders in whom dapsone was discontinued had recurrent thrombocytopenia. Twelve patients had no response, and the remaining 2 patients had to discontinue treatment within 2 weeks because of intolerance. An additional 3 patients had to cease treatment after 6–8 weeks. There were no serious hematologic side effects.

Discussion.—Dapsone appears to be a safe, effective, and economical treatment for some patients with AITP. It is less effective in patients with profound thrombocytopenia, and discontinuation leads to relapse. It is not a good alternative to splenectomy in young patients, but it may be valuable in patients with contraindications to splenectomy.

▶ Autoimmune thrombocytopenic purpura is a classic hematologic disease—not, by the way, a "transfusion medicine" disease. Therapy is very satisfactory when it works, but it doesn't always. Dapsone is clearly another effective agent but probably not a second-line therapy; steroids and splenectomy are the standards. Intravenous IgG is immediately effective and can give some very satisfactory long-term results. Dapsone takes its place with vincristine (not loaded platelets), colchicine, and other tertiary therapies.—D.J. Quesenberry, M.D.

Neonatal Alloimmune Thrombocytopenia Due to a New Platelet-Specific Alloantibody

McFarland JG, Blanchette V, Collins J, Newman PJ, Wang R, Aster RH (Med College of Wisconsin, Milwaukee; Hosp for Sick Children, Toronto)
Blood 81:3318–3323, 1993   116-95-3–13

Background.—Patients with post-transfusion purpura and neonatal alloimmune thrombocytopenia (NAT) have antibodies directed at platelet-specific alloantigens. Serologic studies to date have demonstrated a limited number of platelet alloantigen systems, mostly in cases of post-transfusion purpura and NAT. A case of NAT from maternal antibody specific for a platelet alloantigen not previously reported was presented.

Case Report.—Nonidentical twin was born at 38 weeks' gestation to white woman, 22 years of age; the father was of Filipino descent. The infant had severe NAT. An antibody directed at a new platelet-specific alloantigen, Ca (HPA-6b), was implicated. This allogen, of low frequency in the population, was localized to platelet glycoprotein (GP) IIIa. Immunoprecipitation studies with murine monoclonal antibodies specific for the GP complex IIb-IIIa and GPIIIa alone indicated that the Ca epitope on GPIIIa may be close to the binding site for AP3.

Conclusion.—Cases of NAT associated with Ca are probably as severe as cases resulting from incompatibility for the HPA-1 and HPA-4 platelet alloantigen systems. Each is located on GPIIIa, a densely represented molecule on the platelet surface. Further research is being conducted to identify the genetic basis for the Ca antigen and to study its apparent proximity to the AP3-binding site.

▶ The authors of this report have identified and very thoroughly detailed their observation of a new platelet alloantigen found in an individual with NAT. Instructive is the observation that this antibody appears to be directed at the GPIIIa site. Because this has been recognized, it will now be important to identify the frequency of this platelet-specific alloantibody.—W.R. Bell, M.D.

Chronic Idiopathic Thrombocytopenic Purpura: Splenic Pathologic Features and Their Clinical Correlation

Chang C-S, Li C-Y, Cha SS (Mayo Clinic and Mayo Found, Rochester, Minn)
Arch Pathol Lab Med 117:981–985, 1993   116-95-3–14

Background.—Splenic involvement in chronic idiopathic immune thrombocytopenic purpura (ITP) is characterized by the presence of prominent secondary follicles and foamy macrophages in the spleen. However, few reports have correlated splenic morphology and clinical outcome. A consistent morphologic feature of the spleen in ITP that is predictive of clinical response to splenectomy was sought.

Methods.—Splenectomy was performed in 83 patients with ITP refractory to steroid therapy. Splenic samples were sectioned and stained. The serum platelet count was measured 1 month after surgery to determine the response to splenectomy.

Results.—The splenic weight did not correlate with the presplenectomy platelet count, degree of foamy macrophages, or time from diagnosis to splenectomy. Follicular hyperplasia was found in 23 patients; foamy macrophages in 56; and extramedullary hematopoiesis that was primarily megakaryocytic in 50. Twenty percent of the patients, primarily those with prominent foamy macrophages, had lipogranuloma. Eight patients with no prominent secondary follicles or foamy macrophages had lower splenic weights; the initial response after splenectomy was significantly poorer among these patients compared with the others. The 23 patients with prominent secondary follicles were younger, were more often female, and had higher antiplatelet antibody production compared with the others; all had a greater initial postoperative increase in platelets.

Conclusion.—Follicular hyperplasia or foamy macrophage proliferation, or both, accompanied by some degree of megakaryopoiesis characterized the splenic morphology of most patients with ITP refractory to steroid therapy. Follicular hyperplasia was associated with a better response to splenectomy, and the absence of follicular hyperplasia and foamy macrophages was associated with a poor response.

▶ This paper examined 83 patients with chronic ITP that was refractory to therapy who underwent splenectomy. The authors point out that there are distinct histologic differences in patients with ITP of the splenic tissue. It appears from the data accumulated in this report that those patients without prominent secondary follicles or foamy macrophages and lower splenic weights will not respond to splenectomy. Unfortunately, however, this information cannot be obtained until the spleen has been removed. One must ask whether splenic biopsy before splenectomy would be of any use.—W.R. Bell, M.D.

Infusion of Fcγ Fragments for Treatment of Children With Acute Immune Thrombocytopenic Purpura

Debré M, Bonnet M-C, Fridman W-H, Carosella E, Philippe N, Reinert P, Vilmer E, Kaplan C, Teilaud J-L, Griscelli C (Hôpital Necker-Enfants Malades, Paris; Pasteur Mérieux Sérums & Vaccins, Marcy l'Etolle, France; Hôpital

Saint Louis, Paris; et al)
Lancet 342:945–949, 1993

116-95-3-15

Background.—Blockade of the Fcγ receptor may cause the transient or persistent increase in platelet count associated with intravenous immunoglobulin in acute thrombocytopenic purpura (ITP). Intravenous immunoglobulin slowed reticuloendothelial clearance of radiolabeled RBCs coated with anti-D in patients with ITP, and anti-D increased platelet counts in patients with ITP who were D-positive. This putative mechanism was investigated in acute pediatric ITP.

Methods.—Eleven children with untreated acute ITP received 5 daily intravenous infusions of 150 mg of Fcγ fragments per kg. Platelet counts were performed daily during the first 6 days after Fcγ infusion and subsequently on days 15 and 30; platelet-associated IgG was also measured. Serum concentration of serum CD16 was studied in 5 children.

Results.—Only 1 child did not respond to treatment. In the remaining patients, platelet counts increased rapidly, exceeding $50 \times 10^9/L$ within 24 hours of the second Fcγ infusion. Five responders relapsed, with platelet counts declining below $100 \times 10^9/L$ during the first month. Among 8 patients studied for platelet-associated IgG, the platelet count increased and platelet-associated IgG levels declined. A strong inverse correlation was observed between platelet-associated IgG and platelet count. A transient or stable increase in serum CD16 correlated with the platelet count increase. Serum CD16 was not detected in the Fcγ preparation used.

Conclusion.—Infusion of Fcγ fragments is an efficient treatment for acute ITP in children. The efficacy demonstrated strengthens the hypothesis that Fcγ receptor blockade mediates intravenous immunoglobulin activity in ITP. Nevertheless, the elevated CD16 concentrations in serum may trigger additional immunoregulatory mechanisms that participate in the clinical benefit observed.

▶ The authors of this study point out how intravenous IgG might work in returning thrombocytopenic platelet counts back to normal in patients with immune-mediated thrombocytopenic purpura. Additional studies should be performed before this is widely used. Whether or not there will be toxicity associated with the infusion of these fragments remains to be established. For similar work in this area, please see reference (1).—W.R. Bell, M.D.

Reference

1. Ware RE, Howard TA: *Blood* 82:2137, 1993.

Fetal Thrombocytopenia and Its Relation to Maternal Thrombocytopenia

Burrows RF, Kelton JG (McMaster Univ, Hamilton, Ont, Canada; Canadian Red Cross Blood Transfusion Service Hamilton Centre, Ont, Canada)

N Engl J Med 329:1463–1466, 1993   116-95-3-16

Background.—Severe neonatal thrombocytopenia in an otherwise-healthy infant is rare. However, it can cause major bleeding with intracranial hemorrhage, which may lead to lifelong residual neurologic deficits. A prospective study was performed to determine the frequency of moderate to severe neonatal thrombocytopenia among otherwise-healthy infants, to assess its associated risks, and to examine a number of potential maternal risk factors.

Methods.—During a 7-year period, platelet counts were determined in umbilical cord blood samples from 15,932 neonates and in blood samples from 15,471 mothers. Moderate neonatal thrombocytopenia was defined as a platelet count of 20,000–50,000/mm³ and severe thrombocytopenia as a platelet count of less than 20,000/mm³.

Results.—Nineteen neonates (.12%) had thrombocytopenia, and 1,027 mothers (6.6%) had platelet counts of less than 150,000/mm³. Of the 19 thrombocytopenic infants, 10 were born to mothers with thrombocytopenia, and 9 were born to mothers with normal platelet counts. Eighteen women with 19 pregnancies had maternal-paternal platelet alloantigen discrepancy that placed their infants at potential risk for alloimmune neonatal thrombocytopenia. However, only 6 of 19 infants at risk had severe alloimmune thrombocytopenia. Two of these 6 infants had in utero intracranial hemorrhage, and 1 fetus was stillborn.

Conclusion.—Moderate to severe neonatal thrombocytopenia does occur in otherwise-healthy neonates, but it is rare. Platelet alloimmunization is the most common maternal risk factor for this type of fetal thrombocytopenia.

▶ The reasonably large patient population sampled in this study provides substantial data to suggest that if platelet antibodies are not detected in pregnant females, the neonate will probably not experience thrombocytopenia. Therefore, in such individuals, cesarian section should not be required. However, the number of pregnant patients who experience thrombocytopenia who are antiplatelet-antibody–negative are relatively few when the global population with this problem of thrombocytopenia in pregnancy is considered.—W.R. Bell, M.D.

DRUG-INDUCED THROMBOCYTOPENIA

Acute Thrombocytopenic Purpura in Relation to the Use of Drugs

Kaufman DW, Kelly JP, Johannes CB, Sandler A, Harmon D, Stolley PD, Shapiro S (Boston Univ; Massachusetts Gen Hosp, Boston; Univ of Maryland,

Baltimore)
Blood 82:2714–2718, 1993

116-95-3-17

Introduction.—Recognized causes of thrombocytopenic purpura (TP) include systemic conditions such as collagen diseases, primary bone marrow disorders, cancer chemotherapy, and viral infections. Drugs are thought to have a prominent role among the remaining "idiopathic" cases, often through a process of immune-mediated platelet destruction.

Objective.—In eastern Massachusetts, Rhode Island, and the Philadelphia region during 1983–1991, 62 patients aged 16 and older who had acute TP and recovered rapidly were examined. They were compared with 2,625 hospital controls who were matched for age and gender.

Findings.—On multiple logistic regression analysis, TP was significantly associated with the use of trimethoprim-sulfamethoxazole, quinidine/quinine, dipyridamole, sulfonylureas, or salicylates in the week before the onset of symptoms (table). The overall annual incidence of acute TP was estimated at 18 cases per million population. The estimated excess risk for users of trimethoprim-sulfamethoxazole was 38

Drug Use in the Week Before the Index Day Among 62 Cases of
Acute TP and 2,625 Controls

Drug	Cases	Controls	Multivariate RR Estimate (95% CI)*
Quinidine/quinine	14	13	101 (31-324)
Digoxin	9	73	1.5 (0.4-5.5)
Beta-blockers†	10	190	1.3 (0.5-3.6)
Dipyridamole	8	22	14 (3.5-54)
Furosemide	6	74	2.8 (0.8-10)
Thiazides‡	6	194	0.4 (0.1-1.7)
Sulfonamides§	6	22	40 (10-162)
Sulfonylureas‖	5	51	4.8 (1.5-16)
Salicylates¶	23	466	2.6 (1.3-5.0)
Paracetamol	10	454	0.7 (0.3-1.5)

* Relative to no use during the week before the index day.
† Includes propranolol (4 cases, 52 controls); atenolol (4, 35); metoprolol (2, 40); timolol (0, 28); nadolol (0, 21); betaxolol (0, 10); and labetolol (0, 4).
‡ Includes hydrochlorothiazide (5 cases, 170 controls); methylclothiazide (1, 10); chlorothiazide (0, 8); bendroflumethiazide (0, 2); trichloromethiazide (0, 2); hydroflumethiazide (0, 1); and metolazone (0, 1).
§ Includes trimethoprim/sulfamethoxazole (6 cases, 12 controls); sulfasalazine (0, 6); sulfadiazine (0, 2); sulfacetamide (0, 1); and sulfisoxazole (0, 1).
‖ Includes glyburide (2 cases, 21 controls); tolazamide (2, 9); glipzide (1, 5); chlorpropamide (0, 11); tolbutamide (0, 4); and acetohexamide (0, 1).
¶ Includes aspirin (23 cases, 428 controls); subsalicylate bismuth (0, 15); aspirin + subsalicylate bismuth (0, 7); diflunisal (0, 3); aspirin + salicylamide (0, 2); magnesium choline trisalicylate (0, 2); salicylic acid (0, 2); salicylamide (0, 2); magnesium salicylate (0, 1); sodium salicylate (0, 1); salsalate (0, 1); sweet birch oil (0, 1); and aspirin + magnesium choline trisalicylate (0, 1).
(Courtesy of Kaufman DW, Kelly JP, Johannes CB, et al: *Blood* 82:2714–2718, 1993.)

cases per million per week, and the risk for quinidine/quinine was 26 per million. The risk for users of quinidine specifically was 35 per million per week.

Conclusion.—The low incidence rates attributable to the implicated drugs suggest that TP is not an overriding consideration when contemplating the use of these agents. Even for trimethoprim-sulfamethoxazole, the drug most strongly implicated, the excess risk is relatively low.

▶ This rather large, comprehensive survey over a period of 16 years reminds everyone that the frequency of thrombocytopenia associated with the use of medications remains a significant problem. Of particular interest was the observation that dipyridamole, previously not commonly recognized as an agent associated with thrombocytopenia, is associated with a significant frequency of thrombocytopenia. In 1987, a comprehensive review of dipyridamole (1) revealed that no disease known to afflict humans was therapeutically benefited by its use. In view of the fact that it now has been documented to be associated with a highly undesirable side effect, namely, thrombocytopenia, use of dipyridamole should be thoughtfully reexamined by anyone who prescribes it.—W.R. Bell, M.D.

Reference

1. FitzGerald GA: N Engl J Med 316:1247, 1987.

Increased Expression of Platelet IgG Fc Receptors in Immune Heparin-Induced Thrombocytopenia
Chong BH, Pilgrim RL, Cooley MA, Chesterman CN (Univ of New South Wales, Sydney, Australia; St Vincent's Hosp, Sydney, Australia)
Blood 81:988–993, 1993   116-95-3-18

Background.—About 5% of patients receiving heparin have thrombocytopenia develop. Both a mild, early-onset form and a delayed, more severe form are recognized. The delayed-onset type is a serious immune disorder mediated by IgG heparin-dependent antibody. Previous study indicates that in heparin-induced thrombocytopenia (HIT), heparin-dependent antibodies bind to platelets via platelet IgG Fc receptors (FcRs).

Objective.—The degree of expression of FcRs on platelets was compared in 16 patients with a diagnosis of HIT, 23 patients treated with heparin who did not have thrombocytopenia, and 42 normal controls. The criteria for HIT included a platelet count of less than 140×10^9/L during heparin treatment, resolution of thrombocytopenia after withdrawal of heparin, and presence of a heparin-dependent platelet antibody.

Findings.—Platelet FcRs were substantially increased during the acute phase of HIT, and levels were especially high in patients who had serious thrombotic complications or who died soon after HIT was diagnosed. Platelet FcRs remained elevated for as long as 3 months after the acute illness. Platelets from patients with HIT exhibited increased reactivity to both low concentrations of aggregated IgG, a form of immune complex, and heparin-dependent platelet antibodies.

Conclusion.—The increased expression of platelet FcRs, rather than the premorbid level of FcRs, appears to influence the development of HIT. The increased expression of FcRs on platelets may have relevance for the thrombocytopenia and thrombosis associated with infection and other "immune complex" disorders.

▶ This very detailed study suggests that patients who experience thrombocytopenia in the presence of heparin have an increased expression of FcRs on their platelet membranes, suggesting an increase in platelet reactivity. A concomitant group of patients not receiving heparin also evidenced this phenomenon. Critically important before significant validity can be associated with these findings is that the platelets of patients with HIT need to be studied before administering heparin because their platelets still evidenced increased FcRs on platelet membranes weeks after the heparin was discontinued. This may well be an in vitro observation without in vivo biological significance.—W.R. Bell, M.D.

Can Low Molecular Weight Heparins and Heparinoids Be Safely Given to Patients With Heparin-Induced Thrombocytopenia Syndrome?

Kikta MJ, Keller MP, Humphrey PW, Silver D (Univ of Missouri, Columbia)
Surgery 114:705–710, 1993   116-95-3-19

Background.—Heparin-induced thrombocytopenia syndrome (HIT) is an immune-mediated disorder that develops in .9% to 31% of patients

Platelet Aggregation by LMWH and Heparinoids in the Presence of HAAb

Type	Percent positive reactors (no.)	Lower/upper 95% confidence intervals
LMWH		
Mono-Embolex NM	60.8 (31/51)	47.4%/74.2%
Fragmin	25.5 (13/51)	13.5%/37.5%
Heparinoid		
Org 10172	19.6 (10/51)	8.7%/30.5%

(Courtesy of Kikta MJ, Keller MP, Humphrey PW, et al: *Surgery* 114:705–710, 1993.)

receiving heparin. It occurs when heparin-induced antibodies (usually IgG) that are responsible for platelet activation and aggregation develop. Many patients who take heparin become sensitized, and heparin-associated antiplatelet antibodies (HAAbs) develop. Reanticoagulation of these patients with heparin should be avoided. Low-molecular-weight heparins (LMWHs) and heparinoids have been used to anticoagulate small groups of patients with HIT with mixed results. Some of the patients had HIT in the presence of the unfractionated heparin substitutes. Whether heparin substitute is likely to cause platelets to aggregate in patients with HAAb was investigated.

Methods.—In 51 patients with HIT, HAAb was identified by positive platelet aggregometry testing with commercial unfractionated heparin. Plasma from the patients with HAAbs was tested for the ability to aggregate platelets in the presence of 2 LMWHs, Mono-Embolex NM and Fragmin, and 1 heparinoid, Org 10172.

Results.—Fragmin and Org 10172 aggregated platelets in the presence of HAAbs significantly less often than Mono-Embolex NM. The proportion of plasma reacting to unfractionated heparin substitutes was 60.8% for Mono-Embolex NM, 25.5% for Fragmin, and 19.6% for Org 10172 (table).

Conclusion.—An HAAb that causes platelet aggregation with unfractionated heparin has a substantial likelihood of causing platelet aggregation with a heparinoid or the LMWH. Fragmin, a LMWH, and Org 10172, a heparinoid, aggregated platelets in the presence of HAAb significantly less often than the LMWH Mono-Embolex NM. In vitro testing of the patient's HAAb should be conducted before administering LMWH or heparinoid to ensure that a patient's HAAb will not cause platelet aggregation in the presence of a heparin substitute.

▶ This is a very important topical question. Can LMWH preparations be used in those patients who experience thrombocytopenia while they receive standard unfractionated heparin? In many studies, thrombocytopenia continues to be associated with LMWH preparations. The authors of this article indicate that one can do in vitro testing to see whether the LMWH preparation may be of benefit in those patients who experienced thrombocytopenia with unfractionated heparin. It seems reasonably clear that if the in vitro test indicates that it will not be of benefit, then the LMWH preparation should not be employed.—W.R. Bell, M.D.

Heparin-Induced Thrombocytopenia (HIT): An Overview of 230 Patients Treated With Orgaran (Org 10172)
Magnani HN (Organon Internatl BV, Oss, The Netherlands)
Thromb Haemost 70:554–561, 1993   116-95-3–20

Background.—Heparin-induced thrombocytopenia (HIT) with thrombosis affects 1 in 2,000 patients treated with heparin. Because the arterial or venous thromboses can be life-threatening, an alternative anticoagulation is required. The administration of Orgaran (Org 10172), a low-molecular-weight heparinoid, to patients with HIT was examined.

Methods.—The outcome in 230 patients with HIT who were treated with Orgaran was analyzed during the treatment period plus 2 days. Dosage was dependent on the clinical status of the patient. Criteria for judging the success of Orgaran included an increase of the platelet count in a patient with thrombocytopenia or lack of clinically significant change in a nonthrombocytopenic patient, control of the hemostatic process, stabilization or improvement in ischemia, and no development of cross-reactivity of Orgaran with the antibody.

Results.—Most patients responded well to Orgaran. The overall mortality was 59 of 230 patients treated. Thirty-two of these deaths occurred during Orgaran therapy or within 48 hours of treatment; the remainder occurred in the follow-up period. Mortality was highest in patients undergoing hemofiltration, particularly because of multiple-organ failure. The mortality caused by bleeding (1 patient), thrombosis (5 patients), or septic shock (1 patient) that could be attributed to Orgaran was 3%. The other deaths were attributed to the poor underlying clinical status of the patients. The mortality in patients with an acute thromboembolic event before or secondary to their HIT episode was 19.7%. Nonfatal effects of treatment included bleeding in 40 patients. This was not considered an indicator of treatment failure. A lower cross-reactivity rate (approximately 10%) was seen with the heparin-induced antibody compared with that of the low-molecular-weight heparin.

Conclusion.—The efficacy and safety of Orgaran, along with evidence of its low cross-reactivity with the heparin-induced antibody, indicate that it is a viable alternative to heparin in the treatment or prophylaxis of both arterial and venous thrombosis in patients with HIT.

▶ This report, once again, reconfirms the widespread observation that heparin is associated with thrombocytopenia. Alternatives for standard unfractionated heparin have been sought during the past decade to avoid this problem. The use of the new low-molecular-weight preparations has not eliminated this problem completely, and there is a serious question as to whether a lower frequency of this problem is associated with the low-molecular-weight preparations. In this report, the author studied a heparinoid compound that appears to be a possible alternative for someone who has thrombocytopenia develop while receiving either standard unfractionated heparin or low-molecular-weight heparin. Although the author found an extremely low cross-reactivity rate, thrombocytopenia is, to a very, very low extent, associated with this heparinoid compound. Although it is not completely safe, it may be one of the more viable alternatives at this time.—W.R. Bell, M.D.

Hirudin Therapy for Heparin-Associated Thrombocytopenia and Deep Venous Thrombosis

Nand S (Loyola Univ, Chicago)
Am J Hematol 43:310–311, 1993   116-95-3–21

Background.—The development of thrombocytopenia in association with heparin therapy, which occurs in 5% to 15% of patients, poses a treatment dilemma. Continuing heparin may cause a worsening of platelet counts. In a small number of patients, it may result in the potentially fatal complication of thrombocytopenia with thrombosis. The use of recombinant hirudin in a patient with heparin-associated thrombocytopenia and thrombosis was reported.

Case Report.—Woman, 53, was transferred to a university medical center for deep venous thrombosis (DVT) and thrombocytopenia. Heparin had been started 13 days earlier in a local hospital for DVT of the right leg. On day 7, Coumadin (sodium warfarin) treatment was begun for a mass in the liver. On the third day of Coumadin treatment, heparin was stopped, and the patient experienced extensive DVT of the left lower extremity. Her platelet count was declining. Heparin was begun again before the transfer. On physical examination, she had marked swelling and warmth in both legs to the inguinal region. Her WBC count was 11,400/mm^3; hemoglobin, 7.4 g/dL; and platelet count, 77,000/mm^3. The heparin-associated platelet aggregation test was strongly positive, and venous Doppler assessment revealed acute thrombosis bilaterally to the iliac veins. Heparin was stopped, and dextran 40 was begun in a continuous infusion of 1,000 mL/24 hours. The patient's leg swelling and warmth worsened during the next day. Recombinant hirudin was obtained from Biogen Corporation on compassionate grounds and started at .25 mg/kg/hr in a continuous infusion. This dose was decreased to .2 mg/kg/hr mg the next day and continued for 5 days. Coumadin and aspirin treatment was also initiated after 3 days of hirudin treatment. Factor VII assays were used to monitor Coumadin treatment, because hirudin prolongs prothrombin time. The condition of the patient's legs improved significantly with hirudin. She was able to ambulate in 1 week. Chemotherapy was begun for the hepatoma, which was deemed inoperable by the consulting oncologist. The patient was discharged home on day 23. Hirudin treatment produced no adverse effects.

Conclusion.—The use of hirudin was successful in this patient with heparin-associated thrombocytopenia. The use of recombinant hirudin should be investigated further in such cases.

▶ When anticoagulation is needed, this single-patient report suggests that hirudin may be another alternative that can be employed so that heparin can be promptly discontinued if the platelet count is declining because of the presence of heparin.—W.R. Bell, M.D.

Complications From Heparin-Induced Thrombocytopenia in Patients Undergoing Cardiopulmonary Bypass

Singer RL, Mannion JD, Bauer TL, Armenti FR, Edie RN (Jefferson Med College, Philadelphia)

Chest 104:1436–1440, 1993   116-95-3-22

Introduction.—Heparin-induced thrombocytopenia (HIT) develops when specific heparin-dependent antibodies attach to platelet membranes, leading to platelet activation, aggregation, and degranulation. The occurrence of HIT-related complications was reviewed in 1,500 consecutive patients who had cardiopulmonary bypass between August of 1987 and December of 1991. The great majority of the procedures were coronary artery bypass graft operations or valve replacements or repairs.

Methods.—Cardiopulmonary bypass was done with a clear prime and moderate systemic hypothermia. Patients received bovine lung heparin during bypass, but all previous and postoperative exposure was with porcine mucosal heparin.

Findings.—Heparin-induced thrombocytopenia was diagnosed in 11 patients (.75%), all of whom had previously been exposed to heparin. The mean interval from initial exposure to bypass was 4.5 days. Six of the 11 patients were receiving aspirin just before surgery. The patients had a total of 17 complications, including 6 that required amputation of an extremity, 4 strokes, and 2 instances of pulmonary embolism. Complications occurred a mean of 3.6 days after surgery, when the mean nadir platelet count was 123,000/mm³. Although 9 of the 11 patients had a count of greater than 100,000/mm³, the mean reduction in platelets from the time of first exposure to heparin was 50%. The mean nadir platelet count in 100 consecutive patients with no evidence of HIT was 207,000/mm³, and their mean reduction was 26%.

Discussion.—Heparin-induced thrombocytopenia developed after cardiopulmonary bypass in fewer than 1% of these patients. It could not be related to the duration or amount of heparin treatment, the type of heparin administered, or pretreatment with aspirin. Recombinant hirudin may provide an alternative to heparin for use during cardiopulmonary bypass.

▶ The results of this study should be evaluated by those who think that there is absolutely no association between heparin and the problem of thrombocytopenia. This study also points out the serious nature of this problem. One can also glean from these data that if a patient who has a problem with heparin-associated thrombocytopenia needs cardiopulmonary bypass surgery, this can be accomplished safely because of the relatively short period of time required to carry out such surgery. It is then apparent that as soon as possible after surgery is completed, the patient should be placed on warfarin anticoagulation and that heparin should be discontinued as quickly as possible when the prothrombin time approaches the therapeutic range.—W.R. Bell, M.D.

Thrombotic Thrombocytopenic Purpura

Early Manifestation of Thrombotic Thrombocytopenic Purpura
Lau DH, Wun T (California Davis Cancer Ctr, Sacramento)
Am J Med 95:544–545, 1993   116-95-3–23

Background.—Early diagnosis and prompt plasma exchange greatly decrease mortality caused by thrombotic thrombocytopenic purpura (TTP). A patient may be seen with some or all of the classic signs of fulminant TTP. Two cases in which thrombocytopenia was the earliest laboratory finding preceding full-blown TTP were examined.

Case 1.—Woman, 55, was hospitalized with fever, severe mucositis, and pancytopenia 2 weeks after a third cycle of chemotherapy for inflammatory carcinoma of the breast. After 10 days of antibiotic treatment, the fever and mucositis resolved, and the platelet count and hemoglobin returned to normal levels (Fig 3–4). On day 11, 10 hours after receiving colchicine for acute podagra, her platelet count was 20×10^9/L, and her lactate dehydrogenase (LDH) level was 3.8 μkat/L, but microangiopathic RBC changes were not apparent. On day 14, the hemoglobin level declined sharply and schistocytes appeared on the peripheral smear; serum LDH, total bilirubin, and serum creatinine levels increased suddenly. Thrombotic thrombocytopenic purpura was diagnosed and plasmapheresis was initiated; complete recovery occurred within a month, after 13 sessions of plasmapheresis.

Case 2.—Man, 24, was hospitalized after 7 days of fever, rash, headache, sore throat, and diffuse lymphadenopathy. The admission platelet count was 76×10^9/L; hemoglobin level, 9 mmol/L; serum LDH level, 7.4 μkat/L; total bilirubin level, 22 μmol/L; serum creatinine level, 168 μmol/L; RBC morphology, normal. After 4 days, the platelet count and hemoglobin level declined, and microangiopathic RBCs appeared. The serum LDH was 18.9 μkat/L and the total bilirubin level was 58 μmol/L. Thrombotic thrombocytopenic purpura was diagnosed. Plasmapheresis produced prompt resolution of fever, thrombocytopenia, microangiopathic hemolytic anemia, and renal insufficiency.

Conclusion.—Thrombocytopenia is an early laboratory finding of TTP, preceding microangiopathic RBC changes and serum LDH elevations by 3–4 days. The differential diagnosis of patients seen with an idiopathic isolated low-platelet count should include early TTP.

▶ The authors have demonstrated in 2 patients that in the disease entity of TTP–hemolytic uremic syndrome (HUS), thrombocytopenia appears to present before evidence of microangiopathic RBC changes. This observation needs to be examined by others, particularly by those who have patients with relapsing TTP-HUS. This observation may provide a clue to the etiology of this extremely serious disease entity.—W.R. Bell, M.D.

Patient 1

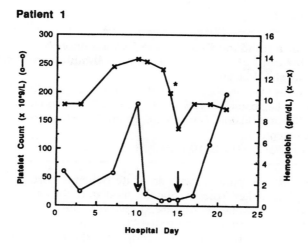

Patient 2

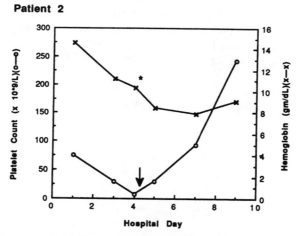

Fig 3–4.—Time courses of platelet count and hemoglobin level during the hospital courses of patient 1 and patient 2. *Open-head arrow* of patient 1 indicates time of colchicine injection. *Blackhead arrows* of patient 1 and patient 2 indicate time of initiation of plasmapheresis. *Time at which microangiopathic changes of RBCs were first observed. (Courtesy of Lau DH, Wun T: *Am J Med* 95:544–545, 1993.)

Coagulation Factors

Evidence for a Rebound Coagulation Phenomenon After Cessation of a 4-Hour Infusion of a Specific Thrombin Inhibitor in Patients With Unstable Angina Pectoris

Gold HK, Torres FW, Garabedian HD, Werner W, Jang I-K, Khan A, Hagstrom JN, Yasuda T, Leinbach RC, Newell JB, Bovill EG, Stump DC, Collen D (Harvard Med School, Boston; Genentech, South San Francisco, Calif; Univ of Vermont, Burlington)
J Am Coll Cardiol 21:1039–1047, 1993   116-95-3–24

Background.—In patients with an acute ischemic coronary syndrome, thrombin plays a key role in platelet-mediated thrombosis associated with atheromatous plaque rupture. However, the efficacy of conventional heparin treatment to prevent ischemic events is limited. Specific thrombin inhibitors have proved superior in experimental models of arterial thrombosis. A phase I clinical trial was initiated to examine the antithrombotic and clinical effects of argatroban, a synthetic competitive thrombin inhibitor, in patients with unstable angina pectoris.

Methods.—Forty-three patients were enrolled. An intravenous infusion of argatroban, .5–5 μg/kg/min, was administered for 4 hours. Monitor-

	Total Group (n = 43)	Patients Without Angina Within 24 Hours (n = 34)	Patients With Angina Within 24 Hours (n = 9)	p Value
Laboratory Variables of the Study Patients				
aPTT(s)				
Baseline	27 ± 2.7	27 ± 2.9	27 ± 1.6	NS
4 h	55 ± 14	52 ± 12	66 ± 15	0.006
6 h	34 ± 1.9	33 ± 5.9	40 ± 12	0.02
In([Arg])*	6.2 ± 0.86	6.1 ± 0.89	6.8 ± 0.40	0.001
In([TAT] + 1)				
Baseline	1.6 ± 0.88	1.60 ± 0.89	1.86 ± 0.83	NS
4 h	1.5 ± 0.90	1.84 ± 0.95	1.41 ± 0.70	NS
6 h	2.39 ± 1.21	2.35 ± 1.17	2.42 ± 1.43	NS
In([FpA] + 1)				
Baseline	3.0 ± 0.60	2.96 ± 0.60	3.15 ± 0.66	NS
4 h	2.34 ± 0.80	2.17 ± 0.74	2.51 ± 1.02	NS
6 h	2.87 ± 1.11	2.97 ± 1.07	2.40 ± 1.30	NS

Abbreviations: aPTT, activated partial thromboplastin time; *FpA,* fibrinopeptide A; *TAT,* thrombin-antithrombin III complex.
* Steady-state plasma argatroban (Arg) levels expressed as In([Arg]) in ng/mL.
(Courtesy of Gold HK, Torres FW, Garabedian HD, et al: *J Am Coll Cardiol* 21:1039–1047, 1993.)

ing consisted of sequential measures of coagulation times, indexes of thrombin activity in vivo, and clinical observation for 24 hours.

Findings.—Significant dose-related increases in plasma drug levels and activated partial thromboplastin times were noted. There was no bleeding time prolongation or spontaneous bleeding. Myocardial ischemia did not occur during treatment. However, 9 patients had an episode of unstable angina a mean 5.8 hours after infusion, which was significantly correlated with a larger argatroban dose and greater prolongation of activated partial thromboplastin time but not with other demographic, clinical, laboratory, or angiographic features (table). Pretreatment plasma levels of thrombin-antithrombin III complex and fibrinopeptide A were increased to 2–3 times normal levels. Thrombin-antithrombin III complex levels were not changed during infusion. However, there was a significant, 2.3-fold decrease in fibrinopeptide A levels. Two hours after infusion, thrombin-antithrombin III complex concentrations increased 3.9-fold above baseline measures, and fibrinopeptide A levels returned to pretreatment values.

Conclusion.—Argatroban inhibits clotting and thrombin activity toward fibrinogen in patients with unstable angina but does not suppress in vivo thrombin formation. Cessation of argatroban infusion is associated with rebound thrombin generation and an early dose-related recurrence of unstable angina.

▶ This study is based on the premise that thrombin is a major contributor to platelet-mediated thrombosis. When the synthetic competitive thrombin inhibitor argatroban was infused, somewhat interestingly, the fibrinopeptide A concentration was reduced but the thrombin-antithrombin III complex levels were not altered. The reduction in the fibrinopeptide A concentration was attributed to the inhibition of thrombin. However, there are other sources of fibrinopeptide A. It is possible that the plasmin generation was also decreased when argatroban was infused. It is also possible that plasminogen production may have been disturbed by this agent. Thus, it has not been definitively identified that the alterations seen were due to the inhibition of thrombin. In addition, when argatroban was discontinued even after only a 4-hour infusion, a rather impressive rebound phenomenon occurred, suggesting that any inhibition by thrombin was very temporary and, apparently, that the production of thrombin was not inhibited.—W.R. Bell, M.D.

Plasma Factor V Activation Is Prevented by Activated Protein C in the Presence of Phospholipid Vesicles, Not Platelets
Solymoss S, Nguyen KTP (McGill Univ, Montreal)
Thromb Haemost 69:124–129, 1993   116-95-3-25

Background.—Protein C is a naturally occurring anticoagulant that catalyzes the inactivation of factor Va and VIIIa, thus playing a significant regulatory role in hemostasis. It is unclear whether the effect of platelets is to enhance or inhibit activated protein C (APC). The effect of APC on factor V activation and Va inactivation in dilute recalcified plasma, phospholipid, and platelets was examined.

Methods.—Serial thrombin and factor V 1- and 2-stage assays were performed along with Western blotting of dilute recalcified plasma containing APC and either phospholipid vesicles or platelets.

Results.—Significantly greater amounts of thrombin were formed at a given APC concentration with platelets than with phospholipid. One-stage factor V levels increased more with platelets and APC than with phospholipid and APC. A substantial decrease in 2-stage factor V values was seen with platelets and 5 nM APC, in contrast to no change seen with phospholipid and 5 nM APC. Western blotting of plasma factor V confirmed factor V activation with platelets and APC but indicated no factor V activation with phospholipid and APC. The introduction of platelets or platelet membrane into phospholipid enhanced rather than inhibited APC catalyzed plasma factor V inactivation. Platelet activation further enhanced factor V activation and inactivation at any given APC concentration.

Conclusion.—These results are consistent with the fact that platelets are more supportive of plasma procoagulant events than phospholipid vesicles are when APC is present. However, this effect is not influenced by a platelet-associated inhibition of APC.

▶ This detailed study suggests that platelet surfaces and platelet membranes may not be the sources of attachment of inert protein C and protein S for their activation. Data support the concept that free phospholipid may be the essential component required for the activation of protein C and protein S complexes in the degradation of activated factor V.—W.R. Bell, M.D.

Dietary Induced Subclinical Vitamin K Deficiency in Normal Human Subjects
Ferland G, Sadowski JA, O'Brien ME (Tufts Univ, Boston)
J Clin Invest 91:1761–1768, 1993   116-95-3–26

Background.—The little research correlating vitamin K_1 intake with vitamin K status has limited usefulness for normal, healthy persons. A subclinical vitamin K deficiency was induced in healthy volunteers 20–40 years and 60–80 years of age.

Methods.—The 32 volunteers initially received a diet containing the recommended daily allowance for vitamin K, equivalent to 80 μg of vitamin K_1. This was followed by a 13-day vitamin K_1 depletion period. After this period, the volunteers entered a 16-day repletion period, consisting of 4 stages of 4 days in which they received 5, 15, 25, and 45 μg of vitamin K_1 per day.

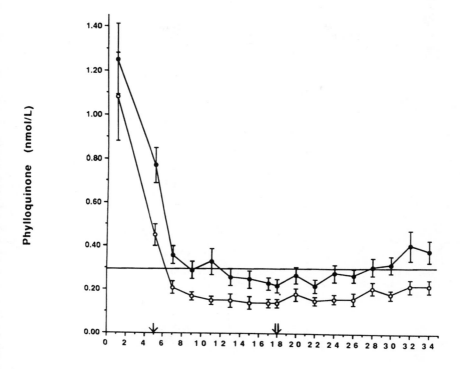

STUDY DAY

Fig 3–5.—Fasting plasma vitamin K_1 concentrations (nmol/L) in young (*open circles*) and elderly (*black circles*) individuals after varying dietary vitamin K_1 intakes. Values are mean ± standard error of the mean, $n = 32$; *arrows* indicate beginning of depletion and repletion periods. During the course of the study, vitamin K_1 levels were significantly affected by vitamin K_1 intake ($P < .0001$) and age ($P < .01$). (Courtesy of Ferland G, Sadowski JA, O'Brien ME: *J Clin Invest* 91:1761–1768, 1993.)

Findings.—Vitamin K_1 depletion significantly decreased plasma vitamin K_1 levels to values 13% to 18% of those on day 1 in both younger and older participants. In the younger volunteers, repletion failed to normalize vitamin K_1 levels. Vitamin K_1 restriction induced different responses in the urinary excretion of γ-carboxyglutamic acid, with values declining significantly in the younger group and remaining unchanged in the older group. Depletion did not significantly affect either prothrombin and activated partial thromboplastin times or factor VII and protein C. Descarboxy prothrombin increased slightly but significantly in younger and older participants during the depletion period (Fig 3–5; table).

Conclusion.—A diet low in vitamin K_1 can produce a functional subclinical vitamin K deficiency without influencing blood coagulation. Fur-

Effect of Dietary Vitamin K_1 Restriction and Repletion on Factor VII and Protein C Antigen Level and Functional Activity

Parameter	Day 1	Day 5	Day 18	Day 34	Normal range
			%		
Factor VII antigen level	88±3	87±3	87±3	89±3	70–130
Factor VII functional activity	105±5	103±4	103±5	104±5	70–130
Protein C antigen level	80±1	78±1	79±1	80±1	70–140
Protein C functional activity	103±4	101±4	105±4	104±3	70–140

Note: Values are expressed as percentage of normal with 100% corresponding to values observed in normal pooled plasma (factor VII, .011 µM; protein C, .048 µM). Mean ± standard error of the mean, n = 32. None of the 4 parameters was significantly affected by dietary vitamin K intake. (Courtesy of Ferland G, Sadowski JA, O'Brien ME: *J Clin Invest* 91:1761–1768, 1993.)

ther research is needed to determine whether pathologic consequences are associated with vitamin K deficiency.

▶ The authors, in a very detailed and careful study, have indicated that less than 2 weeks are required to induce vitamin K deficiency in someone with a nutritionally inadequate diet. Even though coagulation factors were not disturbed at this time, one can realistically expect that if such a deficiency state were continued, a deficiency of coagulation factor function would result. An important feature of this study is the time, which seems relatively short, required to actually induce in humans a deficiency of this substance, which is critically important to normal function of the coagulation system.—W.R. Bell, M.D.

The Activation of Factor X and Prothrombin by Recombinant Factor VIIa In Vivo Is Mediated by Tissue Factor

ten Cate H, Bauer KA, Levi M, Edgington TS, Sublett RD, Barzegar S, Kass BL, Rosenberg RD (Slotervaart Hosp, Amsterdam; Academic Med Ctr, Amsterdam; Beth Israel Hosp, Boston; et al)

J Clin Invest 92:1207–1212, 1993   116-95-3-27

Purpose.—In normal human coagulation, very small amounts of factor Xa and thrombin are produced continuously. There is evidence that basal activation of hemostasis occurs through factor VIIa–dependent activation of factor X. However, there is no direct proof that tissue factor plays a role in this pathway. Chimpanzees were used to address this issue.

Methods and Findings.—High concentrations of recombinant factor VIIa—about 50 µg/kg—were infused into normal chimpanzees. In response, the animals had significant increases in plasma levels of factor IX activation peptide, factor X activation peptide, and prothrombin activation fragment F_{1+2}. According to metabolic turnover studies using radiolabeling, the elevated levels of these activation peptides appeared to result from accelerated conversion of the 3 coagulation system zymogens into serine proteases. Factor X activation and prothrombin mediated by the infused recombinant protein were negated by administration of a monoclonal antibody to tissue factor, which neutralizes function of the factor VIIa–tissue factor complex in vitro. This antibody also suppressed basal activation of factors IX and X.

Conclusion.—Recombinant factor VIIa seems to work as a prohemostatic agent through interaction with endogenous tissue factor sites. Basal activity of the coagulation system appears to depend at least in part on the amount of surface tissue factor in contact with blood components. Previously reported age-dependent elevations in activation peptide markers could result in part from increased biosynthesis of tissue factor in vivo.

▶ In the past 3 to 4 years, factor VIIa has been employed in individuals with circulating anticoagulants to stop hemorrhage. In some, this has been a successful therapeutic modality. It appears from these excellent studies that the prohemostatic effect of this treatment is mediated by way of tissue factor (FIII). This important observation may provide an explanation as to why the activated factor VII material may not work in some individuals. If the recipient has a deficiency in FIII or has an abnormal FIII molecule, the activated factor VII will not mediate hemostasis.—W.R. Bell, M.D.

Coagulation Abnormalities Associated With the Use of Anabolic Steroids
Ansell JE, Tiarks C, Fairchild VK (Univ of Massachusetts, Worcester)
Am Heart J 125:367–371, 1993   116-95-3-28

Introduction.—Competitive athletes continue to abuse anabolic steroids even though studies indicate that they have an increased chance of thromboembolism. The effects of anabolic steroids on the coagulation and fibrinolytic systems of 16 male bodybuilders were assessed to determine whether these drugs produce a hypercoagulable state in this group.

Methods.—Sixteen male bodybuilders who had used or planned to use anabolic steroids participated. None of the participants had a history of a blood clot. Blood values, clotting times, and fibrinolytic systems were monitored during the administration of various anabolic steroids.

Results.—Of the 16 participants aged 20–42 years, 6 provided blood samples during and either before or after receiving anabolic steroids; 10 gave only 1 sample (5 while receiving steroids and 5 while not taking the drugs). The 6 participants with paired samples with and without steroid use demonstrated a significant increase in protein C antigen and free protein S antigen during the period of steroid use. Those participants had a significantly shortened euglobulin lysis time when receiving steroids. Steroids also appeared to increase the platelet count significantly. No liver function abnormalities occurred, whereas total cholesterol levels had a small but significant decrease during steroid use.

Conclusion.—Preliminary studies in bodybuilders indicate that several anabolic steroids do not change the coagulation mechanism nor do these agents promote a hypercoagulable state. More sensitive assays may be required to detect any possible subtle changes in coagulation.

▶ It is frequently asked whether anabolic steroids are associated with hypercoagulability and thrombus formation. The studies carried out by these authors would suggest that there is not a relationship. However, it still remains prudent not to employ these agents in any situation where there is a known risk for thrombus formation.—W.R. Bell, M.D.

Congenital Coagulation Factor Deficiency

Pseudo-von Willebrand Disease: A Mutation in the Platelet Glycoprotein Ibα Gene Associated With a Hyperactive Surface Receptor
Russell SD, Roth GJ (Univ of Washington, Seattle)
Blood 81:1787–1791, 1993   116-95-3-29

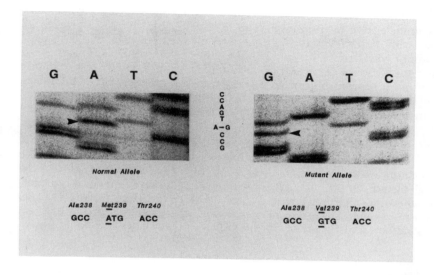

Fig 3–6.—Candidate mutation associated with the pseudo-vWF phenotype in the R family. The sequences of the normal (**left**) and candidate mutant (**right**) alleles differ at the first base of codon 239 of the platelet GP-Ibα gene. The A to G transition (*arrow*) results in the substitution of valine (239-mutant) for methionine (normal) within the region of the GP-Ibα polypeptide that binds to vWF. (Courtesy of Russell SD, Roth GJ: *Blood* 81:1787–1791, 1993.)

Background.—Pseudo–von Willebrand's disease (pseudo-vWD) is an autosomal dominant bleeding disorder brought about by the hyperfunction of a receptor at the platelet surface. Glycoprotein (GP)-Ib is the abnormal receptor, which displays increased affinity for its ligand, vWF. The molecular genetic defect in the pseudo-vWD family was investigated, focusing primarily on the genomic sequence that encodes the vWF-binding region of GP-Ibα.

Method.—Four members of a family afflicted with pseudo-vWD were examined. The mother was normal, but the father and 2 daughters were affected. The affected members experience intermittent thrombocytopenia, enhanced ristocetin-induced platelet aggregation, and a deficiency of high-molecular-weight forms of plasma factor VIII/vWF multimers. Blood samples from the family members were provided, and segments of the platelet GP-Ibα gene were amplified by PCR, cloned, and sequenced.

Results.—A point mutation (A to G, codon methionine to valine) was found in the genomes of the affected family members (Fig 3–6). The mutation results in a single amino acid substitution (valine-mutant for methionine-normal) at residue 239 within the Ibα binding site for vWF. Both the mutant and the normal sequence were found in affected patients, suggesting a heterozygous state. Amplified DNA provided by family members and 58 normal controls was then analyzed by allele-specific oligonucleotide hybridization. The mutant oligonucleotide only hybridized with the DNA of the 3 affected family members (the heterozygotes) and not with that of the unaffected mother or the controls. This suggests that the G for A transition in codon 239 in the R family is a mutation and not a polymorphism. As it is only seen in affected family members, the described mutation is associated with the pseudo-vWD disease phenotype seen in this kindred.

Conclusion.—A novel "hyperfunction" mutation in platelet glycoprotein Ibα that appears to alter the conformation of the vWF-binding site and leads to excessive vWF binding was identified. Single amino acid substitutions within a critical region of either the GP-Ibα receptor or the vWF ligand can produce a significant change in the affinity of 1 molecule for the other. Further research must be done to define the precise relationship between the effects of the mutations and the effects of flow, vasculature, and ristocetin on the individual molecules in vivo and in vitro.

▶ The data presented in this report clearly identify a defect in the GP-Ib receptor on the platelet membrane. Details of this abnormal receptor (which has been recognized for a number of years) have been identified, and the responsible gene mutation has been established. When the etiology of this mutation is identified, hopefully this abnormality can be corrected.—W.R. Bell, M.D.

Recombinant Factor VIII for the Treatment of Previously Untreated Patients With Hemophilia A: Safety, Efficacy, and Development of Inhibitors
Lusher JM, Arkin S, Abildgaard CF, Schwartz RS, and the Kogenate Previously Untreated Patient Study Group (Children's Hosp of Michigan, Detroit; Mount Sinai Med School, New York; Univ of California, Davis; et al)
N Engl J Med 328:453–459, 1993   116-95-3–30

Introduction.—Certain blood-borne viruses can still be transmitted by plasma-derived clotting-factor concentrates despite advances in methods of viral attenuation. These concentrates have been implicated in the transmission of human parvovirus, hepatitis C virus, and HIV. Use of the virus-free recombinant DNA–derived factor VIII would protect patients with hemophilia A from such viruses. A multicenter trial of treatment with recombinant factor VIII was conducted.

Methods.—Patients were 95 infants and children who had not previously been treated with clotting-factor concentrates. The degree of hemophilia A was severe or moderately severe in 59 patients (median age at first treatment, 9.1 months). Eighteen patients (median age, 14.7 months at first treatment) had moderate disease. The 18 patients with mild hemophilia were first treated at a median age of 47 months. After

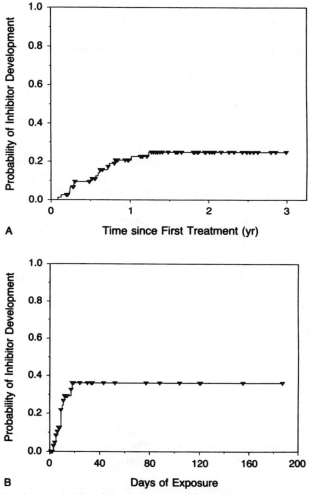

Fig 3–7.—Cumulative probability of the development of factor VIII inhibitor in 77 previously untreated patients with severe or moderate hemophilia from the time of initial treatment with recombinant factor VIII (**A**) and according to the number of days of exposure to treatment with factor VIII (**B**). Each *triangle* denotes a patient without inhibitor formation. Hemophilia was defined as severe or moderate if the plasma factor VIII level was 5% or less. (Courtesy of Lusher JM, Arkin S, Abildgaard CF, et al: N Engl J Med 328:453–459, 1993.)

the start of treatment with recombinant factor VIII, patients were evaluated at least every 3 months.

Results.—To date, the patients have received the concentrate exclusively for a median of 1.5 years; all have responded well. There were only 3 minor adverse reactions reported from a total of 3,315 infusions. Follow-up evaluations showed no elevations in alanine aminotransferase concentrations and no antibody to hamster or murine protein. None of the patients had evidence of any unusual infection or illness. Of 81 patients tested for inhibitor antibodies to factor VIII, 16 had them at a median of 9 days after the start of treatment. The cumulative risk for inhibitor formation is shown in Figure 3-7. Despite continued episodic treatment with the concentrate, inhibitor titers were or became low in 9 patients. Inhibitors disappeared completely in 4 patients receiving episodic treatment and remained at a low level in 5.

Conclusion.—The infants and children who started their treatment for hemophilia A with recombinant factor VIII had generally excellent clinical responses. There was a relatively high prevalence of inhibitors with low titers in the group, but the benefits of recombinant factor VIII appear to outweigh its risks. Transient or low levels of inhibitor might represent part of the natural history of hemophilia in infants.

▶ This excellent study indicates very clearly that recombinant factor VIII is efficacious in the treatment of hemorrhage secondary to hemophilia A. Disturbing, however, is the fact that in 20% of patients treated with this preparation circulating anticoagulants developed. This is unquestionably higher in frequency than with nonrecombinant preparations. In additional studies of patients treated with recombinant factor VIII, circulating anticoagulants approached almost 50% (1). Thus, the newer preparations of factor VIII employed in the treatment of hemophilia A have some serious, undesirable side effects.—W.R. Bell, M.D.

Reference

1. Ehrenforth S, et al: *Lancet* 339:594, 1992.

Homocysteine Inhibits von Willebrand Factor Processing and Secretion by Preventing Transport From the Endoplasmic Reticulum
Lentz SR, Sadler JE (Washington Univ, St Louis, Mo)
Blood 81:683–689, 1993   116-95-3–31

Background.—Homocysteine, a thiol-containing amino acid that is associated with both thrombosis and atherosclerotic disease, selectively inhibits intracellular protein transport in endothelial cells. Hemocysteine has also been shown to decrease the expression of thrombomodulin, a transmembrane glycoprotein, on the cell surface while not affecting the secretion of another endothelial cell protein, plasminogen activator inhibitor-1. The effects of homocysteine on protein transport were further explored by examining its influence on the processing and secretion of vWF, a multimeric glycoprotein, in human umbilical vein endothelial cells.

Findings.—Incubating endothelial cells with 2 mmol of homocysteine per liter resulted in the total loss of vWF multimers and prevented the maturation and secretion of asparagine-linked oligosaccharide. Dimerization was only partially prevented. Pulse-chase incubation studies showed that intracellular protein vWF was degraded before leaving the endoplasmic reticulum of homocysteine-treated cells. Homocysteine inhibited the processing and secretion of a carboxyl-terminal truncation mutant of human protein vWF that is expressed in rat insulinoma cells.

Interpretation.—The intracellular transport of many endothelial cell proteins may be altered in patients with homocystinuria. Selective inhibition of the intracellular transport of vWF and thrombomodulin might predispose to thrombosis by upsetting the balance between procoagulant and anticoagulant proteins. The retention of secretory proteins in the endoplasmic reticulum appears to be regulated by redox mechanisms. Protein transport may also be altered in other processes that affect that intracellular redox potential.

▶ This report, in a very detailed manner, demonstrates that homocysteine actually inhibits the processing of von Willebrand's protein. This may explain why individuals with homocystinuria experience considerable endothelial damage and subsequent thrombus formation. The authors also point out that a number of other intracellularly produced proteins may be altered by the presence of homocysteine. In fact, some of these other proteins may be important for the process of atherogenesis and thrombus formation. Noteworthy is the fact that pigs who are severely deficient in the von Willebrand's protein do not experience atherogenesis, atherosclerosis, or thrombosis.—W.R. Bell, M.D.

Age-Dependent Effect on the Level of Factor IX

Sweeney JD, Hoernig LA (Hemophilia Ctr of Western New York, Buffalo)
Am J Clin Pathol 99:687–688, 1993   116-95-3–32

Background.—Blood coagulation factor levels are influenced by variables such as age, sex, ABO group, and physiologic states such as exercise and pregnancy. Some research has indicated that functional levels of factor IX (IX:C) are lower in children than adults. Other research has found an age-related increase using antigenic measures (IX:Ag). However, there have been no comparisons in a sample with a wide age range using measures of both factor IX:C and IX:Ag. Because IX:C is used as an indicator of hemophilia B, such information is important.

Methods and Findings.—Levels of factor IX:C and IX:Ag were determined in 120 healthy persons, aged 1–67 years. Factor IX:C levels were lowest in prepubertal children, reached a plateau in early adulthood, and had a secondary increase in later adulthood in persons older than 45 years of age. Factor IX:Ag levels demonstrated a similar trend. However, these levels increased disproportionately in early adulthood with a less marked increase in later life, producing a ratio peak in early adulthood.

Conclusion.—Clinicians should use caution in interpreting low-normal factor IX:C levels in prepubertal children. When interpreting the ratio of antigenic to coagulant activity, clinicians may need to consider the patient's age.

▶ The authors of this report have studied a sizable number of apparently healthy normal individuals to identify the influence of age on factor IX. Data generated clearly support the contention that the ratios of antigenic to coagulant activity must be interpreted with respect to the age of the subject from whom the specimen was taken.—W.R. Bell, M.D.

Pharmacokinetics of Monoclonally-Purified and Recombinant Factor VIII in Patients With Severe von Willebrand Disease

Morfini M, Mannucci PM, Tenconi PM, Longo G, Mazzucconi MG, Rodeghiero F, Ciavarella N, De Rosa V, Arter A (Univ of Florence, Italy; Univ of Milan, Italy; Univ of Rome; et al)
Thromb Haemost 70:270–272, 1993   116-95-3–33

Objective.—In plasma, factor VIII and vWF form a noncovalent molecular complex, stabilizing the factor VIII protein by protecting it against intracellular and plasma proteolysis. Recent years have seen the production of purer plasma factor VIII concentrates with little vWF. There are no data on the half-life of monoclonally purified factor VIII in patients with von Willebrand's disease who lack vWF. Whether the small amounts of vWF in monoclonally purified factor VIII can support a normal half-life of factor VIII in 11 patients with severe-type III von Willebrand's disease was determined.

Methods.—The 11 patients all had unmeasurable plasma levels of vWF and low plasma levels of factor VIII. Pharmacokinetic analysis was done after infusion of monoclonally purified factor VIII concentrate, 25 IU/kg. The comparison groups were 10 patients with severe hemophilia A previously infused with the same concentrate and 2 patients with severe von Willebrand's disease who were infused with recombinant factor VIII, which contains no vWF.

Results.—Compared with the patients with hemophilia, the patients with von Willebrand's disease had a significantly shorter half-life and faster plasma clearance of factor VIII. However, there were no significant differences in the in vivo recovery or volume of distribution. The 2 patients who received recombinant factor VIII had a very short half-life and low in vivo recovery, with a larger volume of distribution than monoclonally purified vWF.

Conclusion.—For patients with severe von Willebrand's disease, the small amounts of vWF in monoclonally purified factor VIII concentrate are not enough to stabilize the factor VIII infused. Neither is this amount of vWF sufficient to support the normal circulation of endogenous factor VIII that these patients produce normally. Thus, even when the goal of treatment is correction of the factor VIII defect only, monoclonally purified and recombinant factor VIII products should not be used in the treatment of patients with severe von Willebrand's disease.

▶ This study points out the important observation that purified factor VIII:C concentrates that contain only trace quantities of von Willebrand's protein are inadequate and should not be employed in the treatment of patients with severe von Willebrand's disease. The use of the purified factor VIII:C in this situation will not result in hemostasis, and the problem of hemorrhage will persist.—W.R. Bell, M.D.

Prevalence of von Willebrand Disease in Children: A Multiethnic Study
Werner EJ, Broxson EH, Tucker EL, Giroux DS, Shults J, Abshire TC (Eastern Virginia Med School, Norfolk; Wright-Patterson United States Air Force Med Ctr, Dayton, Ohio; Keesler Med Ctr, Keesler Air Force Base, Miss)
J Pediatr 123:893–898, 1993   116-95-3–34

Background.—The prevalence of von Willebrand's disorder has been estimated at 4–10 cases per 100,000 population. However, a recent survey found a prevalence of .8% in an ethnically homogenous community in northern Italy. The prevalence of von Willebrand's disorder in a heter-

Population Comparisons for vWF Activity (U/dL)

	Blood groups		
	O	**Non-O**	
All*	83 (43-162)	98 (51-190)	
Black	84 (43-182)	98 (63-190)	
White	83 (42-156)	97 (51-188)	} p = NS / p = NS
Male	87 (44-158)	100 (53-211)	
Female	79 (42-182)	93 (49-172)	} p <0.01 / p <0.02

Note: Values are medians, with 95% confidence intervals in *parentheses.* The P values were obtained by using the Wilcoxon rank sum test.
* For blood group O vs. non-O blood groups, $P < .001$.
(Courtesy of Werner EJ, Broxson EH, Tucker EL, et al: *J Pediatr* 123:893–898, 1993.)

ogenous population was determined and whether vWF concentrations differ by blood type, race, or gender was investigated.

Methods.—During routine school physical examinations, vWF was measured using the ristocetin cofactor method in 600 healthy children aged 2–18 years. A questionnaire elicited personal and family bleeding symptoms. Diagnosis of von Willebrand's disorder was based on personal and family history of bleeding symptoms and abnormal vWF activity concentration.

Results.—The prevalence of von Willebrand's disorder was 1.3%, with similar representations among white, black, Hispanic, biracial, and other ethnic groups and between genders. The vWF activity concentrations for children in blood group O differed significantly from those in non-O categories (table). After separation by blood type, black and white populations had similar vWF activity concentrations. Within each blood group, girls had significantly decreased vWF activity compared with boys. The vWF activity concentrations were similar for prepubertal and postpubertal boys, indicating that androgen stimulation had no impact on vWF.

Conclusion.—von Willebrand's disease is the most common congenital hemostatic abnormality and should be considered in any child with a personal or family history of bleeding symptoms. Screening studies are not reliable for identifying patients with von Willebrand's disorder; therefore, vWF activity levels should be included in the laboratory evaluation of mucosal bleeding symptoms in children.

▶ This study, which is relatively small in size, establishes that there is no predilection for race with respect to the frequency of von Willebrand's disease. A prevalence figure of 1.3% was identified from the results of this study. Somewhat instructive was the finding that affected girls had lower von Willebrand's protein concentrations than affected boys. There might be some correlation with the different blood groups. Although this study provides some meaningful data and information, clearly a much, much larger study, hopefully involving many countries, is actually needed before a true prevalence figure can be identified. The authors of this paper were confident that von Willebrand's disease is the most common congenital hemostatic disorder.—W.R. Bell, M.D.

Autopsy Findings in Three Patients With von Willebrand Disease Type IIB and Type III: Presence of Atherosclerotic Lesions Without Occlusive Arterial Thrombi

Federici AB, Mannucci PM, Fogato E, Ghidoni P, Matturri L (Univ of Milan, Italy)

Thromb Haemost 70:758–761, 1993   116-95-3–35

TABLE 1.—Laboratory Values for the 3 Patients With von Willebrand's Disease

Patient (diagnosis)	Bleeding time (min)	Platelet count (× 10⁹/L)	Factor VIII coagulant activity (U/dL)	vWf antigen (U/dL)	Ristocetin cofactor activity (U/dL)	Ristocetin-induced platelet aggregation (mg/ml)
1) F.F. (type IIB vWd)	>30	58–125	19–37	38–49	12–19	0.4–0.6
2) Z. G. (type III vWd)	>30	96–156	1–4	<0.04	<6	>2.5
3) C. G. (type III vWd)	>30	105–122	2–5	<0.04	<6	>2.5

Note: The values given are the ranges of those observed during the follow-up of the patients at the center.
(Courtesy of Federici AB, Mannucci PM, Fogato E, et al: *Thromb Haemost* 70:758–761, 1993.)

TABLE 2.—Morphometric Analysis of Atherosclerosis in the Aortas of 3 Patients With von Willebrand's Disease

Patient	Total aortic area examined (cm²)	No. of atherosclerotic lesions	Area with atherosclerosis (cm²)	Plaques areas (cm²) fibrolipidic	calcified	ulcerated
1	164	54	119 (73%)*	25 (21%)†	83 (70%)	11 (9%)
2	215	39	12 (6%)	12 (100%)	–	–
3	164	67	31 (19%)	25 (81%)	6 (19%)	–

* Percentage of total aortic area.
† Percentage of area with atherosclerosis.
(Courtesy of Federici AB, Mannucci PM, Fogato E, et al: *Thromb Haemost* 70:758–761, 1993.)

Background.—A function of vWF is to support platelet adhesion to the subendothelium and platelet aggregation in conditions of blood flow that cause high shear stress. It has been reported that pigs with severe von Willebrand's disease are protected from spontaneous and diet-induced atherosclerosis of the lower abdominal aorta. Studies also found less arterial thrombus formation in pigs with von Willebrand's disease or normal pigs treated with anti-vWF monoclonal antibodies (MoAbs). Autopsies were performed on 3 men with von Willebrand's disease to determine the extent and localization of atherosclerotic lesions.

Patients.—The men were aged 73, 44, and 52 years at the time of death. One man had the type IIB variant of von Willebrand's disease that is characterized by an abnormal vWF that supports platelet adhesion to the subendothelium normally and has an increased affinity for platelets. The other 2 men had type III von Willebrand's disease, the variant similar to that protecting pigs from atherosclerosis (Table 1). Hemorrhagic diathesis was the most important cause of death in the 3 men.

Autopsy Results.—Severe atherosclerotic lesions were found in every arterial district in the man with type IIB von Willebrand's disease. The 2 men with type III disease had few and slight lesions except for moderately severe atherosclerosis in the coronary district of patient 2. Overall, the lesions were less extensive in the 2 men with severe type III von Willebrand's disease (Table 2). There was no clinical or pathologic evidence of thrombosis in the coronary arteries or other arteries. These findings are consistent with the observations of a decreased prevalence of occlusive thrombi in pigs with von Willebrand's disease and in normal pigs treated with anti-vWF MoAbs. It also appears that vWF is essential for the formation of occlusive thrombi in stenotic arterial vessels under conditions of high shear stress.

Conclusion.—Pigs with severe von Willebrand's disease reportedly are protected from spontaneous and diet-induced atherosclerosis, but there have been few studies in humans. Autopsies in 3 men with von Willebrand's disease revealed atherosclerotic lesions in all patients' although the lesions were less extensive in the patients with type III von Willebrand's disease. These findings indicate that atherosclerosis does develop in individuals with severe von Willebrand's disease. However, any protection from atherosclerosis associated with vWF deficiency may have been offset by lifelong treatment with vWF-containing blood products.

▶ This report clearly identifies the presence of severe and generalized atherosclerotic lesions in patients with severe von Willebrand's disease. This is in contrast to previous speculation in certain animal models that had been advertised to be without atherosclerotic lesions, suggesting a protective effect from a deficiency of von Willebrand's protein. It is rather obvious from this report that the absence of von Willebrand's protein is not a protective measure for the disease process of arterial atherosclerosis. Additional autopsy studies will confirm this finding.—W.R. Bell, M.D.

Incidence of Inhibitor Development in a Group of Young Hemophilia A Patients Treated Exclusively With Lyophilized Cryoprecipitate

Peerlinck K, Rosendaal FR, Vermylen J (Univ of Leuven, Belgium; Univ Hosp Leiden, The Netherlands)
Blood 81:3332–3335, 1993   116-95-3–36

Background.—In patients with hemophilia A, the development of neutralizing antibodies, or inhibitors, to infused factor VIII is a significant treatment problem. The age-dependent cumulative incidence of inhibitor development was analyzed in a cohort of patients with hemophilia A.

Patients and Methods.—Sixty-seven previously untreated patients with hemophilia A were included in this study. All had been born after January 1, 1971 and before April 30, 1990. During this period, patients were treated exclusively with a lyophilized cryoprecipitate distributed by the Belgian Red Cross. Most patients were enrolled in home treatment programs, with transfusions administered at the first sign of hemorrhage or prophylactically 3 times per week. Each year, a factor VIII inhibitor assay was performed, with additional assays done whenever the therapeutic response to transfusions was deemed inadequate. Patients were classified as inhibitors if inhibitor levels exceeded 1 Bethesda unit/mL on 2 separate occasions.

Results.—Forty-eight patients had severe, 10 had moderate, and 14 had mild hemophilia. The incidence of neutralizing isoantibody formation to infused factor VIII in this cohort was 6% (5.3 per 1,000 patient years of observation). The age-dependent cumulative risk at 4 and 8 years of age was 4.6% and 6.7%, respectively.

Conclusion.—The incidence of inhibitor formation is partly product-related and connected with the process of purification and viral inactivation. Each newly introduced factor VIII concentrated must be evaluated separately to determine its propensity to induce neutralizing antibodies in comparison to a reliable reference group. Patient groups such as those studied in this investigation provide a better reference group, as they have been treated with a single factor VIII preparation only. These findings could provide background for additional research on safe, virus-free products associated with a low incidence of inhibitors.

▶ When recombinant factor VIII became available, it was not immediately adopted as routine therapy for a number of reasons, including the relatively high cost and the level of safety of currently available concentrates that had undergone viral inactivation. However, another area of concern is the high reported rates of inhibitor formation in patients receiving the therapy. When this problem is analyzed, a number of factors are identified that made necessary evaluations difficult. A large part of the problem is that previous studies of inhibitor occurrence may not meet current standards. The problems of these studies include the use of different methods to detect inhibitors, mixing of the issues of incidence and prevalence, and inadequate follow-up of patients. This problem could be resolved by a concurrently studied randomized group of previously untransfused patients who receive recombinant factor VIII or human factor VIII concentrate. Such a study would be very difficult in view of the small number of patients available and other factors. The current citation appears to be a carefully performed cohort study of patients receiving cryoprecipitate. It may provide a better estimate of inhibitor incidence for comparison, in the absence of a prospective trial.—P.M. Ness, M.D.

Use of Porcine Factor VIII in the Treatment of Patients With Acquired Hemophilia

Morrison AE, Ludlam CA, Kessler C (Royal Infirmary, Edinburgh, Scotland; George Washington Univ, Washington, DC)
Blood 81:1513–1520, 1993   116-95-3–37

Background.—Acquired hemophilia is characterized by spontaneous development of an autoantibody to plasma coagulation factor VIII. The optimal therapeutic management of this rare disorder has not been established. The use of porcine factor VIII to treat acute bleeding in patients with acquired hemophilia was evaluated.

Methods.—Data were analyzed for 65 patients with acquired hemophilia who had been treated with porcine factor VIII for 74 bleeding episodes.

Results.—The median initial anti–human factor VIII autoantibody inhibitor level was 38 Bethesda units/mL; the mean initial antiporcine factor VIII was 1 Bethesda unit/mL. The mean initial dose of porcine factor VIII of 84 IU/kg increased plasma FVIII:C activity by .85 IU/mL. The mean duration of therapy was 8.5 days, with an average of 11 infusions. Seventy-eight percent of the patients had a good or excellent objective clinical response to porcine factor VIII; only 6 patients did not respond. Subsequent treatment with porcine factor VIII was successful in 5 of 7 patients who re-bled on at least 1 occasion. Side effects were infrequent. Five patients had infusion-related minor rigors or back pain that responded to treatment. One patient discontinued treatment because of major anaphylactic response to porcine factor VIII. Preporcine and postporcine factor VIII platelet counts were measured in 21 patients and were comparable.

Conclusion.—Porcine factor VIII is a safe, clinically effective treatment for bleeding caused by acquired hemophilia. When a patient with this rare disorder is seen, the porcine autoantibody inhibitor level should be measured; if low, porcine factor VIII concentration is a possible first-line treatment.

▶ Acquired hemophilia is an uncommon disorder that can be difficult to manage. In most patients, the antibody activity is greater against human factor VIII than against porcine factor VIII, suggesting the utility of porcine factor VIII for bleeding episodes in this condition. This study confirmed the usefulness of porcine factor VIII in almost 80% of patients. Surprisingly, most of the patients who required second courses of therapy still had good responses; this result was unexpected because the development of antiporcine antibodies is commonly believed to limit the long-term efficacy of this product.—P.M. Ness, M.D.

Hypercoagulable States and Intravascular Coagulation

Complement-Induced Vesiculation and Exposure of Membrane Prothrombinase Sites in Platelets of Paroxysmal Nocturnal Hemoglobinuria

Wiedmer T, Hall SE, Ortel TL, Kane WH, Rosse WF, Sims PJ (Blood Research Inst, Milwaukee, Wis; Duke Univ, Durham, NC)
Blood 82:1192–1196, 1993   116-95-3–38

Background.—Thrombosis developed from a characteristic hypercoagulable state is a common major complication in patients with paroxysmal nocturnal hemoglobinuria (PNH). The hypercoagulability may be attributable to the disorder's platelet defects. The PNH blood cells lack

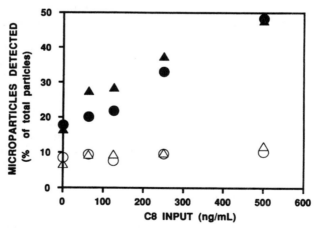

Fig 3–8.—Quantitation of C5b-9-induced platelet microparticles. Platelets were incubated with the C5b-9 proteins. Microparticles were identified by their light-scatter properties and quantitated. Data are shown for 2 normal controls (*open symbols*) and for patients PNH-NY (*black circle*) and PNH-NF (*black triangle*). Data are from a single experiment, representative of 3 performed, using platelets obtained from 4 individuals with PNH. (Courtesy of Wiedmer T, Hall SE, Ortel TL, et al: *Blood* 82:1192–1196, 1993.)

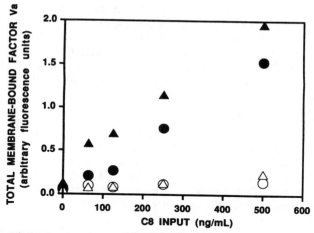

Fig 3–9.—C5b-9-induced exposure of membrane-binding sites for factor Va. Platelets were incubated with the C5b-9 proteins, and FITC-V237 binding to these cells was measured. Total FITC-V237 fluorescence was calculated by multiplying the mean single-particle fluorescence by the total number of particles (platelet or microparticle). Data are shown for 2 normal controls (*open symbols*) and for patients PHN-NY (*black circle*) and PNH-NF (*black triangle*). Data are from a single experiment, representative of 3 performed, using platelets from 4 individuals with PNH. (Courtesy of Wiedmer T, Hall SE, Ortel TL, et al: *Blood* 82:1192–1196, 1993.)

proteins attached to the membrane by glycosylphosphatidylinositol, including those that regulate cell-surface complement activation. An earlier study showed that PNH platelets lack CD59 antigen, making them unusually sensitive to activation by the C5b-9 proteins, which induces abnormally increased procoagulant vesicle production, a possible contributor to thrombosis.

Methods.—In this investigation, PNH platelets lacking CD59 antigen were incubated with the purified complement proteins C5b6, C7, C9, and varying amounts of C8. Factor Va–binding sites in the platelets were monitored with fluorescent-gated flow cytometry to analyze the cells' activation responses.

Results.—The PNH platelets lacking CD59 antigen when compared with controls, produced greatly increased amounts of plasma membrane–derived microparticles and exposed new binding sites for factor Va in the presence of C5b-9 (Fig 3–8). The increase in microparticle formation was complement dose-dependent in PNH platelets as was expression of factor Va–binding sites in both PNH platelets and microparticles (Fig 3–9). Increased expression of Va-binding sites reached a 10-fold increase and was paralleled by increased expression of procoagulant surface, as measured on the prothrombinase complex surface. Activation sensitivity was not affected by either collagen or the calcium ionophore, A23187.

Conclusion.—The deletion of CD59 and its complement inhibitory function makes PNH platelets significantly more sensitive to C5b-9 proteins which generate thrombin, a possible contributor to thrombotic risk in patients with PNH. The PNH platelet's ability to shed C5b-9 complexes by vesiculation may account for its normal survival. The PNH erythrocytes, which also lack CD59, are unable to shed C5b-9 complexes, which may account for their decreased survival.

▶ In addition to hemolytic anemia and pancytopenia, thrombosis is a hallmark of PNH. It is also a vexing management problem; its mechanism has always been arcane. This elegant study demonstrates that the absence of platelet CD59 expression by PNH platelets is associated with the complement-induced induction of procoagulant vesicles and an increased rate of conversion of prothrombin to thrombin. Because PNH platelets are capable of shedding these vesicles, their survival in the circulation is not impaired.

It is noteworthy that thrombosis and hemolysis in PNH are not correlated. It would be of interest and clinical importance if the techniques employed in this study could be used to predict which PNH patients were at risk of thrombosis before something catastrophic occurred.—J.L. Spivak, M.D.

Cyclosporine-Related Hypercoagulability: Fact or Fiction?
Edwards CM, Morgan JDT, Donnelly PK (Leicester Univ, England)
Transplant Proc 24:2616–2617, 1992   116-95-3–39

Background.—Cyclosporine treatment may be responsible for an increased incidence of thromboembolic complications after renal transplantation. Laboratory and clinical evidence of cyclosporine-related hypercoagulability was sought prospectively.

Methods.—In part 1 of the study, thrombelastography was used to quantify the hemostatic derangements after surgery. Twenty-eight consecutive renal transplant recipients receiving high-dose cyclosporine were compared with 20 patients undergoing elective open cholecystectomy. Prophylactic heparin anticoagulation treatment was administered to all patients. In part 2 of the study, 61 consecutive first cadaver renal transplant recipients were randomized preoperatively to 1 of 3 immunosuppressive regimens. Group A received an initial dose of cyclosporine of 17 mg/kg/day, decreased by 2 mg/kg/wk to 7 mg/kg/day. Group B received this regimen plus nifedipine. Group C initially received cyclosporine 10 mg/kg/day, decreased by 2 mg/kg/wk to 4 mg/kg/day, plus azathioprine adjusted to avoid leukopenia. All groups received steroids.

Findings.—In part 1, transplant recipients were significantly hypercoagulable compared with elective surgery patients. In part 2, significantly more patients in group A had thrombotic complications than did those in groups B and C. These complications were pulmonary embolus in 1 patient, deep vein thrombosis in 1, and coronary thrombosis in 1. No thrombotic complications occurred in groups B or C.

Conclusion.—Patients with chronic renal failure have accelerated co-agulation. The immediate postoperative hypercoagulable state in renal transplant recipients may be related to this preexisting pathology and not associated with high cyclosporine dosage. In the long term, renal transplant does seem to exacerbate the effects of chronic renal failure on coagulation. Thus, cyclosporine-related endothelial toxicity may contribute to the post-transplant hypercoagulable state.

▶ This important study points out that the hypercoagulability seen in such patients is almost certainly due to the underlying renal pathology and not the therapeutic effects of cyclosporine.—W.R. Bell, M.D.

Different Incidence of Venous Thrombosis in Patients With Inherited Deficiencies of Antithrombin III, Protein C and Protein S
Finazzi G, Barbui T (Ospedali Riuniti, Bergamo, Italy)
Thromb Haemost 71:15–18, 1994   116-95-3-40

Background.—The management of patients with inherited deficiency of antithrombin III, protein C, or protein S is complex and controversial. Antithrombin III deficiency appears to constitute a greater risk for major thrombosis than protein C or protein S deficiency. However, thus far, only retrospective research demonstrates this. The incidence of thrombosis in patients with inherited deficiency of antithrombin III, protein C, or protein S was compared using a cohort design.

Methods.—A total of 81 patients with a diagnosis of hereditary thrombophilia participated. They were stratified into 3 groups of antithrombotic prophylaxis according to their thrombotic history: group 1 consisted of 53 patients with no history of deep vein thrombosis and no anticoagulant prophylaxis; group 2 included 16 patients with a single episode of deep vein thrombosis associated with a recognized triggering factor, such as surgery or pregnancy; group 3 included 12 patients with spontaneous or recurrent deep vein thrombosis or pulmonary embolism who were receiving lifelong oral anticoagulation. Follow-up was conducted for a total of 160 patient-years. Each participant was seen every 1–6 months as an outpatient, and follow-up visits included anamnesis and a complete physical. End points were deep vein or arterial thrombosis or major bleeding.

Results.—Seven venous thromboses were seen during follow-up, for a total incidence of 4.3% patient-years (table). When comparing age, sex, schedule of antithrombotic prophylaxis, and type of deficiency, younger patients had a slightly lower incidence of thrombosis than older patients had. Patients receiving long-term oral anticoagulation also had a slightly higher incidence of thrombosis. Patients with antithrombin III deficiency had a significantly higher incidence of venous thrombosis than patients with protein C or protein S deficiency, despite the fact that they were often younger and had received more prolonged anticoagulation treatment.

Thrombotic Events Observed During the Follow-Up

Patient	Age/sex	Congenital deficiency	Group of treatment	Follow-up (months)	Site of venous thrombosis
1	23/F	AT III	I	5	Right calf
2	19/M	AT III	III	25	Bilateral femoro-iliac
3	48/F	AT III	I	47	Left popliteal
4	36/M	PC	II	19	Mesenteric
5	33/M	PC	II	33	Left femoro-iliac
6	70/M	PC	I	11	Right femoro-iliac
7	41/F	PS	I	14	Left calf

(Courtesy of Finazzi G, Barbui T: *Thromb Haemost* 71:15-18, 1994.)

Conclusion.—Patients with congenital deficiency of antithrombin III carry a greater thrombotic risk than patients with protein C or protein S deficiency.

▶ The authors of this article report data that suggest that antithrombin III deficiency is much more frequently associated with thrombotic events than either protein C or protein S deficiency. In fact, in this report, patients with antithrombin III deficiency had more thrombotic events than the combined group of patients with protein S or protein C deficiency. This may have been due to the longer duration of treatment in patients who experienced anti-thrombin III deficiency. This, indeed, has not been the experience of other investigators, who have clearly identified a more serious and more frequent problem associated with either protein C or protein S deficiency compared with antithrombin III deficiency. Clearly, more precise studies are needed before a definitive statement can be made.—W.R. Bell, M.D.

Association of Protein S Deficiency With Thrombosis in a Kindred With Increased Levels of Plasminogen Activator Inhibitor-1

Bolan CD, Krishnamurti C, Tang DB, Carrington LR, Alving BM (Walter Reed Army Inst of Research, Washington, DC; Walter Reed Army Med Ctr, Washington, DC)

Ann Intern Med 119:779–785, 1993   116-95-3–41

Background.—Deficiencies of protein S, protein C, and antithrombin III are the most common inherited abnormalities associated with familial venous thrombosis. The role of plasminogen activator inhibitor-1 (PAI-1) in promoting thrombosis has been investigated but has not been established. In 1 North American kindred and 2 European families, increased levels of PAI-1 were the reported cause of familial thrombosis. However, only symptomatic members of these groups were studied and measurements of free protein S were not obtained because the assay was not easily available. The kindred in North America was reevaluated with functional assays of protein C, protein S, and PAI-1 activity. The discovery of protein S deficiency in the kindred and its association with venous thromboembolism was described.

Method.—Plasma levels of total and free protein S antigen and the activities of protein S, protein C, PAI-1, and antithrombin III were measured in 28 adults from 3 generations of the North American kindred. Seven persons had a history of thromboembolism.

Findings.—Protein C activity was normal in all persons with thrombosis. Six of the 7 persons with thrombosis were deficient in total and free protein S compared with 9 of 21 asymptomatic persons. The 6 persons with protein S deficiency and a history of thrombosis tended to smoke and to have higher triglyceride levels than the asymptomatic persons. A history of thrombosis was not correlated with PAI-1 activity. The mean

Clinical and Laboratory Data in Adult Family Members With a History of Thrombosis and in Asymptomatic Members

Variable	Thrombosis Protein S		No Thrombosis Protein S		Reference Range
	Decreased	Normal	Decreased	Normal	
Number, n	6	1	9	12	
Age at onset, y	28 ± 9	41	—	—	
Age, y	45 ± 11	49	35 ± 11	35 ± 18	
Men/total	5/6	0/1	3/9	7/12	
Smoker/Total	4/6	1/1	0/9	7/12	
Protein S					
Functional, %	20 ± 5	105	26 ± 9	100 ± 22	79 to 187 M; 53 to 165 F
Free, %	22 ± 14	61	14 ± 7	100 ± 14	74 to 120 M†; 49 to 129 F
Total, %	61 ± 9	95	58 ± 11	102 ± 8	96 to 124 M†; 83 to 126 F
Protein C, %	96 ± 21	80	—	—	65 to 157
vWF:Ag, %	183 ± 21	225	197 ± 67	177 ± 34	50 to 150
Factor VIII, %	180 ± 25	200	170 ± 78	199 ± 89	50 to 150
PAI-1, AU/mL	6.3 ± 4.7	17	3.3 ± 3.3	14.1 ± 11	0.5 to 14 M; 0.1 to 8 F
Triglycerides, mg/dL	118 ± 29	108	57 ± 23	108 ± 55	40 to 160 M; 35 to 135 F

Note: Values are mean ± standard deviation where indicated. The conversion factor to SI units is .01 for protein S, protein C, vWF:antigen (Ag), and factor VIII. The conversion factor for PAI-1 (kAU/L) is 1 and for triglycerides (mmol/L) is .01129.
† As determined by the enzyme-linked immunosorbent assay procedure.
(Courtesy of Bolan CD, Krishnamurti C, Tang DB, et al: Ann Intern Med 119:779–785, 1993.)

PAI-1 activity in the 7 persons with thrombosis was 7.9 kAU/L compared with 9.3 kAU/L in the 21 asymptomatic persons (table).

Conclusion.—In an evaluation of 28 adults in a North American kindred, a deficiency of total and free or functional protein S was the cause of thrombosis previously attributed to defective fibrinolysis caused by increased levels of PAI-1. Activity of PAI-1 was increased in some persons in the kindred compared with a reference population, but it was not associated with familial thrombosis. The clinical usefulness of routine assays for PAI-1 activity in the evaluation of familial thrombosis has not been established.

▶ The authors of this article make the extremely important point of the importance of comprehensive studies in patients with excessive thrombosis formation. The kindred described was initially thought to experience thrombosis because of increased PAI-1 levels. However, additional studies revealed the presence of impressive protein S deficiency. This represents an important lesson in the thoughtful evaluation of a problem in contrast to the attribution of a problem to a plasma protein whose physiology and function has not been absolutely defined.—W.R. Bell, M.D.

Double-Blind, Placebo-Controlled Trial of Antithrombin III Concentrates in Septic Shock With Disseminated Intravascular Coagulation
Fourrier F, Chopin C, Huart J-J, Runge I, Caron C, Goudemand J (Hôpital B CHRU Lille; Centre Régional de Transfusion Sanguine, Lille, France; Service de Réanimation Polyvalente, CH Valenciennes, France)
Chest 104:882–888, 1993   116-95-3–42

Background.—Disseminated intravascular coagulation (DIC) frequently complicates septic shock by a massive activation of the coagulation system that results in marked increases in thrombin and fibrin production. Antithrombin III is a potent inhibitor of the clotting cascade. In DIC, the magnitude of the initial decrease in antithrombin III is a reliable negative prognostic factor. Uncontrolled clinical studies have suggested that antithrombin III substitution may prevent DIC and death in septic shock. The efficacy of antithrombin III in decreasing the mortality rate and consequences of DIC in septic shock was determined.

Methods.—In a prospective, placebo-controlled trial, 35 patients with septic shock and DIC were randomized to receive intravenous infusion of either antithrombin III concentrates or placebo. The antithrombin III, 90–120 IU/kg, was given in a loading dose, then 90 to 120 IU/kg/day was given for 4 days. Follow-up was for 28 days or until death. Only patients with hemorrhages and severe decreases in prothrombin time, platelet count, and fibrinogen levels received fresh frozen plasma, platelets, and fibrinogen concentrates.

Outcome.—Thirty-two patients were evaluable. In the 17 patients receiving antithrombin III concentrates, antithrombin III levels were rapidly corrected and remained above normal levels until day 10. Circulating protein C and protein S levels were not modified by antithrombin III supplementation. Antithrombin III significantly decreased the duration of DIC. At the end of day 2, 64% of patients receiving antithrombin III and only 11% of those receiving placebo were cured of DIC. At the end of treatment, 71% of those receiving antithrombin III were cured, compared with only 33% of controls. Mortality in the intensive care unit was decreased by 44% in those receiving antithrombin III. Patient care requirements and transfusion requirements were not different in the 2 treatment groups.

Conclusion.—Antithrombin III treatment significantly decreased the duration of DIC in patients with septic shock. The correction of symptoms was evident as early as day 2 after treatment, and antithrombin III levels remained greater than normal until day 10. Antithrombin III supplementation did not affect circulating protein C and protein S levels. Although mortality in those receiving antithrombin was reduced by 44%, the difference compared with controls was not statistically significant. This trend toward improved survival suggests the need for further randomized studies, especially in light of the high cost of antithrombin III supplementation.

▶ Considerable debate continues to exist about whether antithrombin III concentrates are beneficial in patients experiencing DIC. A few excellent trials have been conducted. However, agreement has not been reached concerning the therapeutic efficacy of antithrombin III in this disease process. This study demonstrated that the duration of DIC was significantly reduced in the treatment group vs. the controls. Seventy-one percent of those treated were cured of the DIC process. Mortality, however, was not different between the placebo and antithrombin III–treated groups. Thus, it is clear that antithrombin III is beneficial to some, but not all, patients who receive this treatment. Before absolute statements can be made, additional appropriately controlled, prospective, randomized, and blinded studies are needed.—W.R. Bell, M.D.

Thromboangiitis Obliterans (Buerger's Disease) in Women (A Reevaluation)
Yörükoğlu Y, Ilgit E, Zengin M, Nazliel K, Salman E, Yucel E (Gazi Univ, Ankara, Turkey)
Angiology 44:527–532, 1993   116-95-3–43

Background.—Thromboangiitis obliterans (TAO), also known as Buerger's disease, is defined as a disease of young males associated with heavy tobacco use. The disease has been extremely rare in women, with women accounting for only 1% of the cases. However, the incidence of

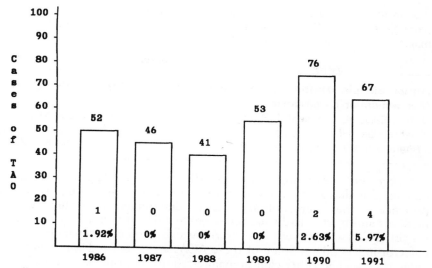

Fig 3–10.—Summary of TAO cases diagnosed between 1986 and 1991 and appearance of female cases during these years. (Courtesy of Yörükoğlu Y, Ilgit E, Zengin M, et al: *Angiology* 44:527–532, 1993.)

TAO among women has increased 10-fold to 20-fold in recent years because of escalating tobacco use in women. Seven cases of TAO in females were reported.

Methods.—During a 6-year period, 314 cases of TAO were diagnosed and angiographically verified; 7 were in women. The appearance, clinical course, and outcome of these 7 cases in women were examined.

Results.—Overall, the male-female ratio of patients with TAO was approximately 47:1, with an incidence of TAO cases in women for the 6 years of 2.09% (Fig 3–10). The mean age of female patients was 32.6 years. The female patients smoked 20–40 cigarettes a day for 7–17 years. The average time between beginning to smoke and diagnosis of TAO was 12 years. All the women were seen with intermittent claudication or ischemia of the affected extremities, with pedal pulses absent in affected extremities. One patient was seen with Raynaud's phenomenon of the upper extremities and mild lower-extremity claudication; in all others, the primary complaint involved the lower extremities. Angiographies of affected extremities revealed abnormalities consistent with TAO. Segments of the tibial and peroneal arteries were occluded in every case.

Conclusion.—The classic definition of TAO should be revised to include women. The true incidence of TAO among women and the male-female ratio remain to be determined.

▶ This report clearly establishes that TAO occurs in females. This is in contrast to years of teaching that indicated this disease only afflicted males. Although tobacco has been known for years to have adverse affects on the pathogenesis of TAO, the precise ingredient that induces this problem remains unknown.—W.R. Bell, M.D.

Anticardiolipin Antibodies and Dependence of a Serum Cofactor: A Mechanism of Thrombosis

Ordi J, Selva A, Monegal F, Porcel JM, Martinez-Costa X, Vilardell M (Vall d'Hebron Gen Hosp, Barcelona)
J Rheumatol 20:1321–1324, 1993   116-95-3–44

Background.—Anticardiolipin antibodies (ACAs) are IgG or IgM class immunoglobulins that react with negatively charged phospholipids. The presence of these autoantibodies can be determined by coagulometric methods and by standard solid-phase enzyme-linked immunosorbent assay (ELISA). Two different types of ACAs exist: cofactor-dependent and cofactor-independent. Some of these ACAs are associated with autoimmune diseases and other clinical manifestations, but others are not. The serum cofactor dependency of ACAs in infectious and autoimmune diseases was evaluated.

Methods.—Patients were divided into 4 groups based on etiology and clinical manifestations. Group 1 patients had ACAs and an autoimmune disease—either systemic lupus erythematosus or the primary antiphospholipid syndrome. Group 2 patients had ACAs without symptoms, underlying infection, or autoimmune disease. Group 3 patients had ACAs

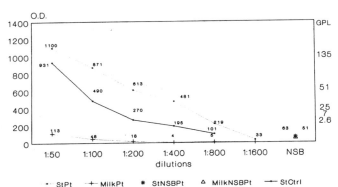

Fig 3–11.—*Abbreviations: StPt*, aCL activity in standard ELISA; *MilkPt*, aCL activity in a modified ELISA; *StNSBPt*, nonspecific binding in standard ELISA; *MilkNSBPt*, nonspecific binding in modified ELISA; *StCtrl*, international control. Anticardiolipin antibody (*aCL*) activity and dependence of the cofactor in a patient with primary antiphospholipid syndrome (PAPS). (Courtesy of Ordi J, Selva A, Monegal F, et al: *J Rheumatol* 20:1321–1324, 1993.)

and infectious diseases (syphilis, leprosy, HIV infection, or Q fever). Group 4 patients were controls. The presence of ACAs was determined by ELISA and a modified ELISA in which bovine serum albumin, gelatin, and skim milk powder were substituted for fetal calf serum.

Results.—There was a significant association between patients with cofactor-dependent ACAs and thrombotic risk. All except 1 patient in group 1 had cofactor-dependent ACAs (Fig 3–11). Three of 4 patients in group 2 had cofactor-independent ACAs and 1 had cofactor-dependent ACA activity. In group 3, 17 of 19 patients were cofactor-independent; 2 patients with infections and ACAs were cofactor-dependent and had mild thrombocytopenia. There were significant associations between cofactor-dependent and autoimmune diseases and cofactor-independent ACAs with infectious diseases.

Conclusion.—There was a significant association between patients with cofactor-dependent ACAs and thrombotic risk. The dependence or independence of the cofactor helps differentiate infectious from autoimmune ACAs. The association between cofactor-dependent and autoimmune diseases and cofactor-independent ACAs and infectious diseases was also significant.

▶ The mechanism whereby ACAs or circulating inhibitors in patients with systemic lupus erythematosus and allied conditions experience thrombosis remains unknown. The authors of this manuscript, however, have shown that there is a cofactor, the nature of which is undefined in serum, that seems to be important for correlation with the presence of thrombus formation in patients with these various connective tissue disorders. The nature of this serum cofactor needs to be identified.—W.R. Bell, M.D.

Increased Thrombin Generation and Activity in Patients With Systemic Lupus Erythematosus and Anticardiolipin Antibodies: Evidence for a Prothrombotic State
Ginsberg JS, Demers C, Brill-Edwards P, Johnston M, Bona R, Burrows RF, Weitz J, Denburg JA (McMaster Univ, Hamilton, Ont, Canada)
Blood 81:2958–2963, 1993   116-95-3–45

Objective.—Whether patients with systemic lupus erythematosus (SLE) and anticardiolipin antibodies (ACAs) have biochemical evidence of an ongoing prothrombotic state was determined.

Patients and Methods.—Forty-three consecutive patients referred to a SLE clinic during a 5-month period were included. Patient age ranged from 19 to 75 years, and all met standard diagnostic criteria for SLE. Clinical and laboratory evaluations were performed on 2 separate occasions at least 3 months apart. During clinical evaluation, information concerning ongoing use of warfarin was obtained. In addition, the presence of earlier venous and arterial thromboembolic disease was determined by history, critical review of objective tests, and examination for reflux in the deep veins of the legs. Disease-related activity was assessed by performing a lupus activity criteria count. The laboratory evaluation included taking blood on both visits and assaying these samples for prothrombin fragments (F1 + 2) and fibrinopeptide A, as well as ACAs. Patients were classified as ACA+ or ACA− depending on assay results. The ACA+ patients included those with abnormal assays on both visits; ACA− patients were those with either negative assays on both visits or negative assays on 1 occasion and positive assays on the other.

Results.—A significantly higher mean level of F1 + 2 was noted for ACA+ patients, at 1.07 nmol/L compared with .79 nmol/L and .47 nmol/L for ACA− patients and those receiving warfarin, respectively. In addition, ACA+ patients had a significantly higher mean level of fibrinopeptide A at 1.01 nmol/L vs. .45 nmol/L for ACA− patients. When excluding patients with earlier thromboembolism, significant differences in the mean levels of F1 + 2 and fibrinopeptide A continued to be noted between ACA+ and ACA− patients, whereas when those with earlier thromboembolism or active disease were excluded, the analysis revealed a significant difference in the mean level of fibrinopeptide A and a nonsignificant trend in the mean level of F1 + 2.

Conclusion.—In patients with SLE, the presence of ACAs is associated with an ongoing prothrombotic state.

▶ The authors of this article have demonstrated in a detailed manner that patients with ACAs and SLE have increased quantities of prothrombin fragment F1+2, prothrombin fragments F1+2, and fibrinopeptide A. Although thrombin can mediate the release of these components into the circulating blood, it is also possible for plasmin to release these same components into the circulating blood. The fact that warfarin anticoagulation results in a reduction in the presence of prothrombin F1+2 and fibrinopeptide A supports the contention that this may be thrombin but does not eliminate plasminogen as the possible agent releasing these components into the circulating blood.—W.R. Bell, M.D.

Systemic Lupus Erythematosus–Like Illness Associated With Syndrome of Abnormally Large von Willebrand's Factor Multimers
Cockerell CJ, Lewis JE (Univ of Texas, Dallas; Holt-Krock Clinic, Fort Smith, Ark)
South Med J 86:951–953, 1993   116-95-3–46

Objective.—Systemic lupus erythematosus (SLE) is associated with a wide range of cutaneous findings and systemic manifestations. It can occur in association with congenital complement deficiencies or circulating antiphospholipid antibodies. A patient with clinical signs similar to those of SLE—including cutaneous manifestations—in association with abnormally large vWF multimers was described.

Case Report.—Woman, 29, with a family history of circulating abnormally large vWF multimers, had microangiopathic hemolytic anemia during pregnancy. She had a left hemispheric transient ischemic attack 2 years later and had 3 different cerebrovascular accidents and an acute myocardial infarction during the next 6 years. Eight years after her initial presentation, she consulted a dermatologist for an eruption of macules, papules, and plaques with associated periungual erythema and telangiectasia. She had an antinuclear antibody titer positive at a level of 1:160 and a homogenous pattern. Analysis of a skin biopsy specimen demonstrated changes compatible with cutaneous lupus erythematosus. These lesions were thought to represent a SLE-like diathesis associated with the patient's thrombotic disorder. The patient has had no further episodes and is being treated with aspirin and dipyridamole.

Discussion.—A SLE-like illness with skin lesions in patients with circulating, abnormally large vWF multimers is reported. Patients with this rare hematologic syndrome are at risk for catastrophic thrombotic thrombocytopenic purpura. The hematologic evaluation of patients with SLE and vasculitis or coagulation disorders should include a search for circulating abnormal vWF multimers.

▶ This is another disease entity where abnormally large von Willebrand's multimers have been identified in the circulating blood. It is now being recognized that in several diseases, these abnormally large multimeric von Willebrand's proteins can be observed. Thus, it is becoming clearer that abnormally large von Willebrand's multimers are not specific for thrombotic thrombocytopenic purpura/hemolytic uremic syndrome (TTP-HUS). It is noteworthy that none of these other disease entities have the classic features of TTP-HUS, such as red cell fragmentation, severe thrombocytopenia, and striking elevations in serum lactate dehydrogenase.—W.R. Bell, M.D.

Mechanisms of Thrombin Generation During Surgery and Cardiopulmonary Bypass
Boisclair MD, Lane DA, Philippou H, Esnouf MP, Sheikh S, Hunt B, Smith KJ (Charing Cross and Westminster Med School, London; Radcliffe Infirmary, Oxford, England; Harefield Hosp, Middlesex, England; et al)
Blood 82:3350–3357, 1993   116-95-3–47

Background.—In vivo studies have contributed greatly to the understanding of the complex biochemistry of blood coagulation. However, the mechanisms of the in vivo response to hypercoagulable stimuli are still unclear. Plasma-based enzyme-linked immunosorbent assays (ELISAs) were used to investigate the mechanisms that activate the coagulation system in vivo during cardiopulmonary bypass surgery.

Method.—A novel immunoassay for factor XIIa was used to detect activation of the contact system; factor IX activation peptide (FIXAP) was used as a marker for the activation of factor IX; and prothrombin fragment F1 + 2 was used as a marker for the generation of thrombin.

Results.—Levels of F1 + 2 increased in response to surgical intervention even before blood was diverted into an external circuit. From then on, F1 + 2 levels increased significantly during surgery and bypass to a maximum of 448.5 ng/mL. Levels of factor XIIa increased slightly in response to surgical intervention before the establishment of extracorporeal circulation. However, no evidence was found to support the belief that exposure of blood to foreign surfaces in the bypass machine brings activation of the contact system of coagulation. Levels of FIXAP increased later in surgery from 4.98 ng/mL to a maximum of 10.2 ng/mL. The increase began at the time of near-maximum F1 + 2 levels. There was no correlation between activation of the contact system (factor XIIa levels) and the generation of thrombin (F1 + 2 levels). However, a strong correlation was found between the generation of thrombin (F1 + 2 levels) and FIXAP levels, despite a delay in the time between the activation of prothrombin and factor IX.

Conclusion.—These results do not support the accepted view that contact activation resulting from exposure of blood to foreign surfaces is the principal procoagulant stimulus in cardiopulmonary bypass surgery. Instead, they suggest that the major trigger to coagulation during this surgery is the tissue factor–factor VIIa mechanism response to the cutting of blood vessels, which directly activates factor X and then prothrombin. Late activation of factor IX, which probably contributes to maximal prothrombin activation, may have arisen because of direct tissue factor–factor VIIa action because of secondary feedback activity of thrombin on the intrinsic system.

▶ Boisclair et al. have clearly and very carefully identified that thrombin generation does occur during cardiopulmonary bypass. This may be why there is a greater propensity for thrombotic obstruction of bypass tubing. It also may provide an explanation for the observation that thrombocytopenia occurs during this procedure. It will be important to repeat these studies in patients receiving hirudin in contrast to those undergoing bypass while receiving heparin anticoagulation. This is particularly important because hirudin has a greater capacity to prevent the activation of, as well as to neutralize, thrombin than does heparin.—W.R. Bell, M.D.

Thrombosis and Hormone Replacement Therapy in Postmenopausal Women
Saleh AA, Dorey LG, Dombrowski MP, Ginsburg KA, Hirokawa S, Kowalczyk C, Hirata J, Bottoms S, Cotton DB, Mammen EF (Grace Hosp, Detroit; Hutzel Hosp, Detroit; Pontiac Gen Hosp, Detroit; et al)
Am J Obstet Gynecol 169:1554–1557, 1993   116-95-3–48

TABLE 1.–Results of Multivariate Analysis of Covariance Comparing Levels of Prothrombin Fragment 1 + 2 and Thrombin–Antithrombin III Complex in 68 Postmenopausal Women Receiving Hormonal Replacement Therapy and 38 Postmenopausal Controls

	Controls (n = 38)	Hormone replacement therapy (n = 68)	F ratio	Significance
Age as a covariate				
Prothrombin fragment 1 + 2 (nmol/L)	1.0 ± 0.4	1.3 ± 0.8	1.45	NS
			1.06	NS
Thrombin–antithrombin III complex	3.0 ± 4.8	2.2 ± 0.9	3.27	NS

* Age was used as a covariate. Results are expressed as mean ± standard deviation. NS, nonsignificant difference, $P > .05$.
(Courtesy of Saleh AA, Dorey LG, Dombrowski MP, et al: Am J Obstet Gynecol 169:1554–1557, 1993.)

Introduction.—Postmenopausal hormone replacement has clearly benefited women with respect to cardiovascular status, osteoporosis, cholesterol changes, and genitourinary disturbances, but its effects on thrombosis remain uncertain.

TABLE 2.—Results of Multivariate Analysis of Variance Comparing the Levels of Prothrombin Fragment 1 + 2 and Thrombin–Antithrombin III Complex in 26 Postmenopausal Women Receiving Estrogen Alone and 42 Postmenopausal Women Receiving Estrogen and Progestin

	Estrogen alone (n = 26)	Estrogen and progestin (n = 42)	Significance
Age (yr)	55 ± 6	54 ± 6	NS*
Prothrombin fragment 1 + 2 (nmol/L)	1.3 ± 0.6	1.3 ± 0.9	NS†
Thrombin–antithrombin III complex (µg/L)	2.0 ± 0.6	2.4 ± 1.0	NS†

Note: Age was not used as a covariate because the Student's t-test did not show significant differences between the 2 groups. Results are expressed as mean ± standard deviation.
* Nonsignificant difference by Student's t-test, P > .05.
† Nonsignificant difference by multivariate analysis of variance, P > .05.
(Courtesy of Saleh AA, Dorey LG, Dombrowski MP, et al: Am J Obstet Gynecol 169:1554–1557, 1993.)

Study Design.—Clotting status was examined using new markers in a prospective series of 106 postmenopausal women, 68 of whom were receiving hormone replacement therapy. Forty-two of these women received estrogen and progestin cyclically, whereas 26 received only estrogen. Almost all of the women used conjugated estrogens in the form of

Premarin in a daily dose of .625 or 1.25 mg. The progestin, medroxyprogesterone acetate, was administered orally for 10 days in each cycle. Plasma levels of prothrombin fragment 1 + 2 and thrombin-antithrombin III complex were measured by enzyme-linked immunosorbent assay.

Results.—When controlling for age, there were no significant differences in the levels of either marker between the postmenopausal women receiving hormone replacement therapy and the controls (Table 1). There were also no significant differences between the postmenopausal controls and a group of 29 healthy, nonpregnant younger women receiving no medication. Marker levels were comparable in postmenopausal women receiving both estrogen and progestin and those receiving estrogen alone (Table 2).

Implications.—These findings allay concern that postmenopausal administration of estrogen and progesterone promote hypercoagulability, but some patients clearly do have thromboembolic problems while receiving hormone replacement. These patients might have other risk factors predisposing them to thrombosis, such as hyperactive platelets, atherosclerotic disease, or lupus anticoagulant.

▶ This study, which examined a relatively small population of postmenopausal women receiving hormone replacement with relatively low doses of estrogen compounds, indicated that there was no evidence of activation of the coagulation system in these women in comparison to controls. These data support the contention that hormone replacement in an attempt to prevent the development or progression of osteoporosis can be safely administered in postmenopausal women. However, it may be reasonable to screen such women, before hormone replacement is administered, for the presence of a lupus-like inhibitor. When tests for lupus inhibitor are positive, there may be an enhanced tendency to form thrombosis when hormone replacement is employed.—W.R. Bell, M.D.

Plasminogen Activators, Plasminogen Activator Inhibitors and Markers of Intravascular Coagulation in Pre-Eclampsia

Koh SCL, Anandakumar C, Montan S, Ratnam SS (Natl Univ of Singapore)
Gynecol Obstet Invest 35:214–221, 1993   116-95-3-49

Background.—Widespread fibrin deposition is a prominent histologic finding in fatal cases of eclampsia. Significantly decreased levels of plasminogen activator (PA) inhibitor (PAI)-2 have been associated with preeclampsia, whereas PAI-1 levels appear to be unchanged. Levels of PAs, PAIs, and markers of intravascular coagulation in preeclampsia and their relation to pregnancy outcomes were investigated.

Methods and Findings.—Data on 23 women with preeclampsia were analyzed. Decreased levels of plasma urokinase–like PA and PAI-2 were noted in these women with preeclampsia. Levels of plasma tissue-type

Plasminogen Activators, PAIs, and Intravascular Coagulation Markers and Platelets in Patients With Moderate and Severe Preeclampsia As Compared With Normal Pregnant Individuals

	Gestation weeks	t-PA IU/ml	ng/ml	uPA IU/ml	ng/ml	PAI-1 AU/ml	ng/ml	PAI-2 ng/ml [a]	D-dimer ng/ml	β-TG ng/ml	TAT µg/l	PLT ×10⁹/l
Normal pregnancy												
n	14	14	14	14	14	14	14	14	14	14	13	13
Mean	30.6	0.84	6.66	9.79	2.36	23.75	29.16	105.2	875.9	91.7	17.0	267.5
SD	3.76	0.32	2.79	9.95	2.38	10.56	18.54	22.0	983.2	127.8	11.0	77.2
Range	26–37	0.43–1.6	2.3–12.6	0.45–33.0	0.8–	5–43.5	14.8–90.4	62–144	112–3.700	18–480	4.8–32.8	168–440
Moderate and severe PE												
n	14	14	14	14	14	14	13	14	14	14	14	10
Mean	30.2	1.14	14.55	3.91	1.61	43.61	35.95	58.4	704.7	104.9	17.7	211.7
SD	5.2	0.88	5.66	5.32	0.62	32.89	18.99	34.9	477.4	58.5	13.0	71.9
Range	21–37	0.34–3.7	4.2–26.0	0.62–13.8	0.9–3.1	12–140	14–88	13–112	250–2,150	38–220	4.2–41.3	130–380
p	NS	NS	0.001	<0.05	0.05	<0.05	NS	<0.001	NS	NS	NS	NS

Abbreviations: n, number of samples; *PLT*, platelets.
(Courtesy of Koh SCL, Anandakumar C, Montan S, et al: *Gynecol Obstet Invest* 35:214–221, 1993.)

PA antigen were increased. Most of the women with moderate and severe preeclampsia delivered preterm. Those with moderate and severe preeclampsia had significantly lower concentrations of PAI-2 and urokinase-like PA antigen than patients with mild preeclampsia. Also, women with moderate and severe preeclampsia had significantly increased tissue-type PA antigen compared with those with mild preeclampsia. Compared with normal pregnancy values, the PAI-1 activity was significantly increased only in moderate and severe preeclampsia. No significant differences were seen in levels of thrombin–antithrombin III complexes, D-dimer, or β-thromboglobulin between women with preeclampsia and those with normal pregnancies. However, these values were above nonpregnant levels. Platelets in women with preeclampsia were within the normal pregnancy range (table).

Conclusion.—The measurement of urokinase-like PA and PAI-2 levels in preeclampsia may have a prognostic value in determining pregnancy outcomes. Further research is needed to confirm these findings.

▶ These authors have indicated that there is, indeed, evidence of activity of the fibrinolytic system in this disease state. It appears relatively clear that the greatest center of activity results from disturbance or alteration of endothelial cells. These data suggest that this disorder may largely be caused by endothelial cell damage or perhaps that endothelial cell damage is a secondary phenomenon in this disease entity. These data add more support for the contention that this disease process is related to the disease entity of thrombotic thrombocytopenic purpura/hemolytic uremic syndrome (TTP-HUS). It would be important to assay for additional endothelial cell–associated proteins such as thrombomodulin and unusually large von Willebrand's multimers. Such information may help to understand why this disease process is self-limiting and why it terminates with the delivery of the uterine contents without going on to a more full-blown spectrum of the disease process designated TTP-HUS.—W.R. Bell, M.D.

Features of Thrombi and Diagnostic Accuracy of Impedance Plethysmography in Symptomatic and Asymptomatic Deep Vein Thrombosis
Agnelli G, Cosmi B, Radicchia S, Veschi F, Boschetti E, Lupattelli L, Rinonapoli E, Nenci GG (Università di Perugia, Italy)
Thromb Haemost 70:266–269, 1993   116-95-3–50

Background.—For patients with symptomatic deep venous thrombosis (DVT), impedance plethysmography (IPG) is a highly sensitive and specific diagnostic procedure. However, it is insufficiently sensitive in high-risk asymptomatic patients. Whether differing features of thrombi such as location, size, and occlusiveness could account for the differing accuracy of IPG in patients with symptomatic DVT and those with asymptomatic DVT was investigated.

Comparison of the Accuracy of IPG in the Diagnosis of DVT in
Symptomatic and Asymptomatic Patients

	Symptomatic patients	Asymptomatic patients	p
Sensitivity	84% (27/32)	18% (26/149)	0.0001
95% CL	70%–98%	12%–24%	
Specificity	83% (45/54)	92% (270/294)	n. s.
95% CL	72%–94%	88%–95%	
P.P.V.	75% (27/36)	52% (26/50)	0.03
95% CL	59%–90%	38%–66%	
N.P.V.	94% (47/50)	92% (270/293)	n. s.
95% CL	87%–100%	89%–95%	

Abbreviations: 95% CL, 95% confidence limits; P.P.V., positive predictive value; N.P.V., negative predictive values.
(Courtesy of Agnelli G, Cosmi B, Radicchia S, et al: *Thromb Haemost* 70:266–269, 1993.)

Methods.—Two groups of patients were studied: 1 group included 117 consecutive outpatients with clinical suspicion of DVT, and the other included 246 consecutive patients scheduled for hip surgery. All of the symptomatic patients underwent IPG on the day of referral and then venography. The asymptomatic patients underwent IPG as part of a DVT surveillance program and then bilateral venography.

Results.—Venography documented DVT in 37% of the symptomatic and 34% of the asymptomatic limbs. Impedance plethysmography was much more accurate in the symptomatic group (table). Symptomatic patients were more likely than asymptomatic patients to have proximal DVTs, 78% vs. 46%. As a marker of thrombus size, the mean Marder score was higher in the symptomatic than the asymptomatic group, 19 vs. 10. Sixty-nine percent of DVTs in the symptomatic group were occlusive, compared with 36% in the asymptomatic group.

Conclusion.—In patients with asymptomatic DVT, the low accuracy of IPG may result from the high prevalence of small, distal, nonocclusive thrombi. Because these thrombi do not cause critical obstructions of venous outflow, they do not result in positive IPGs. For high-risk asymptomatic patients, venography is the only reliable technique for detecting DVT.

▶ This thoughtful study is one of a growing number of recently published reports that establish the unsatisfactory diagnostic accuracy of IPG. This information is not new to a host of investigators in the area of DVT. However, many physicians have continued to use this technique, as have some internationally recognized experts who have reported this technique to be highly accurate. It is disconcerting that such a prolonged period of time has been necessary before the truth finally emerged. Particularly disconcerting is the fact that some investigators who strongly recommended this technique now condemn it. For additional information on this topic, please see the references (1, 2).—W.R. Bell, M.D.

References

1. Anderson DR, et al: *Ann Intern Med* 118:25, 1993.
2. Davidson BL, et al: *Ann Intern Med* 117:735, 1992.

A Comparative Analysis of D-Dimer Assays in Patients With Clinically Suspected Pulmonary Embolism

van Beek EJR, van den Ende B, Berckmans RJ, van der Heide YT, Brandjes DPM, Sturk A, ten Cate JW (Univ of Amsterdam; Slotervaart Hosp, Amsterdam)

Thromb Haemost 70:408–413, 1993   116-95-3–51

Background.—Sensitive and specific assays are available for the detection of fibrinogen degradation or activation products or, in the case of the D-dimer assay, fibrin split products. These tests have come into use as a means of indirectly confirming or rejecting the diagnosis of venous thromboembolic diseases, and D-dimer assays using enzyme-linked immunosorbent assay (ELISA)/EIA and latex methods have been recommended. A comparative analysis of D-dimer assays in patients with clinically suspected pulmonary embolism was conducted focusing on patients with nondiagnostic lung scans.

Methods.—The sample included 151 consecutive patients with clinically suspected pulmonary embolism. Forty-three had normal lung scan results, 48 had high-probability scans, and 60 had nondiagnostic scans. Of the latter group, 43 underwent angiography, which demonstrated pulmonary emboli in 12 patients. Six commercially available D-dimer kits were assessed, including 4 ELISAs and 2 latex agglutination–based assays. These tests were compared for reproducibility, cutoff values, specificity, and percentage of patients in whom angiography could be avoided at a sensitivity of 100%.

Results.—At a cutoff point of 500 µg/L, the latex assays agreed with the corresponding ELISAs in 81% to 83% of patients. Fifteen percent of patients had a normal latex assay and abnormal ELISA, whereas 7% had a normal latex assay and abnormal ELISA. With the ELISAs, intraassay variation was 2% to 17%, and interassay variation was 12% to 26%. Cutoff values for the ELISAs were 25 µg/L for the Behring test, 50 µg/L for the Agen test, 300 µg/L for the Stago test, and 550 µg/L for the Organon test, with specificities ranging from 14% to 38%. It was possible to avoid angiography in only 4% to 15% of patients.

Conclusion.—In patients with clinically suspected pulmonary embolism, latex D-dimer assays are not useful, and ELISA techniques are of only limited value in excluding the diagnosis. Some diagnostic test with the accuracy of an ELISA/EIA and the performance properties of a latex test is urgently needed. If they were standardized and calibrated, D-dimer assays would be more clinically useful.

▶ In this rather extensive and carefully detailed study, 6 commercially available D-dimer kits were used to detect the presence of fibrin fragment D-dimer in patients with suspected pulmonary emboli. The amount of testing that was done was absolutely extensive and comprehensive. The authors were easily able to conclude that this particular diagnostic test was useless in identifying the presence of pulmonary emboli. This particular technique of looking for various fragments of fibrinogen or fibrin, or both, has been thoroughly studied in the past. Although 1 or 2 reports suggested its utility, most reports, including a rather extensive study (1), concluded that this test was completely useless for identifying the presence of pulmonary emboli. It is absolutely amazing to see the same type of technique repeatedly employed over 20 years, identified time after time to be without any usefulness, but yet somehow still studied. During the next 20 years, how many times will the same technique be employed in an attempt to make the diagnosis of endogenous thrombose formation? For similar work in this area, please see references 2 and 3.—W.R. Bell, M.D.

References

1. Light RW, Bell WR: *Arch Intern Med* 133:372, 1974.
2. Gogstad GO, et al: *Clin Chem* 39:2070, 1993.
3. Trofatter KF Jr, et al: *South Med J* 86:1017, 1993.

Blood Viscosity, Fibrinogen, and Activation of Coagulation and Leukocytes in Peripheral Arterial Disease and the Normal Population in the Edinburgh Artery Study

Lowe GDO, Fowkes FGR, Dawes J, Donnan PT, Lennie SE, Housley E (Glasgow Royal Infirmary, Scotland; Univ of Edinburgh, Scotland; MRC/Scottish Natl Blood Transfusion Service Blood Components Assay Group, Edinburgh, Scotland)
Circulation 87:1915–1920, 1993   116-95-3-52

Background.—Previous studies have reported that patients with claudication experience increased blood and plasma viscosity, hematocrit, fibrinogen, and activation of coagulation and leukocytes. The relationship between these factors and symptomatic and asymptomatic peripheral artery disease was examined.

Patients and Methods.—A random sample of 1,581 men and women aged 55–74 years in Edinburgh, Scotland participated. Measurements of blood and plasma viscosity, hematocrit, fibrinogen urinary fibrinopeptide A, plasma leukocyte elastase, and uric acid were taken. These were then related to peripheral arterial stenosis via ankle-brachial systolic pressure index (ABPI) and to lower-limb ischemia via intermittent claudication questionnaire and reactive hyperemia tests.

Results.—With the exception of fibrinopeptide A, each variable was significantly associated with prevalent symptomatic and asymptomatic peripheral arterial disease. Multivariate analysis revealed that blood viscosity and fibrinogen were independently associated with peripheral arterial narrowing (ABPI). In addition, a positive interaction was noted between fibrinogen and smoking in the association with ABPI. In the presence of a given degree of arterial narrowing, plasma viscosity was correlated with claudication. Finally, leukocyte elastase and uric acid were associated with reactive hyperemia independently of arterial narrowing.

Conclusion.—In the general population, blood rheologic factors, leukocyte activation, and arterial narrowing are related to lower-limb ischemia, and may play a role in its pathogenesis.

▶ This sizable study supports previous observations that plasma fibrinogen may be a very important marker for the presence of peripheral arterial intraluminal narrowing, ischemia, and eventual obstruction. Elevated fibrinogen results in increase in plasma viscosity, and with increase in viscosity there is actual activation of coagulation proteins in white cells. The question must be raised whether fibrinogen will actually become a marker for atheromatous disease, a position that has been occupied by cholesterol for the past several decades.—W.R. Bell, M.D.

Fibrinogen and the Albumin-Globulin Ratio in Recurrent Stroke
Beamer N, Coull BM, Sexton G, de Garmo P, Knox R, Seaman G (Oregon Health Sciences Univ, Portland)
Stroke 24:1133–1139, 1993   116-95-3–53

Background.—In patients initially enrolled in a cross-sectional study of blood viscosity in ischemic cerebrovascular disease, those having a low albumin-globulin ratio seemed to experience most of the subsequent vascular events. Patients were placed in a high- or low-albumin globulin cohort, and the association between a low albumin-globulin ratio, clinical risk factors for stroke, and the incidence of subsequent stroke, myocardial infarction, or vascular death was evaluated.

Patients and Methods.—A total of 126 patients with acute ischemic stroke (group 1), 109 individuals matched with group 1 for age, medications, and recognized clinical risk factors for stroke (group 2), and 84 healthy volunteers matched with groups 1 and 2 for age (group 3) were included. The average follow-up was 1.5 years. At enrollment, the median albumin-globulin ratio for group 1 was 1.45. This ratio was used to categorize patients into 2 cohorts: those with ratios of 1.45 or less were

TABLE 1.—Distribution of Recurrent Vascular Events

Type of event	Group 1		Group 2		Group 3		Total
	Low* (n=65)	High† (n=61)	Low* (n=29)	High† (n=80)	Low* (n=9)	High† (n=75)	
New stroke	15	8	2	1	0	0	26
Vascular death	11	3	2	2	0	1	19
Myocardial infarction	1	1	1	0	0	3	6
Total	27	12	5	3	0	4	51

* Albumin-globulin (A-G) ratio ≤ 1.45.
† A-G ratio > 1.45.
(Courtesy of Beamer N, Coull BM, Sexton G, et al: Stroke 24:1133–1139, 1993.)

placed in the low albumin-globulin group, whereas those with ratios greater than 1.45 were assigned to the high albumin-globulin cohort. Subsequent hospitalizations, outpatient visits, and telephone interviews with patients and providers were used to verify the incidence of vascular end points.

TABLE 2.—Relative Risk for a Vascular Event (Univariate)

Factor	Group 1	Group 2	Groups 1 and 2
Low A-G ratio	2.1*	4.6	3.2
(≤1.45)	1.2-3.8†	1.2-18.0	1.8-5.6
	<.01‡	<.03	<.0001
High fibrinogen	1.9	0.4	2.0
(≥397 mg/dL)	1.1-3.3	0.05-2.8	1.2-3.3
	<.03	NS	<.02
Diabetes	1.6	3.4	2.1
	1.0-2.8	0.08-14.1	1.2-3.5
	NS	NS	<.01
History of prior stroke	1.6	1.4	1.9
	1.0-2.7	0.4-5.5	1.1-3.1
	NS	NS	<.02
Ischemic heart disease	1.3	6.3	1.6
	0.8-2.2	0.8-51.0	1.0-2.8
	NS	<.06	NS
Hypertension	1.1	2.1	1.2
	0.6-1.8	0.5-10.0	0.7-2.0
	NS	NS	NS

Abbreviations: A-G, albumin-globulin; NS, not significant.
* Relative risk.
† 95% confidence level.
‡ P determined by Fisher's exact test.
(Courtesy of Beamer N, Coull BM, Sexton G, et al: *Stroke* 24:1133–1139, 1993.)

Results.—Overall, 51 vascular events occurred, including 39 in group 1, 8 in group 2, and 4 in group 3 (Table 1). Patients in groups 1 and 2 in the low albumin-globulin cohort had at least twice the risk for a subsequent vascular event when compared with those in the high albumin-globulin cohort. In addition, significantly more group 1 patients in the low albumin-globulin cohort had a history of previous stroke, compared with the high albumin-globulin cohort. A Cox proportional-hazards analysis revealed that both low albumin-globulin ratios and diabetes had a significant independent association with increased risk for subsequent vascular events when groups 1 and 2 were combined (Table 2).

Conclusion.—In patients with stroke and those with clinical risk factors for stroke, shifts in blood protein concentrations to a prothrombotic environment characterized by lower levels of albumin and increased globulin and fibrinogen concentrations are associated with significantly increased risks for subsequent vascular events.

Plasma Fibrinogen and Its Correlates in Children From a Biracial Community: The Bogalusa Heart Study

Bao W, Srinivasan SR, Berenson GS (Tulane Univ, New Orleans, La)
Pediatr Res 33:323–326, 1993   116-95-3-54

Background.—The relationships of fibrinogen to other risk factors for coronary heart disease have been studied extensively in adults. Information on children is limited. The Bogalusa Heart Study revealed that coronary atherosclerosis and racial differences in cardiovascular risk begin in childhood. The association between fibrinogen and other cardiovascular risk factors in children was examined.

Methods.—Fibrinogen levels were measured in 3,047 children aged 5–17 years; 40% of the children were black and 49% were girls. Questionnaires elicited information about health habits, including cigarette smoking, alcohol consumption, and oral contraceptive use, as well as parental history of cardiovascular disease, stroke, and diabetes mellitus.

Results.—There were no significant race and sex differences in fibrinogen levels, although levels increased with age or sexual maturation in black girls. After adjustment for age, fibrinogen concentration correlated with ponderal index, triceps skinfold thickness, and subcapsular skinfold thickness for all race-sex groups, with the strongest correlation in white girls. Fibrinogen correlated significantly with increased WBC count for white children. Step-wise regression revealed an independent association between fibrinogen and ponderal index, WBC count, and high-density lipoprotein cholesterol (table). Children with the highest fibrinogen concentration were more likely to have increases in other risk factors and a significantly higher prevalence of maternal diabetes mellitus and paternal hypertension.

Significant Predictors of Fibrinogen by Race and Sex:
The Bogalusa Heart Study

	Caucasian males (n = 905)	Caucasian females (n = 851)	Black males (n = 597)	Black females (n = 567)
	PI	PI	PI	Height
	−HDL-C	WBC	WBC	PI
	WBC	Height		−HDL-C
		LDL-C		
R^2	0.0416	0.0903	0.0296	0.076

Abbreviations: PI, ponderal index (weight/height³); HDL-C, high-density lipoprotein cholesterol; LDL-C, low-density lipoprotein cholesterol.
(Courtesy of Bao W, Srinivasan SR, Berenson GS: *Pediatr Res* 33:323–326, 1993.)

Discussion.—The relationship of fibrinogen levels to myocardial infarction, stroke, and peripheral vascular disease cannot be determined in children. Nevertheless, childhood fibrinogen levels may continue into adulthood and contribute to arterial intimal atherosclerotic changes. Because obesity is a risk factor for peripheral thrombosis and obesity strongly correlates with higher fibrinogen levels, the genetic factors that control obesity may also regulate fibrinogen levels. Thus, control of the accepted adult risk factors (e.g., weight, exercise, diet, and smoking) should also apply to children.

▶ These 2 reports (Abstracts 116-94-3–53 and 116-95-3–54) add to the growing list of articles that are providing progressively more evidence to indicate that plasma fibrinogen concentration is an important risk factor for adverse cardiovascular events, and, in addition, an important predictor for future cardiovascular events. It is perhaps no surprise that fibrinogen is critically important with respect to cardiovascular events, because without it, thrombus formation does not occur.—W.R. Bell, M.D.

Fibrinogen in Relation to Personal History of Prevalent Hypertension, Diabetes, Stroke, Intermittent Claudication, Coronary Heart Disease, and Family History: The Scottish Heart Health Study

Lee AJ, Lowe GDO, Woodward M, Tunstall-Pedoe H (Ninewells Hosp and Med School, Dundee, Scotland; Royal Infirmary, Glasgow, Scotland; Reading Univ, Scotland)
Br Heart J 69:338–342, 1993   116-95-3–55

Introduction.—Recent reports of 5 epidemiologic studies relate the plasma fibrinogen concentration to the incidence of coronary heart dis-

TABLE 1.—Mean (Standard Error) Plasma Fibrinogen (g/L) by Indicators of Myocardial Infarction

Indicators of myocardial infarction	Men	Women
Medical history	2·55 (0·05)***	2·80 (0·11)***
	n = 209	n = 58
Rose chest pain questionnaire	2·40 (0·04)***	2·56 (0·06) ***
	n = 306	n = 181
Electrocardiogram (Q/QS)	2·61 (0·09) ***	2·62 (0·12)*
	n = 90	n = 24
No cardiovascular or related disease	2·27 (0·01)	2·34 (0·01)
	n = 3367	n = 3096

* $P < .05$.
*** $P < .001$ for indicator vs. no disease group (t-tests).
(Courtesy of Lee AJ, Lowe GDO, Woodward M, et al: *Br Heart J* 69:338–342, 1993.)

TABLE 2.—Mean (Standard Error) Plasma Fibrinogen (g/L) by
Indicators of Angina and Ischemia

Indicators of angina	Men	Women
Medical history	2·53 (0·05)***	2·57 (0·05)***
	n = 236	n = 157
Rose chest pain	2·48 (0·05)***	2·50 (θ·05)***
questionnaire	n = 248	n = 299
Electrocardiogram	2·44 (0·05)***	2·42 (0·03)**
(Whitehall-ischaemia)	n = 363	n = 391
No cardiovascular or	2·27 (0·01)	2·34 (0·01)
related disease	n = 3367	n = 3096

* P < .01.
*** P < .001.
(Courtesy of Lee AJ, Lowe GDO, Woodward M, et al: Br Heart J 69:338–342, 1993.)

ease, but only 2 of them have correlated baseline plasma fibrinogen levels with prevalent coronary disease.

Study Population.—Plasma fibrinogen levels were related to a number of factors in 8,824 middle-aged men and women aged 40–59 years who were entered in the Scottish Heart Health Study, a random population survey in local governmental districts in Scotland.

Findings.—Participants who had a parent or sibling with premature heart disease had significantly higher fibrinogen levels than others, as did those with a self-reported history of high blood pressure, diabetes, stroke, or intermittent claudication. Men and women with indicators of myocardial infarction (history, chest pain, ECG abnormalities) had significantly higher plasma fibrinogen levels than others (Table 1). In addition, persons with any evidence of angina had significantly increased plasma fibrinogen levels (Table 2). After adjusting for other coronary risk factors, the risk for both myocardial infarction and angina increased linearly with the fibrinogen concentration.

Conclusion.—This large population study affirms that the plasma fibrinogen concentration is a risk factor for coronary heart disease.

▶ This is yet another large study that strongly suggests that plasma fibrinogen concentration is a risk factor for the development of coronary heart disease and stroke, as well as hypertension, diabetes, and peripheral vascular disease. These data, along with many additional data from studies done during the past 5 years, strongly support the contention of plasma fibrinogen concentration as an important cardiovascular risk factor and deserve serious attention and consideration.—W.R. Bell, M.D.

Haematocrit: A Predictor of Cardiovascular Mortality?

Erikssen G, Thaulow E, Sandvik L, Stormorken H, Erikssen J (Akershus Cen-

tral Hosp, Nordbyhagen, Norway; Natl Univ Hosp, Oslo, Norway)
J Intern Med 234:493–499, 1993   116-95-3-56

Background.—There appears to be a positive link between blood viscosity and peripheral vascular disease. Because 75% of blood viscosity is accounted for by hematocrit, it seems likely that there is a similar association between hematocrit and cardiovascular disease (CVD). Such an association was assessed.

Methods.—An extensive examination program was carried out on 2,014 apparently healthy men with no suspected symptoms of heart disease. The examination involved blood tests, spirographic studies, resting ECG, and a symptom-limited bicycle test. Hematocrit measurements were also done in a 25% random subsample. Sequential, cause-specific mortality was monitored prospectively for 16 years.

Results.—Hematocrit measures were taken in 488 men aged 40–59 years. The mean hematocrit obtained was 47.2%. After corrections were made for differences in age, plasma cholesterol, systolic blood pressure, erythrocyte sedimentation rate, and smoking habits, an increase in hematocrit by 2 SDs was associated with an increase in CVD mortality by a factor ranging from 2.9 at 10 years and 1.9 at 16 years of follow-up (Fig 3–12). No association was seen between hematocrit and non-CVD mortality.

Conclusion.—Hematocrit apparently acts as an independent risk factor for death from CVD. Because of the ease of measuring hematocrit, it is suggested that it be included systematically in future epidemiologic

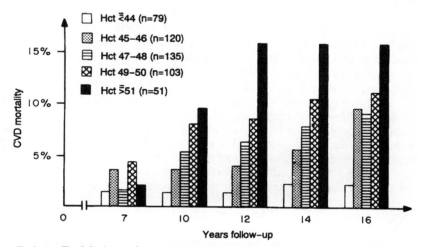

Fig 3–12.—Total death rates from CVD by hematocrit (Hct) groups after 8, 10, 12, 14, and 16 years of follow-up. (Courtesy of Erikssen G, Thaulow E, Sandvik L, et al: *J Intern Med* 234:493–499, 1993.)

studies, and, if these results are confirmed by others, it should become an integral part of future screening for risk of CVD in middle-aged men.

▶ This potentially important study provides reasonably convincing evidence that elevated hematocrit values are associated with an increased risk for CVD. It is unfortunate in this otherwise thoroughly comprehensive study that plasma fibrinogen concentrations were not measured. In the minds of many investigators, plasma fibrinogen has recently been shown to be more predictive than cholesterol for risk of premature death from CVDs. Perhaps the investigators have specimens that could be retrospectively employed to measure plasma fibrinogen.—W.R. Bell, M.D.

Anticoagulation Therapy

Risk Factors for Complications of Chronic Anticoagulation: A Multicenter Study
Fihn SD, for the Warfarin Optimized Outpatient Follow-Up Study Group (Seattle Veterans Affairs Med Ctr)
Ann Intern Med 118:511–520, 1993   116-95-3–57

Background.—An increasing number of patients are currently receiving warfarin therapy. The risk factors for complications associated with this treatment were investigated.

Methods.—Five anticoagulation clinics participated in a retrospective cohort study. Data on the occurrence of hemorrhagic and thromboembolic complications in 928 consecutive patients receiving a total of 1,003 courses of warfarin were analyzed.

Findings.—In 1,950 patient-years of follow-up, 1,332 bleeding events occurred. Four were fatal; 31 were life-threatening; 226 were serious; and 1,071 were minor (Tables 1 and 2). At 1 and 3 years, the cumulative incidences of fatal bleeding were 1% and 2%, respectively. The cumulative incidences of first episodes of life-threatening and serious bleeding were, respectively, 1% and 12% at 1 year, 2% and 20% at 2 years, 5% and 28% at 4 years, and 9% and 40% at 8 years. Of the 156 patients with serious or life-threatening hemorrhage, 32% had a recurrence, usually within 1 year. Independent predictors of a first episode of serious hemorrhage were a mean prothrombin time ratio (PTR) of 2 or more during treatment, recent initiation of warfarin treatment, variability of PTR with time, and 3 or more co-morbid conditions. Factors unassociated with risk for bleeding were age, reason for anticoagulation, use of interfering drugs, and hypertension. The risk associated with a thromboembolic complication at a PTR of less than 1.3 was 3.6 times higher than that at PTRs of 1.3 to 1.5.

Conclusion.—Attention to modifiable risk factors, frequent monitoring early in treatment, and careful patient selection may decrease the incidence of warfarin-related bleeding complications. Older age does not appear to be a risk factor.

TABLE 1.—Frequency of Bleeding Complications

Severity Classification	First Bleeding Complications		All Bleeding Complications	
	Number	Rate *events/100 patient-years*	Number	Rate *events/100 patient-years*
Minor	337	17.3	1071	54.9
Serious	147	7.5	226	11.6
Life-threatening	22	1.1	31	1.6
Fatal	4	0.2	4	0.2
Total	510		1332	

(Courtesy of Fihn SD, for the Warfarin Optimized Outpatient Follow-Up Study Group: *Ann Intern Med* 118:511–520, 1993.)

TABLE 2.—Sites of Bleeding Complications

Type	First Bleeding Complications			All Bleeding Complications		
	Serious	Life-Threatening	Fatal	Serious	Life-Threatening	Fatal
	n					
Epistaxis or gingival bleeding	18	0	0	35	0	0
Hematoma	9	0	0	13	0	0
Uterine bleeding	5	2	0	7	2	0
Hematuria	31	0	0	47	0	0
Hemoptysis	10	1	0	14	1	0
Gastrointestinal bleeding	24	14	4	35	23	4
Cerebral bleeding	3	2	0	3	2	0
Retinal bleeding	5	0	0	5	0	0
Excessive bleeding with trauma	7	1	0	7	1	0
Other or multiple sites	35	2	0	60	2	0
Total	147	22	4	226	30	4

(Courtesy of Fihn SD, for the Warfarin Optimized Outpatient Follow-Up Study Group: *Ann Intern Med* 118:511–520, 1993.)

▶ This thoroughly detailed study provides some valuable information regarding the risk of bleeding associated with warfarin anticoagulation. One of the most revealing findings in this excellent study was that patients who have a less-than-therapeutic PTR have a fourfold greater frequency of thromboembolic complications than if their PTR was in the therapeutic range. Not surprising is the frequency of hemorrhage in those patients whose PTRs were frequently out of control. Attention to detail will clearly result in a lower frequency of hemorrhage associated with such anticoagulation.—W.R. Bell, M.D.

Unexpectedly High Rate of Phlebographic Deep Venous Thrombosis Following Elective General Abdominal Surgery Among Patients Given Prophylaxis With Low-Molecular-Weight Heparin

Bounameaux H, Huber O, Khabiri E, Schneider P-A, Didier D, Rohner A (Univ Hosp, Geneva)

Arch Surg 128:326–328, 1993   116-95-3–58

Background.—Administration of subcutaneous low-molecular-weight heparin after general abdominal surgery has been shown by fibrinogen-uptake tests to decrease the frequency of deep venous thrombosis (DVT) by 65%. The diagnostic accuracy of 2 possible alternatives to the fibrinogen uptake test was assessed, and the frequency of phlebographically documented postoperative DVT was examined.

Methods.—A total of 194 patients undergoing general abdominal surgery were randomized in a single-blind study to receive either 1 daily subcutaneous injection of 2,500 IU of dalteparin sodium, or 3,075 IU of nadroparin calcium. Both of these regimens are currently used in Europe to prevent DVT. Liquid crystal contact thermography was performed postoperatively and every second day after surgery. Bilateral ascending phlebography was planned for the ninth postoperative day, together with blood sampling for plasma measurement of D-dimers.

Results.—Bilateral ascending leg phlebography revealed the presence of DVT in 45 of 185 patients tested. Thirty of these were in the group who received the lower dose compared with 15 in the higher-dose group.

Conclusion.—An unexpectedly high rate of phlebographically documented DVT after abdominal surgery was found despite prophylaxis with 2 approved regimens of low-molecular-weight heparin. The high rate of DVT seen here contrasts with past research rates of around 5% where fibrinogen uptake tests were used as the end point. The results indicate that the doses of low-molecular-weight heparin used may not confer sufficient protection in high-risk patients. They also suggest that the sensitivity of the fibrinogen uptake test may be much less than the 90% reported in the past. Caution should therefore be exercised when observing rates of DVTs derived using the fibrinogen uptake test as a single diagnostic tool. The findings indicate that the efficacy of prophylaxis was related to dose: fewer cases of DVT were seen in the group receiving a higher dose. However, the high rate of DVT in both groups suggests that an even greater dose may be required or that different low-molecular-weight heparin fractions should be investigated.

▶ The results of this appreciably sized patient population study indicate that there is a nearly 25% failure rate with the use of the newer low-molecular-weight heparin preparations. These results are in sharp contrast to a number of studies that reported a much lower frequency of postoperative DVT when such preparations are employed. It is unfortunate that in this study, another treatment arm did not contain standard unfractionated heparin. Critically important would be for this group of investigators to do a second study employing, in addition, unfractionated heparin. Ideal, also, would be a control group not receiving prophylactic heparin anticoagulation. Apparently both new preparations of low-molecular-weight heparin were equally ineffective.—W.R. Bell, M.D.

Prospective Comparative Study of Computer Programs Used for Management of Warfarin
Poller L, Wright D, Rowlands M (Withington Hosp, Manchester, England)
J Clin Pathol 46:299–303, 1993   116-95-3-59

Background.—Interest is increasing in the use of computer-based dosage programs to assist in managing outpatients receiving warfarin therapy. Previous research suggests that such programs can improve the control of long-term warfarin treatment and decrease demands on medical and secretarial personnel. The feasibility of computerized dosing during the critical early phase of warfarin treatment—and in the long term—was examined.

Results Obtained from New Patients or Those Receiving Long-Term Treatment

	Percentage of visits under anticoagulated	Percentage of visits within range	Percentage of visits over anticoagulated	Mean appointment interval (weeks)
New Patients				
Traditional	35.9	50.8	13.3	2.6
Charles	29.0	55.7	15.3	2.6
Coventry	29.6	54.3	16.0	3.1
Hillingdon	34.9	55.8	9.3	2.1
Long term warfarin				
Traditional	18.9	49.1	32.1	4.9
Charles	23.1	59.0	17.9	3.9
Coventry	17.0	51.1	31.9	3.4

(Courtesy of Poller L, Wright D, Rowlands M, et al: *J Clin Pathol* 46:299–303, 1993.)

Methods.—One hundred eighty-six patients who were receiving long-term treatment or who had just begun therapy were included. Three dosage programs were compared: the Hillingdon system AC version 3.1, the Charles Anticoagulant Clinic Manager, and the Coventry program. All 3 were examined in a pilot investigation, and 2 were included in a follow-up trial.

Findings.—Compared with traditional dosing methods, all 3 systems seemed to provide satisfactory control. The computerized programs provided significantly better control for patients receiving more intensive therapy with an assigned target range of 3–4.5 International Normalized Ratio (INR). By contrast, the medical staff undertreated these patients almost half of the time (table).

Conclusion.—For both early and long-term treatment, computer-based programs can assist outpatient anticoagulant control with warfarin. In most patients, the control achieved is as good as that obtained using traditional dosing methods by experienced clinic physicians. Medical staff tend to be too conservative in determining proper dosages for patients within the intense target range of 3–4.5 INR.

▶ This is a critically important and topical area for the management of patients who need anticoagulation on an outpatient basis. Although this system of employing computer programs theoretically sounds optimal, one must seriously question whether this effort will result in a reduction in the problem of hemorrhage, which is inherent in 7% to 12% of patients who take warfarin anticoagulation. Also, one must ask whether this system will result in patients more frequently being in the therapeutic range as opposed to under-coagulated.—W.R. Bell, M.D.

Low-Dose Warfarin Decreases Coagulability Without Affecting Prothrombin Complex Activity

Holm J, Berntorp E, Carlsson R, Erhardt L (Lund Univ, Malmö, Sweden)
J Intern Med 234:303–308, 1993 116-95-3–60

Background.—Full-dose warfarin treatment has been proved to have a preventive effect on cardiovascular mortality after myocardial infarction. However, full-dose anticoagulant therapy also brings a significantly higher risk of bleeding and the subsequent need for frequent and expensive prothrombin controls. The potential of fixed, low-dose warfarin in combination with aspirin in lowering factor VII coagulant activity (FVII:C) and its effects on the plasma coagulation cascade were investigated by measuring prothrombin fragment 1+2 (F1 + 2), protein C, and prothrombin.

Methods.—Included were 12 men with a history of myocardial infarction at least 3 years previously. All patients received 75 mg of aspirin daily. The study was performed during a 12-week period, starting with a daily dose of 1.25 mg of warfarin for the first 4 weeks, then an increased dose of 2.5 mg daily for the remaining 8 weeks. At baseline, prothrombin, coagulation factors VII and X, protein C, protein S, and F1 + 2 were measured twice with a 2-week interval. These measurements were then repeated every 2 weeks during treatment and for 4 weeks after cessation of warfarin. Blood hemoglobin analysis was also done at baseline and 4 weeks after treatment ended.

Results.—A daily dose of 1.25 mg of warfarin within a period of 4 weeks reduced the mean values of FVII:C from 113 units dL^{-1} at baseline to 107 units dL^{-1}. A similar decrease of F1 + 2 from 1.6 nmol 1^{-1} to 1.27 nmol 1^{-1} was seen. However, no significant change in protein C or P-prothrombin complex activity level was seen at this stage. Increasing the warfarin dose to 2.5 mg daily brought a further decrease in FVII:C and a decrease in protein C from 116% to 99%. P-prothrombin complex activity levels also decreased from 107% to 81%. Blood hemoglobin remained stable throughout warfarin treatment.

Conclusion.—A fixed dose of warfarin combined with a low dose of aspirin are a safe and effective treatment against arterial thrombotic disease and require only initial monitoring of prothrombin levels. Treatment with low-dose warfarin should be investigated further.

Effect of Low-Intensity Warfarin Anticoagulation on Level of Activity of the Hemostatic System in Patients With Atrial Fibrillation
Kistler JP, for the Boston Area Anticoagulation Trial for Atrial Fibrillation Investigators (Massachusetts Gen Hosp, Boston)
Stroke 24:1360–1365, 1993   116-95-3–61

Background.—In previous work, the Boston Area Anticoagulation Trial for Atrial Fibrillation (BAATAF) has demonstrated that low-intensity warfarin anticoagulation can safely decrease the stroke rate in patients with nonvalvular atrial fibrillation. It was presumed that this beneficial effect was caused by a decrease in clot formation in the cardiac atria. To examine this possibility, the effect of warfarin therapy on in vivo clotting was assessed in 125 patients in the BAATAF.

Methods.—Plasma samples were obtained from 62 patients in the warfarin treatment group and 63 in the control group. The plasma level of prothrombin activation fragment F1 + 2 was measured in each sample.

Results.—In the warfarin group, the mean level of this activation fragment was 71% lower than in the control group across all age groups and in both sexes. Approximately half of all controls were taking aspirin, but their activation fragment level was similar to controls not taking aspirin.

Conclusion.—Prothrombin activation was significantly suppressed in vivo by warfarin, but not aspirin, among patients in the BAATAF. These findings correlate with the significant decrease in ischemic stroke among patients treated with warfarin in the BAATAF.

▶ Both Abstracts 116-95-3–60 and 116-95-3–61 strongly support the use of low-dose warfarin anticoagulation; a dose of warfarin that does not prolong the prothrombin time may be efficacious in prophylactic prevention of thrombus formation. A mechanism whereby this may occur is postulated with a reduction in the concentration of the coagulant fraction of factor VII, designated factor VII:C. These observations may represent a very important advance in the therapeutic use of warfarin anticoagulation. Additional studies are obviously needed. If future studies support the present findings, then these findings may represent a very important advance in the therapeutic efficacy of warfarin anticoagulation, essentially avoiding the major undesirable side effect of this form of therapy, namely, hemorrhage.—W.R. Bell, M.D.

Mechanism of the Anticoagulant Effect of Warfarin as Evaluated in Rabbits by Selective Depression of Individual Procoagulant Vitamin K–Dependent Clotting Factors

Zivelin A, Rao LVM, Rapaport SI (Univ of California, San Diego)
J Clin Invest 92:2131–2140, 1993   116-95-3–62

Objective.—There have been only a few animal studies on the mechanism of the antithrombotic effect of warfarin. A rabbit model was used to determine how depression of each of the procoagulant vitamin K–dependent clotting factors relates to the function of warfarin as an anticoagulant.

Methods.—Rabbits were given a vitamin K–depleted diet beginning at various times before administration of warfarin. Warfarin was injected intravenously in a dose of .5 mg/kg/day for 5 days. Intravascular coagulation was induced by infusing a solution containing about 20 ng/mL of reconstituted tissue factor (TF) within 4 hours. Activities of individual procoagulation factors were estimated in assays using rabbit substrates.

Results.—In animals achieving a protective degree of anticoagulation from warfarin, the mean activities were 12% for factor VII, 7% for factor IX, 14% for factor X, and 13% for prothrombin. Immunodepletion of plasma factor X or prothrombin protected rabbits against TF-induced coagulation, but factor VII and factor IX had no such effect. When either factor X or prothrombin was selectively restored before infusing TF, the protective effect of warfarin was eliminated. In addition, selectively restoring prothrombin had the effect of sensitizing warfarin-treated animals to more marked coagulation.

Implications.—It appears that depression of both factor X and prothrombin is necessary for warfarin to be clinically effective. Suppression of plasma prothrombin is especially important. When both heparin and warfarin are administered to treat acute thrombosis, heparin should be continued for several days after starting warfarin, regardless of the prothrombin time. In view of the intravascular half-clearance time of factor X (about 40 hours) and prothrombin (about 60 hours) in humans, an overlap of 6 days would seem appropriate in patients with extensive venous thrombosis.

▶ This study, which employed techniques to identify the selective inhibition of vitamin K–dependent factors, suggests that the main mechanism for the inhibitory effect of warfarin anticoagulation is mediated via the depression of factors X and II. The authors emphasize the importance of the inhibition of factor II. This is somewhat intriguing because when standard doses of warfarin anticoagulation are administered, the last of all the vitamin K–dependent factors to be depressed is factor II. In many patients with therapeutically efficacious doses of warfarin in their circulation, factor II is frequently not seriously depressed below normal. In those studies where low-dose warfarin is employed and considered to be therapeutically efficacious, factor II is only minimally depressed below the upper limits of normal. One must ask whether this study is meaningful only in the rabbit or whether these results can be extrapolated to humans.—W.R. Bell, M.D.

Influence of Long Term Oral Anticoagulants Upon Prothrombin Fragment 1 + 2, Thrombin-Antithrombin III Complex and D-Dimer Levels in Patients Affected by Proximal Deep Vein Thrombosis

Elias A, Bonfils S, Daoud-Elias M, Gauthier B, Sié P, Boccalon H, Boneu B (Hôpital de Rangueil, Toulouse, France; Centre de Transfusion, Toulouse, France)

Thromb Haemost 69:302–305, 1993   116-95-3–63

Background.—Conventional doses of oral anticoagulants (OACs) decrease the plasma level of prothrombin fragment 1 + 2 (F1 + 2) far below the lower normal limit. Low-dose regimens are able to decrease or normalize previously increased F1 + 2 levels, suggesting that conventional doses of OACs may be excessively high.

Study Plan.—The effects of long-term OAC treatment on plasma levels of F1 + 2, thrombin–antithrombin III complexes, and D-dimer were examined in 20 patients with a Duplex ultrasound diagnosis of deep venous thrombosis. Measurements were made at the start of OAC treatment, 1–6 days after diagnosis and full heparinization and, subsequently, after 1, 7, and 13 weeks. The results were compared with those obtained in blood donors and age-matched healthy participants.

Findings.—All patients had a favorable clinical outcome. Highly significant variations in levels of the 3 markers were observed (table). After 1 week of OAC therapy, increased levels of thrombin–antithrombin III complexes were associated with subnormal levels of F1 + 2, suggesting a persistent hypercoagulable state. Subsequently, thrombin–antithrombin III complex levels were normal, whereas levels of F1 + 2 were far below normal. Levels of D-dimer declined continuously, reflecting an ongoing fibrinolytic process.

Evolution of the Levels of D-Dimers, F1 + 2, and Thrombin-Antithrombin Complexes in Patients Treated for 3 Months by Oral Anticoagulants

	Patients days of OAC treatment				Controls blood donors	age-matched
	1	8 ± 2	35 ± 5	92 ± 12		
n	20	20	20	20	40	40
Age	63 ± 17	63 ± 17	63 ± 17	63 ± 17	39 ± 10	63 ± 19
INR	–	2.8 ± 0.7	2.9 ± 0.9	2.8 ± 0.6	–	–
Factor II (%)	–	32 ± 12	22 ± 11	21 ± 6	–	–
D-Dimer ($\mu g\ l^{-1}$)	3,235 (1,412 – 7,413)	1,891 (870 – 3,980)	635 (245 – 1,620)	377 (165 – 831)	119 (32 – 426)	317 (46 – 2,290)
F1 + 2 ($nMol\ l^{-1}$)	0.79 (0.45 – 1.41)	0.47 (0.32 – 0.70)	0.26 (0.15 – 0.46)	0.20 (0.12 – 0.37)	0.65 (0.4 – 1.4)	0.98 (0.3 – 2.4)
TAT ($\mu g\ l^{-1}$)	5.2 (3.1 – 8.7)	3.3 (2.2 – 4.8)	2.2 (1.8 – 2.7)	2.0 (1.7 – 2.3)	1.7 (1.1 – 2.6)	2.6 (1.1 – 5.8)

Note: The values are expressed as mean ± 1 SD. For D-dimer, F1 + 2, and thrombin-antithrombin, the statistical evaluations were performed on log-transformed data (log-normal distribution); this accounts for the assymetrical standard deviation. In the blood donor and age-matched population, the *numbers in brackets* correspond to the mean ± 2 SD (normal range distribution). (Courtesy of Elias A, Bonfils S, Daoud-Elias M, et al: *Thromb Haemost* 69:302–305, 1993.)

Conclusion.—Prospective clinical trials will be needed to determine whether it is possible to decrease the intensity of anticoagulant therapy after 1 month on the basis of very low levels of F1 + 2.

▶ This study suggests that warfarin anticoagulation is simply not adequate for inhibition of thrombin generation. These data indicate that the doses of warfarin employed are not preventative for the conversion of prothrombin to thrombin. Another possibility that very definitely can exist is that the F1 + 2 originates from the action of plasmin on prothrombin, leading to the generation of these fragments, and that this is a well-recognized pathway that is not influenced by the presence of warfarin anticoagulation. For additional information on this matter, please see the reference (1).—W.R. Bell, M.D.

Reference

1. Sobel M, et al: *Circulation* 88:IIa426, 1993.

A Comparison of Subcutaneous Low-Molecular-Weight Heparin With Warfarin Sodium for Prophylaxis Against Deep-Vein Thrombosis After Hip or Knee Implantation

Hull R, Raskob G, Pineo G, Rosenbloom D, Evans W, Mallory T, Anquist K, Smith F, Hughes G, Green D, Elliott CG, Panju A, Brant R (Univ of Calgary, Alta, Canada; Chedoke-McMaster Hosps, Hamilton, Ont, Canada; Ohio State Univ, Columbus; et al)

N Engl J Med 329:1370–1376, 1993   116-95-3-64

Introduction.—Without prophylactic anticoagulation, postoperative deep venous thrombosis may develop in as many as 60% of patients who undergo hip or knee replacement. Approaches to preventing this complication have included warfarin anticoagulation, pneumatic compression, and subcutaneous heparin. The latter method has the advantage over warfarin of not requiring frequent monitoring. In a multicenter study, warfarin prophylaxis was compared with use of a low-molecular-weight heparin fraction.

Study Design.—A randomized, double-blind trial was performed in 1,436 adult patients scheduled for total hip or total knee arthroplasty. Either daily subcutaneous treatment with low-molecular-weight heparin, 75 international factor Xa inhibitory units/kg, or adjusted-dose warfarin therapy was begun after surgery and continued for 2 weeks, when venography was performed, or until discharge. The warfarin dose was adjusted each day to maintain equivalence with an international normalized ratio of 2–3.

Results.—Warfarin was administered to 721 patients, and heparin to 715 others. Interpretable venograms were available for 617 and 590 patients, respectively. Deep venous thrombosis developed in 37% of the warfarin-treated patients and in 31% of those receiving heparin, repre-

TABLE 1.—Outcomes, by Location of Surgery

Type of Event	Hip Surgery			Knee Surgery		
	Warfarin Sodium (N = 397)	Low-Molecular-Weight Heparin (N = 398)	Difference* (95% CI) %	Warfarin Sodium (N = 324)	Low-Molecular-Weight Heparin (N = 317)	Difference* (95% CI) %
	no. with event/no. studied (%)			no. with event/no. studied (%)		
Successful venography†	335 (84.4)	330 (82.9)	—	268 (82.7)	249 (78.6)	—
Deep-vein thrombosis						
All	79/340 (23.2)	69/332 (20.8)	2.4 (−3.8 to 8.7)	152/277 (54.9)	116/258 (45.0)	9.9 (1.5 to 18.3)‡
Proximal	13/340 (3.8)	16/332 (4.8)	−1.0 (−4.1 to 2.1)	34/277 (12.3)	20/258 (7.8)	4.5 (−0.5 to 9.6)
Bleeding						
Major	6/397 (1.5)	11/398 (2.8)	−1.3 (−3.3 to 0.8)	3/324 (0.9)	9/317 (2.8)	−1.9 (−4.0 to 0.2)
Minor	9/397 (2.3)	5/398 (1.3)	—	5/324 (1.5)	5/317 (1.6)	−0.1 (−2.0 to 1.9)
Wound hematoma	10/397 (2.5)	23/398 (5.8)	−3.3 (−6.0 to −0.5)§	19/324 (5.9)	28/317 (8.8)	−2.9 (−7.0 to 1.1)
	mean ±SD			mean ±SD		
Postoperative blood loss (ml)	515±365	520±386	—	616±540	649±563	—
Postoperative blood replacement (ml)	197±294	275±393	—	245±331	299±456	—

Abbreviations: CI, confidence interval; SD, standard deviation.
* Calculated by subtracting the percentage for the heparin group from that for the warfarin group.
† Reasons for unsuccessful venography: patient refusal (52, hip; 27, knee); inability to perform the procedure (42, hip; 33, knee); inadequate results (20, hip; 45, knee); and other (16, hip; 19, knee).
‡ P = .02 for the difference between treatment groups for the patients who underwent knee surgery.
§ P = .03 for the difference between treatment groups for the patients who underwent hip surgery.
(Courtesy of Hull R, Raskob G, Pineo G, et al: N Engl J Med 329:1370–1376, 1993.)

senting a 16% risk reduction. Deep vein thrombosis was more common in patients who underwent knee surgery (Table 1). Major bleeding occurred in 1.2% of those receiving warfarin and in 2.8% of heparin-treated patients. Wound hematomas developed more frequently in heparin-treated patients (Table 2).

Discussion.—Low-molecular-weight heparin seems to be at least as effective as warfarin in preventing venous thrombosis after hip or knee implantation surgery. Venous thrombosis actually was less frequent in

TABLE 2.—Complications Involving Bleeding

Type of Bleeding	Warfarin Sodium (N = 721)	Day after Surgery*	Low-Molecular-Weight Heparin (N = 715)	Day after Surgery*
	no. of patients		no. of patients	
Major bleeding				
At surgical site	7	1, 2, 3, 3, 4, 7, 10	18	1, 1, 1, 1, 2, 2, 2, 2, 2, 2, 2, 2, 3, 4, 4, 5, 5, 6
Hematemesis	2	1, 8	2	1, 2
Minor bleeding				
At surgical site	1	5	—	—
Hematemesis	2	1, 3	5	1, 2, 2, 4, 5
Hematochezia	2	10, 15	—	—
Hematuria	1	1	2	1, 5
Melena	1	6	—	—
Miscellaneous trivial bleeding†	7	4, 5, 5, 6, 8, 9, 12	3	2, 4, 10

* Numbers in roman type indicate patients with knee surgery; numbers in italic type indicate patients with hip surgery.

† Seven patients in the warfarin group had trivial bleeding, as follows: hematochezia (2 patients), epistaxis (2 patients), subconjunctival bleeding (2 patients), and hemoptysis (1 patient). Three patients in the heparin group had trivial bleeding: epistaxis (2 patients) and mucocutaneous lip bleeding (1 patient).

(Courtesy of Hull R, Raskob G, Pineo G, et al: N Engl J Med 329:1370–1376, 1993.)

heparin-treated patients, but they more frequently had wound hematoma and bleeding complications. Whether preoperative or postoperative prophylaxis is superior remains to be established.

▶ This study is another one of many employing this newer low-molecular-weight heparin preparation for the treatment of deep vein thrombosis. The study compares the new low-molecular-weight heparin with sodium warfarin. Results of previous studies all concluded that the low-molecular-weight heparin preparation was as efficacious as standard unfractionated heparin. All of these previous studies emphasized that because low-molecular-weight heparin is simpler to employ—a once- or twice-daily subcutaneous injection, no monitoring, and complete safety—this newer preparation was most likely the treatment of choice. However, this study points out that there is an appreciable amount of bleeding associated with low-molecular-weight heparin even when administered in a prophylactic regimen. It is somewhat disconcerting that this observation was not made earlier. If this observation of increased frequency of bleeding is confirmed in other studies, it may represent a distinct disadvantage for this new form of therapy. The authors also commented on the fact that the low-molecular-weight heparin is much more expensive than currently available standard therapy. The authors concluded that even though this increased expense is somewhat offset by the absence of the need to monitor treatment, they could not make a final statement as to which was more cost-effective.—W.R. Bell, M.D.

Efficacy and Cost of Low–Molecular-Weight Heparin Compared With Standard Heparin for the Prevention of Deep Vein Thrombosis After Total Hip Arthroplasty

Anderson DR, O'Brien BJ, Levine MN, Roberts R, Wells PS, Hirsh J (McMaster Univ, Hamilton, Ont, Canada; Hamilton Civic Hosps Research Centre, Hamilton, Ont, Canada)

Ann Intern Med 119:1105–1112, 1993   116-95-3–65

Background.—Low-molecular-weight heparin is more effective than standard heparin in preventing deep venous thrombosis (DVT) after or-

Estimated Costs of Prophylactic Management and
Management of Deep Vein Thrombosis and
Bleeding Complications

Management	Cost, $
Prophylaxis	
Drug/dose	
Low–molecular-weight heparin (enoxaparin)	3.83
Heparin	1.48
Dose administration	2.92
Management of deep vein thrombosis	
Proximal	
Ward (5 days hospitalization)	1078.00
Laboratory	53.00
Heparin	23.00
Physician	142.00
Outpatient	98.00
Total	1394/event
Distal	
Ward (2.9 days hospitalization)	638.00
Laboratory	45.00
Heparin	14.00
Physician	112.00
Outpatient	51.00
Total	860/event
Management of bleeding	
Major bleeding	
Direct cost	2040.00
Prolonged hospitalization (3.2 days)	751.00
Total	2791/event
Minor bleeding	
Total	189/event

(Courtesy of Anderson DR, O'Brien BJ, Levine MN, et al: *Ann Intern Med* 119:1105–1112, 1993.)

thopedic surgery without increasing bleeding complications but is expected to cost more than standard heparin. The cost-effectiveness of low-molecular-weight heparin depends on its price in relation to standard heparin in addition to treatment costs for thrombotic and bleeding complications associated with its use. This meta-analysis compared the efficacy, safety, and cost-effectiveness of the heparin formulations in postsurgical DVT prophylaxis.

Methods.—Data were extracted from 6 randomized, controlled trials directly comparing low-molecular-weight heparin and standard heparin in DVT prophylaxis after total hip arthroplasty. Hospital expenses for treating DVT and bleeding complications were estimated by using retrospective data from 447 patients in a randomized, controlled DVT prevention study.

Results.—Low-molecular-weight heparin was significantly more effective in preventing proximal DVT and symptomatic pulmonary embolism. The agents had comparable rates of distal DVT and major or minor bleeding. The incidence of major bleeding and DVT correlated with extended hospitalization. The price per dose was $3.83 for low-molecular-weight heparin and $1.48 for standard heparin (table). The estimated cost of managing proximal DVT was $1,394; of distal DVT, $860; of a major bleeding event, $2,791; of a minor bleeding event, $189. On the basis of a drug price ratio of 2.6 in the French market, use of low-molecular-weight heparin would cost only $48 more per patient than standard heparin. This cost is more than offset by the expenses avoided for treating DVT and bleeding.

Conclusion.—Low-molecular-weight heparin is more effective than and at least as safe as standard heparin in preventing DVT after total hip arthroplasty. Use of low-molecular-weight heparin should lead to overall cost savings; however, the relative cost-effectiveness depends on the price ratio between the drugs.

▶ Although only 1 preparation of low-molecular-weight heparin has been approved for commercial availability in North America, the price of this material is considerably higher than standard unfractionated heparin—approximately 20–30 times more expensive. However, as pointed out in this article, if this agent can be given without the need for any monitoring, if it can be given in such a way with such a degree of efficacy that the patient does not need to be hospitalized, and if it prevents the complications of thrombosis from occurring, one can reasonably understand that it will be more than cost-effective. Only time will provide the answer to whether the efficacy of this preparation can be realized.—W.R. Bell, M.D.

Therapy of Venous Thromboembolism in Patients With Brain Metastases
Schiff D, DeAngelis LM (Mem Sloan-Kettering Cancer Ctr, New York; Cornell

Univ, New York)
Cancer 73:493–498, 1994

116-95-3–66

Background.—Deep venous thrombosis (DVT) and pulmonary embolism (PE) are common in patients with brain metastases, yet optimal treatment for these conditions is still unknown. Anticoagulation brings potentially catastrophic risks of hemorrhage, whereas the placement of inferior vena cava filters has been shown to bring a high rate of recurrent PE as well as recurrent DVT and filter thrombosis. The efficacy of these different therapies was evaluated.

Methods.—A review was carried out of 51 patients with brain metastases who experienced DVT or PE and were treated at 1 center between January of 1980 and July of 1992. Attention was paid to age, sex, the primary tumor, evidence of hemorrhage in the brain metastases before therapy was begun, history of radiation therapy or surgery for the tumor, history of seizures, chemotherapy, the nature of the initial venous thrombolytic event, initial therapy, dosage and duration of anticoagulation, neurologic deterioration, and date of last follow-up or death.

Results.—Two patients received no treatment for DVT and died of PE. Ten patients initially received Greenfield filters; 4 of them had recurrent venous thromboembolism diagnosed within 1 month of filter placement (Table 1). Three of these patients then received anticoagulation and were grouped with 39 patients initially treated with anticoagulation. This treatment lasted for a mean of 100 days. Two patients in this group experienced devastating cerebral hemorrhages. A third patient had a mild deterioration that may have been caused by hemorrhage. This gave a 7% incidence of serious CNS complications. Three patients receiving anticoagulants were asymptomatic but revealed new hyperdensity of metastases on a noncontrast CT scan. Three patients who were taking warfarin experienced recurrent DVT with prothrombin times between 15.1 and 17.7 seconds. Minor systemic bleeding complications related to or exacerbated by anticoagulation occurred in 8 of 42 patients (Table 2).

Conclusion.—Anticoagulation effectively prevents recurrent thromboembolism. Only 12% of patients who received anticoagulation experienced nonfatal recurrent DVT or PE when coagulation values were in the low, therapeutic, or normal range. In contrast, 40% of patients receiving filters sustained recurrent thromboembolic disease. Although there was evidence of systemic bleeding in 19% of patients receiving anticoagulation, the bleeding was generally minor. Such findings indicate that anticoagulation is more effective than inferior vena cava filters in patients with brain metastases and venous thromboembolism.

▶ This thoughtful article points out the utility and danger of the placement of inferior vena cava filters in patients with metastatic carcinoma. The overwhelming majority of patients with metastatic carcinoma, particularly those with metastatic carcinoma of the brain, are experiencing Trousseau's syn-

TABLE 1.—Patients With Complications of Greenfield Filters

Age (yr)	Sex	Tumor	Reason for filter	Complication	Time after filter placement (d)	Subsequent anticoagulation
52	F	NSCLC	DVT, hemorrhagic brain metastasis	Bilateral leg swelling, probable contralateral DVT (clinical diagnosis)	18	No
53	M	Renal	DVT 2 days after craniotomy for resection of metastasis	Contralateral DVT with phlegmasia cerulea dolens (positive venogram)	21	Yes
63	M	NSCLC	PE, required bronchoscopy for tissue diagnosis	Recurrent PE (high-probability ventilation-perfusion scan)	5	Yes
50	M	Melanoma	PE, metastasis hemorrhagic by MRI though not by CT	Recurrent PE (high-probability ventilation-perfusion scan)	31	Yes

Abbreviation: NSCLC, non-small-cell lung cancer.
(Courtesy of Schiff D, DeAngelis LM: *Cancer* 73:493–498, 1994.)

TABLE 2.—Complications of Anticoagulation in 42 Patients

Complication	Therapeutic coagulation parameter* (%)	Supratherapeutic coagulation parameters† (%)	Total (%)
Systemic bleeding			
Major	0	0	0
Minor			
Guaiac-positive stool with stable hematocrit level	3 (7)	1 (2)	4 (10)
Gastrointestinal bleeding (present before anticoagulation)	1 (2)‡	0	1 (2)
Thigh hematoma	0	1 (2)‡	1 (2)
Hemoptysis	1 (2)	1 (2)	2 (4)
Brain hemorrhage			
Symptomatic	1 (2)	2 (4)	3 (7)
Asymptomatic	3 (7)	0	3 (7)

* Defined as prothrombin time (PT) ≤ 2 times control and partial thromboplastin time (PTT) < 2.5 times control.
† Defined as PT > 2 times control or PTT > 2.5 times control.
‡ Required blood transfusion.
(Courtesy of Schiff D, DeAngelis LM: *Cancer* 73:493–498, 1994.)

drome. The classic features of Trousseau's syndrome are migratory recurrent arterial and venous thromboses. By no means are the thrombotic disorders in these patients only inferior to the vena cava. In actuality, the filter may be a nidus for thrombus formation in such patients. Our experience would certainly concur with those of the authors of this publication: anticoagulation is the more effective and intelligent choice for the management of patients with neoplasm and thrombotic disorders.—W.R. Bell, M.D.

Fibrinolysis

A Comparison of Immediate Angioplasty With Thrombolytic Therapy for Acute Myocardial Infarction
Grines CL, for the Primary Angioplasty in Myocardial Infarction Study Group (William Beaumont Hosp, Royal Oak, Mich)
N Engl J Med 328:673–679, 1993   116-95-3-67

Introduction.—The success of thrombolytic therapy for acute myocardial infarction is limited by failure to reperfuse all occluded coronary arteries, serious bleeding complications, and recurrent myocardial ischemia. Because of these limitations, there is an increasing interest in the use of immediate percutaneous transluminal coronary angioplasty (PTCA) as an alternative to thrombolytic therapy.

Study Design.—In a prospective, multicenter study, 395 patients who were seen within 12 hours of the onset of ischemic chest pain were initially treated with intravenous heparin and aspirin and then randomly assigned to undergo immediate PTCA without previous thrombolytic therapy or to treatment with intravenous tissue plasminogen activator (t-PA) followed by conservative care. Radionuclide ventriculography was performed within 24 hours and at 6 weeks.

Outcome.—Of the 195 patients assigned to the PTCA group, 90% underwent the procedure with a success rate of 97%; none of the patients required emergency coronary artery bypass surgery after unsuccessful PTCA. Compared with intravenous t-PA, PTCA was associated with a lower rate of nonfatal reinfarction or death, both in the hospital and at 6 months (Table 1). The beneficial effect of immediate PTCA was observed mainly in patients classified as "not low risk," i.e., those older than 70 years of age and those who had an anterior infarction or a heart rate greater than 100 beats/min on admission (Table 2). The left ventricular ejection fraction at rest and during exercise was similar in both treatment groups. Intracranial bleeding occurred more frequently in patients who received t-PA. In patients treated with t-PA, PTCA was performed for failure of thrombolysis in 7%, recurrent unstable ischemia in 17.5%, and positive exercise test in 7.5%.

Conclusion.—Immediate PTCA is an attractive alternative to intravenous thrombolysis for acute myocardial infarction and may even be preferable for high-risk patients. Immediate angioplasty results in a high rate of patency in infarct-related vessels, with lower rates of intracranial bleeding and nonfatal reinfarction or death but similar left ventricular systolic function when compared with t-PA therapy.

▶ This study in patients with acute myocardial infarction indicates that results of survival are better with the technique of immediate angioplasty than

TABLE 1.—Clinical Events Occurring During Hospitalization

EVENT*	PTCA GROUP (N = 195)	t-PA GROUP (N = 200)	P VALUE
Stroke — no. (%)			
Hemorrhagic	0	4 (2.0)	0.05
Nonhemorrhagic	0	3 (1.5)	0.09
Bleeding			
Transfusions — no. (%)			
Overall	24 (12.3)	16 (8.0)	0.16
Excluding CABG	12 (6.2)	10 (5.0)	0.62
Transfusions per pint — mean ±SD	3.9±2.0	5.3±6.0	0.13
Primary site of bleeding or indication for transfusion — no. (%) *			
Intracranial	0	4 (2.0)	—
Access site	4 (2.1)	1 (0.5)	—
Retroperitoneal	2 (1.0)	0	—
Gastrointestinal	1 (0.5)	5 (2.5)	—
Other sites	2 (1.0)	2 (1.0)	—
CABG †	12 (6.2)	6 (3.0)	—
Decrease in hematocrit ‡	3 (1.5)	1 (0.5)	—
Pulmonary edema — no. (%)	7 (3.6)	7 (3.5)	0.96
Intubation — no. (%)	7 (3.6)	11 (5.5)	0.36
Hypotension — no. (%)			
Transient	63 (32.3)	67 (33.5)	0.80
Sustained	24 (12.3)	22 (11.0)	0.69
Arrhythmias — no. (%)			
Nonsustained VT	55 (28.2)	54 (27.0)	0.79
Sustained VT	4 (2.1)	8 (4.0)	0.26
VF	13 (6.7)	4 (2.0)	0.02
Supraventricular	4 (2.1)	8 (4.0)	0.26
AV block	12 (6.2)	10 (5.0)	0.62
Pericarditis — no. (%)	3 (1.5)	3 (1.5)	0.98
Vascular surgical repair — no. (%)	4 (2.1)	0	0.05
Dialysis — no. (%)	1 (0.5)	0	0.31

Abbreviations: CABG, coronary artery bypass grafting; VT, ventricular tachycardia; VF, ventricular fibrillation; AV, atrioventricular.

* Includes only bleeding considered serious or requiring transfusion.

† In patients who underwent CABG.

‡ Transfusion was given for decreased hematocrit; no site of bleeding was identified.

(Courtesy of Grines CL, for the Primary Angioplasty in Myocardial Infarction Study Group: N Engl J Med 328:673–679, 1993.)

with thrombolytic therapy. Noteworthy is the fact that the thrombolytic agent employed was the t-PA. Associated with the t-PA agent was a 6.5% inhospital mortality, largely from intracranial hemorrhage. One must consider these results in view of the fact that if a thrombolytic agent without such a high

TABLE 2.—In-Hospital Reinfarction and Death

EVENT	PTCA GROUP (N = 195)		t-PA GROUP (N = 200)		P VALUE
	no.	% (95% CI)	no.	% (95% CI)	
Reinfarction	5	2.6 (0.4–4.8)	13	6.5 (3.1–9.9)	0.06
Death					
Overall	5	2.6 (0.4–4.8)	13	6.5 (3.1–9.9)	0.06
Low risk *	3	3.1 (0–6.6)	2	2.2 (0–5.2)	0.69
Not low risk *	2	2.0 (0–4.7)	11	10.4 (4.6–16.2)	0.01
Nonfatal reinfarction or death	10	5.1 (2.1–8.1)	24	12.0 (7.5–16.5)	0.02

Abbreviation: CI, confidence interval.
Note: Patients defined as being at "low risk" had no high-risk factors. Those in the "not low risk" category were older than 70 years of age, had an anterior infarction, or had a heart rate of more than 100 beats/min on admission.
† Percentages are of the patients in the category.
(Courtesy of Grines CL, for the Primary Angioplasty in Myocardial Infarction Study Group: N Engl J Med 328:673–679, 1993.)

rate of associated mortality had been employed, the outcome might have been considerably different. However, this study supports the contention that immediate angioplasty is better than t-PA thrombolytic therapy in the management of acute myocardial infarction. For additional studies, please see the references (1–3).—W.R. Bell, M.D.

References

1. Zijlstra F, et al: N Engl J Med 328:680, 1993.
2. Gibbons RJ, et al: N Engl J Med 328:685, 1993.
3. Granger CB, et al: J Am Coll Cardiol 21:920, 1993.

Prehospital Thrombolytic Therapy in Patients With Suspected Acute Myocardial Infarction

The European Myocardial Infarction Project Group (Unité de Pharmacologie Clinique, Lyon, France)
N Engl J Med 329:383–389, 1993   116-95-3–68

Background.—The efficacy of thrombolytic therapy for acute myocardial infarction depends in part on how soon after the onset of symptoms it is administered. The delay in treatment could be reduced if thrombolytic therapy were administered before admission to the hospital. The benefits and risks of prehospital thrombolytic therapy compared with therapy administered at the hospital were investigated.

Methods.—In this double-blind study, patients seen within 6 hours of the onset of symptoms who underwent 12-lead ECG were admitted.

The patients were randomly treated with either anistreplase before admission, followed by placebo in hospital (prehospital group), or placebo before admission and anistreplase in hospital (hospital group).

Results.—A group of 2,750 patients received prehospital treatment, and 2,719 were assigned to the hospital group. The prehospital group received therapy a median of 55 minutes earlier than the hospital group. The prehospital group showed a reduction in the overall mortality at 30 days that was not statistically significant. The mortality rate from cardiac causes was significantly lower in the prehospital group than in the hospital group. More adverse effects were seen in the prehospital group in the time before admission. In particular, there was an excess of ventricular fibrillation, shock, symptomatic hypotension, and symptomatic bradycardia. However, these adverse effects were offset by a greater incidence of these complications in the hospital group during the inhospital period.

Conclusion.—Prehospital thrombolytic therapy appears to decrease the mortality rate from cardiac causes. Although the net gain of 15 lives for every 1,000 patients treated in this study was not statistically significant, it is consistent with the hypothesis that earlier thrombolytic treatment would result in a decreased mortality rate. The administration of prehospital thrombolytic therapy for patients with suspected myocardial infarction within 6 hours of the onset of the symptoms is feasible and safe when done by an experienced and well-equipped staff. However, it is strongly recommended that a defibrillator be available in the ambulance.

▶ There is little question in the minds of students of the process of coronary thrombosis and myocardial infarction that the earlier one can bring about resolution of thrombus, establish patency, and reconstitute blood flow to the myocardium, the more efficacious the final result will be for the patient. This study indicated a nonsignificant reduction in overall mortality at 30 days in the patients treated before they arrived at the hospital, and clearly, death from cardiac causes was significantly less frequent in those treated before they reached the hospital as opposed to those treated only after arriving in the emergency room. It is apparent from this study that prehospital thrombolytic therapy can be administered safely and that current education should stress the importance of this strategy in management.—W.R. Bell, M.D.

An International Randomized Trial Comparing Four Thrombolytic Strategies for Acute Myocardial Infarction

The GUSTO Investigators (Cleveland Clinic Found, Ohio)
N Engl J Med 329:673–682, 1993

116-95-3–69

Introduction.—Since the survival benefit of intravenous streptokinase in acute myocardial infarction was established in 1986, there has been no proof that any other thrombolytic regimens provide further benefits, except for aspirin. Questions remain about the relative efficacy of strepto-

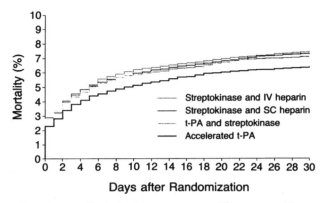

Fig 3–13.—Thirty-day mortality in the 4 treatment groups. The group receiving accelerated treatment with t-PA had lesser mortality than the 2 streptokinase groups (P = .001) and than each individual treatment group: streptokinase and subcutaneous (SC) heparin (P = .009), streptokinase and intravenous (IV) heparin (P = .003), and t-PA and streptokinase combined with intravenous heparin (P = .04). (Courtesy of the GUSTO Investigators: N Engl J Med 329:673–682, 1993.)

kinase and tissue plasminogen activator (t-PA) and the role of adjunctive therapy with intravenous vs. subcutaneous heparin. Some of the newer thrombolytic regimens for the treatment of acute myocardial infarction were compared by the Global Utilization of Streptokinase and Tissue Plasminogen Activator for Occluded Coronary Arteries (GUSTO) investigators.

Methods.—The GUSTO trial included 41,021 patients with evolving myocardial infarction at 1,081 hospitals in 15 countries. The patients were randomized to receive streptokinase plus intravenous heparin, streptokinase plus subcutaneous heparin, accelerated t-PA and intravenous heparin, or a combination of streptokinase plus t-PA with intravenous heparin. In the accelerated t-PA group, the thrombolytic was administered during 1.5 hours, with two thirds of the dose administered within the first 20 minutes. Whether these newer thrombolytic therapies that produce earlier and sustained reperfusion could improve survival was determined.

Results.—The 30-day mortality was 7.2% with streptokinase plus subcutaneous heparin, 7.4% with streptokinase with intravenous heparin, 6.3% with accelerated t-PA and intravenous heparin, and 7% for the combination regimen (Fig 3–13). Thus, accelerated t-PA decreased mortality by 14% compared with the 2 streptokinase-only regimens. Hemorrhagic stroke rates were .49%, .54%, .72%, and .94%, respectively, showing a significant excess for the accelerated t-PA and combination regimens. Death or disabling stroke occurred in 6.9% of the accelerated t-PA group vs. 7.8% of the streptokinase-only groups.

Conclusion.—This large-scale, international, randomized trial suggests that accelerated t-PA plus intravenous heparin offers a significant survival benefit vs. previous thrombolytic regimens. It carries a small excess risk of stroke, but the odds of survival without a stroke are best with accelerated t-PA. Its cost-effectiveness is likely to be another important advantage.

▶ This study comparing different regimens of streptokinase and t-PA planned to study 54,000 patients. The study was apparently stopped after 41,021 patients for reasons, at this juncture, that remain unclear. Differences between streptokinase and intravenous heparin, streptokinase and subcutaneous heparin, t-PA and streptokinase, and accelerated t-PA and intravenous heparin were essentially imperceptible. The greatest difference was identified by a combined end point of death or disabling stroke with a difference of .9% favoring the patients receiving accelerated t-PA. With this barely perceptible difference, one must know that if a few additional patients were studied—a very few—and experienced results favoring streptokinase like many others did in the trial, this barely perceptible difference of .9% would not be visible. The slightest change in outcome with a few additional patients could change the entire meaning of the study. Not mentioned in the results or discussion of this report are factual data found within indicating that streptokinase was actually superior if the patient received treatment greater than 2 hours following the time of infarction and was also more successful in patients older than 70 years of age. This report is essentially consistent with 7 previous reports demonstrating essentially no difference between these various thrombolytic agents or regimens.—W.R. Bell, M.D.

Streptokinase, But Not Tissue Plasminogen Activator, Attenuates Platelet Aggregation in Patients With Acute Myocardial Infarction

Karlberg K-E, Chen J, Hagerman I, Bergström K, Wallin R, Saldeen T, Sylvén C (Huddinge Univ Hosp, Sweden; Uppsala Univ, Sweden)
J Intern Med 234:513–519, 1993   116-95-3–70

Background.—Research has shown that reocclusion is more common after tissue plasminogen activator (t-PA) than after streptokinase use in patients with acute myocardial infarction. Whether t-PA and streptokinase administered during acute myocardial infarction have different effects on platelet aggregation that may contribute to the higher reocclusion rate after t-PA was investigated.

Methods.—Twenty patients with chest pain and ST elevations suggesting acute myocardial infarction were enrolled. Ten received t-PA, 100 mg over 3 hours, and 10 received streptokinase, 1.5×10^6 over 1 hour. Platelet aggregation was estimated using filtragometry and whole blood aggregometry before, just after, and 24 hours after fibrinolytic treatment.

Findings.—Immediately after treatment, streptokinase prolonged aggregation time and decreased conductance, indicating inhibited platelet function. Fibrinogen declined by a mean 2.5 g/L^{-1}. In the group receiving t-PA, the corresponding changes were nonsignificant. There was no significant decrease in fibrinogen. After 24 hours, when all patients were receiving acetylsalicylic acid, aggregation was inhibited in both groups. Just after fibrinolytic treatment, neutrophils were activated comparably in the 2 groups, with increments of elastase and Bβ 30–43 by a mean of 26 μg/L^{-1} and 280 pmol/L^{-1}, respectively.

Conclusion.—Although streptokinase and t-PA have similar degrees of platelet and leukocyte activation, the former appears to inhibit platelet aggregation. One possible mechanism is streptokinase-induced reductions in fibrinogen and increases of fibrinogen split products. Further development of adjuvant antiplatelet treatment may therefore be clinically important.

▶ This carefully performed study clearly demonstrates that after streptokinase is employed as a thrombolytic agent in the treatment of acute myocardial infarction, there is a definite inhibition of platelet aggregation. However, when t-PA was employed, there was no inhibition of platelet aggregation. This observation may be critically important. This may be the explanation for the well-known and long-known observation that there is a greater frequency of early reocclusion associated with the use of t-PA in contrast to all other thrombolytic agents. The most likely reason for the inhibition of platelet aggregation seen in association with the use of streptokinase is the quantity of fibrinogen-fibrin degradation products that is produced. One cannot eliminate the possibility that a different type of degradation product is produced with streptokinase in contrast to t-PA. Further studies are needed to delineate this possibility.—W.R. Bell, M.D.

The Effects of Tissue Plasminogen Activator, Streptokinase, or Both on Coronary-Artery Patency, Ventricular Function, and Survival After Acute Myocardial Infarction

The GUSTO Angiographic Investigators (George Washington Univ, Washington, DC)
N Engl J Med 329:1615–1622, 1993   116-95-3-71

Background.—Thrombolytic treatment enhances survival after acute myocardial infarction, but it is not clear whether the rate at which coronary patency is restored influences the outcome. It is far from clear whether more rapid restoration of blood flow in the infarct vessel ensures better ventricular function or an improved chance of patient survival.

Study Plan.—A total of 2,431 patients seen at 75 centers within 6 hours of the start of chest pain were randomly assigned to 1 of 4 regimens: streptokinase with subcutaneous or intravenous heparin; accelerated doses of tissue plasminogen activator (t-PA) combined with intravenous heparin; or a combination of both activators with intravenous heparin. Patients were also randomized to undergo angiography 90 minutes, 3 hours, 24 hours, or 5–7 days after the start of thrombolytic treatment. Patients examined at 90 minutes had repeat angiography after 5–7 days.

Observations.—Early patency of the infarct-related vessel was most frequent in patients receiving t-PA with heparin. Coronary blood flow at 90 minutes was normal in 54% of these patients and in 29% to 38% of the other treatment groups. Reocclusion occurred in 5% to 7% of the various treatment groups. Regional ventricular wall motion was best preserved in patients receiving t-PA with heparin and those who received combined thrombolytic treatment. Mortality at 30 days was lowest (4.4%) in patients with normal early coronary blood flow and highest (8.9%) in those with no flow at this stage.

Conclusion.—More rapid and more complete return of coronary blood flow in the infarct-related vessel is associated with better ventricular performance and decreased mortality.

▶ The authors conclude that accelerated t-PA produced the most favorable outcome in this study. However, what the authors do not comment on, even though the data are available within the report, is that the dose intensity of the t-PA employed was considerably higher than in either regimen of streptokinase. It should also be noted that the t-PA was administered continuously until the post-treatment angiogram was obtained. With streptokinase, however, the agent was stopped for 30 or more minutes before the post-treatment angiogram was performed. Thus, these 2 features might possibly skew the results in favor of the t-PA compound. Also not mentioned in this article or in its companion predecessor, Abstract 116-95-3–69, is that a mortality benefit was only seen in the patients treated in the United States. In all patients outside the United States, no mortality benefit was seen between streptokinase and t-PA. Also not pointed out is that bypass was required significantly more frequently in those patients receiving t-PA than in those patients receiving streptokinase. Not considered in the overall cost is the cost of the surgical procedures involved and their associated frequency in those patients receiving t-PA therapy. In view of so many patients requiring surgery who were treated with t-PA, the survival rate that was reported to be more favorable for t-PA may actually be related to the fact that they had a surgical procedure rather than the thrombolytic therapy. In this study, the time interval between the onset of symptoms and the institution of therapy was less than 6 hours in the overwhelming majority of patients. However, it must be noted that in those whose treatment was begun more than 6 hours from the time of onset of symptoms, the streptokinase was more efficacious than t-PA. On more detailed analysis of the data, it is apparent that the only group that definitely showed an improvement with t-PA more favorable than with streptokinase was patients seen within 2 hours of the onset of symptoms. One must ask how many patients actually are seen within 2 hours of the onset of their symptomatology. Unless a study is being conducted, the number who fall into this category is exceedingly small. Thus, the number of patients who will actually have the opportunity to receive this benefit credited to t-PA is very, very small on a worldwide basis.—W.R. Bell, M.D.

Thrombolytic Therapy in Acute Ischemic Stroke: A Danish Pilot Study

Overgaard K, Sperling B, Boysen G, Pedersen H, Gam J, Ellemann K, Karle A, Arlien-Søborg P, Olsen TS, Videbæk C, Knudsen JB (Univ Hosp, Rigshospitalet, Copenhagen; Bispebjerg Hosp, Denmark; Univ Hosp, Odense, Denmark; et al)

Stroke 24:1439–1446, 1993   116-95-3–72

Background.—The value of thrombolytic treatment of acute ischemic stroke has not been established definitively. The feasibility and safety of recombinant tissue plasminogen activator (rt-PA) in patients with acute ischemic stroke were assessed in a pilot study. Cerebral ischemia and regional cerebral blood flow (rCBF) were studied in a patient subgroup before and after thrombolytic therapy.

Methods and Findings.—Twenty-three patients were treated with 100 mg of rt-PA infused intravenously for 1 hour. Thrombolytic treatment was begun 78 to 355 minutes after symptom onset. In 17 patients, angiography performed 16–24 hours after treatment indicated patent intracranial arteries in 12 patients, partial occlusion of the middle cerebral artery in 3, and total occlusion of the middle cerebral artery in 2. In 12 patients, technetium-99m hexamethylpropyleneamine oxime administered intravenously was measured 5 minutes before and within 24 hours after thrombolytic treatment. In 10 of these patients, brain tissue reperfusion was noted. Two patients with angiographically documented middle cerebral artery occlusion had no reperfusion. These findings indicate a relationship between reperfusion measured by rCBF and angiographic patency. There were 3 deaths. Patients with reperfusion within 24 hours had greater clinical improvement on the Scandinavian Stroke Scale the sooner treatment was begun and the more severe the neurologic deficits were.

Conclusion.—Acute cerebral ischemia can be documented by measurement of rCBF without delaying thrombolytic treatment. Repeated measurements can show whether cerebral reperfusion has occurred. Early reperfusion in this series was associated with clinical improvement.

▶ This study provided considerable information that supports the contention that cerebral vascular occlusions can be resolved with thrombolytic therapy. When rCBF returns, there is an associated dramatic clinical improvement in the status of the patient. Repeat studies 5 weeks after the initial treatment indicate that those patients who successfully experienced reperfusion did well subsequently. Somewhat disturbing is the fact that the investigators selected the thrombolytic agent associated with the greatest frequency of CNS hemorrhage to perform this study. Better results might have been obtained if a more appropriate thrombolytic agent had been employed.—W.R. Bell, M.D.

The St. Jude Valve: Thrombolysis As the First Line of Therapy for Cardiac Valve Thrombosis

Silber H, Khan SS, Matloff JM, Chaux A, DeRobertis M, Gray R (Cedars-Sinai Med Ctr, Los Angeles)
Circulation 87:30–37, 1993

116-95-3–73

Objective.—Thrombotic complications are a major problem among patients with prosthetic heart valves. Initial results suggest that thrombolytic therapy may be a useful alternative to valve replacement in the management of these complications. The medical and surgical management of thrombosed St. Jude heart valves was evaluated in a 13-year study.

Patients.—A total of 988 St. Jude prosthetic valves were implanted during the study. Prosthetic valve thrombosis developed in 17 patients. The mean patient age was 67 years; 11 of the involved valves were aortic and 6 were mitral. Thirteen of these patients had congestive heart failure, 2 had syncope and fatigue, 1 had a cerebrovascular accident, and 1 was asymptomatic. Cinefluoroscopy was used for diagnosis and monitoring of therapy. Treatment was medical in 12 patients, with thrombolytic therapy in 10 and heparin in 1, and surgical in 2. In 2 patients, diagnosis was made at autopsy.

Outcome.—Of 12 patients treated with thrombolysis, 9 showed striking improvement in leaflet movement and symptoms within 12 hours of treatment. One showed symptomatic improvement with only partial improvement in leaflet motion. Two had no change in leaflet motion but were stabilized by conservative therapy. Overall, 83% of patients responded at least partially to medical treatment, and none of this group died or had any major complication. There were 4 minor complications, including 2 patients with hematoma, 1 with transient facial weakness, and 1 with epistaxis. Repeat thrombolytic therapy was successful in 2 patients with late rethrombosis, and all patients were alive and well at 3 months. All 3 patients treated with surgery recovered uneventfully.

Conclusion.—Excellent results with initial thrombolytic therapy were reported for patients with thrombotic complications involving St. Jude valves. The success rate is high and the risk of permanent side effects is low. Surgery is usually not needed unless the patient fails to respond to thrombolysis. A urokinase protocol that induces a longer but less intense thrombolytic state than for treatment of acute myocardial infarction was used.

▶ These authors point out the growing enthusiasm and interest in the use of thrombolytic therapy to bring about resolution of thrombotic material that has accumulated on artificial cardiac valves. Although one is immediately concerned about the possibility of embolization in this situation, in actual fact this is a relatively rare experience. If thrombolytic therapy can be employed successfully, this avoids the need for a serious degree of surgery.—W.R. Bell, M.D.

Safety of Thrombolytic Therapy in Elderly Patients With Massive Pulmonary Embolism: A Comparison With Nonelderly Patients

Meneveau N, Bassand J-P, Schiele F, Bouras Y, Anguenot T, Bernard Y, Schultz R (Hôpital Universitaire Saint-Jacques, Besançon, France)
J Am Coll Cardiol 22:1075–1079, 1993   116-95-3–74

Background.—Thrombolytic treatment can lyse thrombi faster than conventional heparin therapy in patients with massive pulmonary embolism, but elderly patients are at an increased risk of bleeding. At the same time, elderly patients might especially benefit from the more rapid results achievable with thrombolytic agents.

Objective.—The safety of thrombolysis was examined in a prospective series of 89 patients with a diagnosis of massive pulmonary embolism. Thirty-six of the patients were 71 years of age or older (average age, 78 years), whereas 53 younger patients had an average age of 54 years.

Treatment.—Patients received a loading dose of 250,000 IU of streptokinase in 15 minutes, followed by infusion of 100,000 IU/hour for 12 hours. Heparin was started 12 hours after the start of thrombolytic treatment. Urokinase or tissue-type plasminogen activator was used only if there was a contraindication to streptokinase.

Results.—The early course was comparable in the older and younger patients (Table 1). Fifteen and 10 patients, respectively, underwent partial interruption of the inferior vena cava. One elderly and 2 nonelderly patients died while hospitalized. Bleeding complications occurred in 28% of the elderly patients and 15% of the younger group (Table 2). No patient in either group had intracranial bleeding. Three fourths of the 8 episodes of major bleeding were related to early invasive procedures.

TABLE 1.—Clinical Course After Thrombolytic Therapy

	Nonelderly (≤70 yr)	Elderly (>70 yr)	p Value
Uncomplicated course	42 (79)	24 (67)	
Death	2 (3.7)	1 (2.7)	NS
Recurrence	1 (fatal) (1.8)	1 (fatal) (2.7)	NS
Embolectomy	3 (5.6)	1 (2.7)	NS
Filter insertion	10 (19)	15 (42)	0.03
Bleeding	8 (1 fatal)	10	NS
Hospital stay (days)	11.4 ± 4.5	13 ± 5.7	NS
MPA (mm Hg)	13 ± 9	13 ± 10	NS
Miller (/34)	8 ± 2.1	7.3 ± 4	NS

Abbreviations: *Miller (/34)*, Miller score; *MPA*, mean pulmonary artery pressure.
Note: Values presented are mean value ± standard deviation or number (%) of patients.
(Courtesy of Meneveau N, Bassand J-P, Schiele F, et al: *J Am Coll Cardiol* 22:1075–1079, 1993.)

TABLE 2.—Bleeding Complications

	Nonelderly (≤70 yr)	Elderly (>70 yr)	p Value
Total	8 (15)	10 (28)	0.14
Minor	5 (9.4)	5 (13.8)	0.74
Major	3 (5.6)	5 (13.8)	0.29
Cerebral	0	0	
Gastrointestinal	1	1	NS
Hematoma	0	2*	NS
Due to filter insertion	2 (1 fatal)	2	NS

* Hematomas linked to femoral access. Values presented are number (%) of patients.
(Courtesy of Meneveau N, Bassand J-P, Schiele F, et al: *J Am Coll Cardiol* 22:1075–1079, 1993.)

Conclusion.—Thrombolytic treatment is a reasonable approach in elderly patients with massive pulmonary embolism, providing that contraindications are carefully sought. Early caval interruption and pulmonary angiography via a femoral approach carry a high risk of excessive bleeding.

▶ A frequently posed question is whether or not the elderly are more at risk for bleeding when receiving thrombolytic therapy. This study specifically raised this question and was unable to identify a risk for elderly individuals. However, the number of patients is relatively small. I think the most helpful comment is that thrombolytic therapy is not necessarily more risky in elderly individuals. However, for thrombolytic therapy, it is absolutely clear that it remains critically important to consider the generalized body biochemistry and physiology in an individual patient rather than strictly age.—W.R. Bell, M.D.

Deep Venous Insufficiency: The Relationship Between Lysis and Subsequent Reflux
Meissner MH, Manzo RA, Bergelin RO, Markel A, Strandness DE Jr (Univ of Washington, Seattle)
J Vasc Surg 18:596–608, 1993
116-95-3-75

Background.—Venous valvular insufficiency is known to be the most important causal mechanism in the development of the post-thrombotic syndrome. However, the factors contributing to valve incompetence after deep venous thrombosis (DVT) are not well understood. The relationship between recanalization and valve competence was investigated.

Methods and Findings.—One hundred thirteen patients with acute DVT were assessed with serial duplex ultrasonography. The median lysis times for segments developing reflux were 214 to 474 days—2.3 to 7.3 times longer than for corresponding segments (all but the posterior tibial vein) in which reflux did not develop. The median lysis times for those with and without reflux in the posterior tibial vein were nearly identical. The median time to reflux onset was significantly shorter than the median lysis time in the middle and distal superficial femoral veins. It occurred simultaneously with recanalization in all other segments.

Conclusion.—In all but the posterior tibial segment, early recanalization is important in preserving valve integrity. However, the small number of patients with reflux despite lysis before 1 month or without reflux despite a delay in lysis until 9–12 months indicates that other factors may contribute to valvular incompetence. Such factors may be especially important in the posterior tibial vein, in which the lysis time is not strongly associated with the ultimate reflux development.

▶ This very thoughtfully and thoroughly performed study points out that early recanalization and restoration of blood flow after DVT are indeed important factors in maintaining venous valve function. However, the authors have identified a small number of patients who do have venous valve damage despite early, rapid, and complete lysis, as well as a sizable number of patients who do not have venous valve damage despite relatively late lysis of the thrombi. These observations suggest that other factors may contribute to venous valvular incompetence.—W.R. Bell, M.D.

Thrombolytic Therapy in Paroxysmal Nocturnal Haemoglobinuria Complicated by Hepatic Vein Thrombosis
Frawley KJ, MacKechnie SG, Taylor KM (Mater Hosp, Brisbane, Queensland, Australia)
Australas Radiol 37:396–398, 1993   116-95-3–76

Background.—Hepatic vein thrombus, a common complication of paroxysmal nocturnal hemoglobinuria, is often fatal. Thrombolytic treatment in a patient with paroxysmal nocturnal hemoglobinuria (PNH) complicated by hepatic vein thrombosis was reported.

Case Report.—Man, 50, was given a diagnosis in 1988 of PNH after a 2-year history of recurrent abdominal pain. Warfarin was begun in 1989 because of continuing episodic abdominal pain thought to be caused by mesenteric ischemia. This treatment was discontinued in 1990 after it failed to control the patient's symptoms, and dipyridamole, verapamil, and theophylline were tried without success. Later in 1990, when clinical features and tests suggested a large splenic hematoma, he underwent splenectomy. A massive splenic infarct was found at surgery. After surgery, a central line–related axillary vein thrombosis developed, and anticoagulant treatment was begun again. Four months later, a right femoral artery thrombosis developed and was treated with an embolectomy. A calf hematoma then developed, and anticoagulation therapy was discontinued. In August of 1991, the patient reported malaise, low-grade fever, and abdominal distention. Ultrasonography and CT showed ascites and occlusion of the inferior vena cava with probable hepatic vein involvement. A thrombus was also seen in the superior mesenteric vein. The liver had a heterogenous appearance at CT with patchy contrast uptake. The extent of the thrombus was seen with venography. Thrombolytic treatment, with streptokinase infused at 40,000 units/hr through a catheter in the inferior vena cava was begun. Partial lysis of the thrombus was seen the next day. Streptokinase was increased to 50,000 units/hr, and another cavogram showed contrast passage to the right atrium. Selective catheterization of the hepatic veins revealed the typical spider web pattern associated with hepatic venous thrombosis. The treatment was changed to recombinant tissue plasminogen activator (rt-PA). Venography on day 3 showed some flow from the proximal hepatic veins, and the rt-PA was stopped and heparin begun. At 1 week, CT showed a reduction in the size of the inferior vena cava thrombus. However, the inferior vena cava and superior mesenteric thrombus and patchy liver changes persisted. The patient's symptoms also continued. Warfarin was begun again. Intermittent abdominal pain continued. A trial of chemotherapy was tried but was complicated by neutropenic sepsis and massive ascites, respiratory insufficiency, and renal failure. In August of 1992, the patient died.

Conclusion.—In patients with PNH complicated by hepatic vein thrombus, rapid diagnosis with ultrasound, CT, or venography may improve the prognosis. Thrombolytic agents may be more beneficial than heparin in the early management of such patients.

▶ This encouraging report indicates that if thrombolytic therapy is employed early and successfully in hepatic vein thrombosis, it is the optimal treatment of choice. If hepatic vein thrombosis cannot be resolved with thrombolytic therapy, alternative treatments are unsatisfactory. These alternative treatments include various intra-abdominal venous-to-venous shunts, the duration of which is short-lived at longest, and, finally, hepatic transplantation. One of the most important features in successful resolution of hepatic vein thrombosis is to employ thrombolytic therapy directly into the substance of the thrombus or thrombi as early as possible.—W.R. Bell, M.D.

Combined Effects of Urokinase and Heparin on PTT Values During Thrombolytic Therapy
Sheiman RG, Phillips DA (Univ of Massachusetts, Worcester)
Angiology 44:114–122, 1993   116-95-3–77

Background.—The local infusion of heparin and urokinase in inhibiting thrombosis and clot propagation is often complicated by hemorrhage. Maintaining fibrinogen levels above 100 mg/dL during therapy is the only criterion that currently exists to minimize this risk. However, it is thought that elevated partial thromboplastin time (PTT) may also play a role in such bleeding complications. The relationship between increasing PTT values and declining fibrinogen levels during thrombolytic therapy with urokinase and heparin was quantified.

Methods.—All patients who underwent treatment of acute arterial or venous thrombosis with urokinase and heparin between January of 1989 and December of 1990 were reviewed. Eleven patients were identified who had been receiving a steady-state heparin dose for at least 24 hours before the addition of high-dose urokinase and who maintained the same steady-state heparin dose throughout their course of thrombolytic therapy. Changes in PTT values were therefore considered to be secondary to the addition of urokinase in this group. Examination of the fibrinolytic and coagulation states was carried out on the 11 patients, along with laboratory monitoring of fibrinogen levels, prothrombin times, and PTT values, every 4 hours during concomitant urokinase and heparin administration. Prothrombin times and PTT values were checked every 8 hours during the period before and after urokinase administration.

Results.—Four patients experienced minor bleeding problems, and 1 had a major bleeding complication that led to termination of therapy. Three of the 5 patients with bleeding had PTT levels greater than 150 seconds. None had fibrinogen levels less than 100 mg/dL at any time. Urokinase enhanced the effect of heparin on PTT values as a result of decreasing fibrinogen levels. In 10 of the 11 patients, this effect brought a doubling of PTT values when compared with heparin alone. The significant increase in PTT levels occurred only after fibrinogen levels approached 200 mg/dL in 8 patients.

Conclusion.—Complications during thrombolytic therapy with urokinase and heparin could not be attributed solely to decreased fibrinogen levels resulting from urokinase. In 3 of 5 patients, bleeding complications resulted from unanticipated elevations in PTT values resulting from the added effect of depressed levels of fibrinogen on the PTT values in patients already receiving heparin, once urokinase was begun. When fibrinogen levels declined below 200 mg/dL, PTT values increased by 100% or more. Familiarity with this relationship may allow better control of PTT values and avoidance of extreme elevations during combined therapy.

▶ The authors of this manuscript suggest that when the plasma fibrinogen level declines to 200 mg/dL or less activated PTT (APTT) is prolonged. That APTT is not influenced by a decrease in fibrinogen per se until the level decreases to less than 25 mg/dL is well known, and this phenomenon has been studied for many years. Thus, the fibrinogen level of 200 mg/dL is not responsible. Most likely responsible for prolonging the APTT are the degradation products of fibrinogen that have been degraded from the initial value to a lower value of 200 mg/dL. It should be pointed out that when 2 agents such as heparin and a thrombolytic are capable of prolonging the APTT, it is not possible to decide which is exerting the influence that is responsible.

Also, a concentration of plasma fibrinogen of 200 mg/dL per se is not associated with bleeding. This is a perfectly fine level.—W.R. Bell, M.D.

α_2-Antiplasmin Supplementation Inhibits Tissue Plasminogen Activator-Induced Fibrinogenolysis and Bleeding With Little Effect on Thrombolysis

Weitz JI, Leslie B, Hirsh J, Klement P (McMaster Univ, Hamilton, Ont, Canada)

J Clin Invest 91:1343–1350, 1993

116-95-3–78

Background.—Tissue plasminogen activator (t-PA) causes fibrinogen proteolysis when α_2-antiplasmin concentrations decline, which may contribute to t-PA–induced bleeding. Clot-bound plasmin is protected from α_2-antiplasmin inhibition. Thus, it is possible that α_2-antiplasmin supplementation blocks t-PA–induced fibrinogenolysis and hemorrhage without affecting thrombolysis. Added to human or rabbit plasma, α_2-antiplasmin inhibits t-PA–induced fibrinogenolysis, but it does not affect the lysis of ^{125}I-fibrin clots.

Methods and Findings.—Rabbits with preformed ^{125}I-labeled jugular vein thrombi were randomly assigned to t-PA, t-PA and α_2-antiplasmin, or saline. The α_2-antiplasmin infusion modestly reduced t-PA–induced thombolysis. However, it decreased fibrinogen consumption from 87% to 27% and blood loss from ear incisions from 5,594 to 656 μL.

Conclusion.—α_2-Antiplasmin appears to limit t-PA–induced bleeding by inhibiting fibrinogenolysis and subsequent fragment-X formation. Both sodium dodecylsulfate–polyacrylamide gel electrophoresis and immunoblot analysis show less fragment-X formation in animals treated with α_2-antiplasmin, and when added to a solution of fibrinogen and plasminogen clotted with thrombin in the presence of t-PA, fragment X shortens lysis time in a concentration-dependent manner. Fragment-X incorporation into hemostatic plugs, therefore, appears to contribute to t-PA–induced hemorrhage. The α_2-antiplasmin supplementation may improve the safety of fibrin-specific plasminogen activators by blocking t-PA–mediated fibrinogenolysis.

▶ This carefully detailed study suggests that infusion of α_2-antiplasmin may prevent bleeding when thrombolytic therapy is employed. In the overwhelming majority of patients who receive thrombolytic therapy, α_2-antiplasmin levels are not dramatically reduced below normal. In view of the fact that when the α_2-antiplasmin was administered there was a decrease in the ability of the thrombolytic agent to induce thrombolysis, one must be concerned about the possibility that the administration of α_2-antiplasmin in humans may enhance thrombus formation, a highly undesirable side effect.—W.R. Bell, M.D.

Congenital Plasminogen Deficiency Caused by a Ser[572] to Pro Mutation

Azuma H, Uno Y, Shigekiyo T, Saito S (Univ of Tokushima, Japan)
Blood 82:475–480, 1993   116-95-3-79

Background.—Plasminogen, the proenzyme of the serine protease plasmin, is a 791–amino acid residue single-chain glycoprotein. Its gene spans approximately 52.5 kb on chromosome 6q26-27 and consists of 19 exons. Plasminogen deficiencies are associated with reduced plasma plasmin levels, which leads to a disruption in normal recanalization and tissue repair processes. This, in turn, can result in thrombotic tendencies. To date, the mutations responsible for plasminogen deficiency have not been established. The precise genetic abnormality in a Japanese family with plasminogen deficiency has been identified.

Methods and Findings.—Polymerase chain reaction and restriction fragment polymorphism analysis were used to assess all 19 exons of the plasminogen gene, including the exon-intron boundaries, in a Japanese woman, 43 years of age with cerebral infarction, and her family members. All exons were individually amplified with 19 sets of primers and then were subcloned into a M13 vector and single-stranded DNA sequencing. A single T-to-C transition in exon 14, which changed a Ser[572] codon (TCC) to Pro[572] codon (CCC), was noted. This mutation generated a new *Fok* I site. Therefore, the *Fok* I digestion patterns of the PCR-amplified exon 14 fragments from each family member were investigated. In each instance, the patterns were consistent with the activities and antigen levels of plasma plasminogen in these individuals. Moreover, *Fok* I endonuclease failed to restrict any of the PCR-amplified exon 14 fragments taken from 15 normal individuals.

Conclusion.—A T-to-C transition in exon 14 is responsible for the inherited plasminogen deficiency found in this Japanese family with a history of thrombotic episodes.

▶ The authors have clearly demonstrated a mutation that can induce congenital plasminogen deficiency. Such techniques can be employed in the future on other individuals to see exactly how many different types of mutations actually exist in those who have low circulating plasminogen levels.—W.R. Bell, M.D.

The Influence of the Nature of the Asparagine 289-Linked Oligosaccharide on the Activation by Urokinase and Lysine Binding Properties of Natural and Recombinant Human Plasminogens

Davidson DJ, Castellino FJ (Univ of Notre Dame, Ind)
J Clin Invest 92:249–254, 1993   116-95-3-80

Background.—To further contribute to the understanding of protein structure-function relationships, several strategies were used to obtain recombinant human plasminogens (HPgs) containing different oligosaccharide side chains on its sole N-linked glycosylation site, present at Asn289.

Methods.—Approaches used included expression of the complementary DNA for HPg in insect cell lines under differing conditions, addition of glycosidase inhibitors during expression, and purification of specific glycoforms of HPg using affinity chromatography in an insolubilized lectin column. The activation kinetics for urokinase of each of the purified HPgs were then assessed, as were their relative abilities to bind to the ligand ϵ-aminocaproic acid (EACA).

Results.—When N- and O-linked oligosaccharides were removed from HPgs, a slight increase in the k_{cat}/k_m was noted for their activation. A glycoform containing tetrasialyl-tetra-antennary complex oligosaccharide on Asn289 was a somewhat poorer substrate for urokinase compared with plasma HPg, which contains bisialyl-biantennary complex carbohydrate on Asn289. Human plasminogens with high mannose-type glycans on Asn289 revealed the most striking differences. Approximately 6% of the k_{cat}/K_m of plasma HPg was found in $(Man_9GlcNAc_2)$-HPg, whereas $(Glc_3Man_9GlcNAc_2)$-HPg did not undergo an activation at a significantly rate by urokinase. Differences were also noted in the relative abilities of the HPg glycoforms to interact with EACA. The HPgs containing complex-type glycans demonstrated the most effective interactions, whereas HPgs with high mannose-type oligosaccharides demonstrated the least effective binding abilities. A fourfold difference between HPg containing tetrasialyl-tetra-antennary glycan and HPg with $(Glc_3Man_9GlcNAc_2)$ assembled on Asn289 represented the full range of binding effects.

Conclusion.—The nature of the N-linked glycan assembled on HPg markedly influences its ability to be activated by urokinase and to bind to ω-amino acid effector molecules.

► This study, which was very neatly performed, convincingly indicates the importance of carbohydrate moieties associated with human plasminogen. These carbohydrate moieties are critically important for alteration by various thrombolytic agents and the resulting generation of plasmin.—W.R. Bell, M.D.

39-kD Protein Inhibits Tissue-Type Plasminogen Activator Clearance In Vivo

Warshawsky I, Bu G, Schwartz AL (Washington Univ, St Louis, Mo)
J Clin Invest 92:937–944, 1993 116-95-3–81

Introduction.—The plasma serine protease tissue plasminogen activator (t-PA) catalyzes the first rate-limiting step in the fibrinolytic cascade.

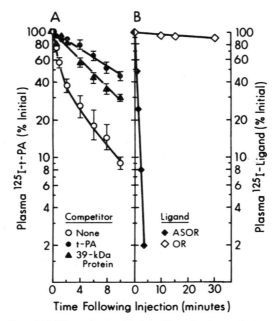

Fig 3–14.—A, effect of 39-kD protein or unlabeled t-PA on the plasma clearance of ^{125}I-t-PA in rats. Rats were injected with 30 pmol of ^{125}I-t-PA without (*open circle*) (8 rats) or with preinjection of 250 nmol of unlabeled 39-kD protein (*triangle*) (4 rats) or 12 nmol of unlabeled t-PA (*filled circle*) (3 rats). Blood samples were collected at the indicated times and trichloroacetic acid–insoluble radioactivity was determined. Each *symbol* represents the mean ± SEM. **B,** plasma clearance of control proteins. Rats were injected with 5 pmol of ^{125}I-orosomucoid (OR) (*open diamond*) or 5 pmol of ^{125}I-asialoorosomucoid (ASOR) (*filled diamond*). Samples were processed as described above. (Courtesy of Warshawsky I, Bu G, Schwartz AL: *J Clin Invest* 92:937–944, 1993.)

The liver clears it rapidly from the circulation after intravenous administration, limiting its use as a thrombolytic agent after acute myocardial infarction. Studies in both rat and human hepatoma cells have demonstrated that binding of t-PA to its clearance receptor—the low-density lipoprotein receptor-related protein/α_2-macroglobulin receptor—is inhibited by a 39-kD protein that co-purifies with the receptor. A Rats were used to determine whether giving purified recombinant 39-kD protein could alter in vivo t-PA clearance.

Findings.—Rats given purified 39-kD protein had a significant prolongation in the plasma half-life of ^{125}I-t-PA from 1 to 5 or 6 minutes. A similar prolongation in the plasma half-life of t-PA enzymatic activity was also seen. The protein was rapidly cleared from the circulation in a biphasic process, with half-lives of 30 seconds and 9 minutes. The liver was the primary organ of clearance. The ^{125}I-39-kD protein clearance was slowed in dose-dependent fashion by preadministration of excess unlabeled 39-kD protein, suggesting that specific clearance receptors were responsible for this process (Fig 3–14). When increasing doses of unlabeled and labeled 39-kD protein were administered together, the amount of labeled 39-kD protein associating with the liver decreased as the amount associating with the kidney increased, suggesting the existence of 2 clearance mechanisms.

Conclusion.—Recombinant 39-kD protein can significantly decrease clearance of t-PA. The mechanism of this effect is inhibition of the hepatic t-PA receptor. The 39-kD protein, which is rapidly cleared from the circulation, is taken up by both the liver and kidney.

▶ Tissue-type plasminogen activator is exceedingly expensive. The half-life of this agent is less than 5 minutes inside the human body. If the half-life of this agent can be prolonged, as is suggested by this report, then the amount of t-PA that needs to be administered could be reduced, and, thus, the cost of a treatment could be considerably less. However, these studies were performed in rats and must therefore be confirmed in humans. One must also be cautious because this 39-kD protein may, inside the human body, diminish the activity of the t-PA. The 39-kD protein might also act as an antigen and induce antibodies, thereby causing additional unneeded problems.—W.R. Bell, M.D.

Treatment With Tranexamic Acid During Pregnancy, and the Risk of Thrombo-Embolic Complications
Lindoff C, Rybo G, Åstedt B (Univ of Lund, Sweden; Univ of Gothenburg, Sweden)
Thromb Haemost 70:238–240, 1993   116-95-3–82

Background.—Tranexamic acid (AMCA) inhibits fibrinolysis and is used to treat fibrinolytic bleeding and to prevent bleeding at surgery. Its potential to predispose to thrombosis by depressing the fibrinolytic system has been debated. Pregnant women, especially those who have had cesarean section, are at an increased risk for thromboembolic effects of antifibrinolytic treatment. The occurrence of arterial and venous throm-

TABLE 1.—Distribution of Controls and Patients According to Diagnosis, Mode of Delivery, and Thromboembolic Complications

| | | Patients Duration of treatment with AMCA | | |
Diagnosis	Controls	1–3 days	3–7 days	>7 days
Abruptio placentae	212 (186/2)	67 (51)	27 (4)	41/1 (36)
Placenta praevia	89 (68)	12 (7)	11 (7)	52 (44/1)
Non-spec. bleeding	1,545 (189/2)	25 (13)	8 (–)	13 (7)
Total	1,846 (443/4)	104 (71)	46 (11)	106/1 (87/1)

Note: Figures in parentheses denote numbers of patients delivered by cesarean section, and figures after the oblique denote the occurrence of thromboembolism.
(Courtesy of Lindoff C, Rybo G, Åstedt B: *Thromb Haemost* 70:238–240, 1993.)

TABLE 2.—The Relationship Between the Occurrence of Thromboembolism
(TE) and the Use of AMCA During Pregnancies Complicated by Different
Bleeding Disorders

| | Number of cases | | | |
	AMCA	controls	O. R.	95% C. L.
TE	2	4	3.6	0.7–17.8
No TE	254	1,842		

Abbreviations: O.R., odds ratio; C.L., confidence limits.
(Courtesy of Lindoff C, Rybo G, Åstedt B: *Thromb Haemost* 70:238–240, 1993.)

boembolic complications in pregnant women treated with AMCA was
examined retrospectively.

Methods.—The case records of 2,102 patients with bleeding disorders
during pregnancy were analyzed retrospectively; AMCA had been administered until delivery in 256 patients. Of the patients treated with AMCA,
169 were delivered by cesarean section. The control group comprised
the 1,846 patients not treated with AMCA. The relationship between the
use of AMCA and the occurrence of thromboembolism was calculated.

Findings.—In the AMCA group, 2 patients had pulmonary embolism,
1 of them after a vaginal delivery. In the control group, 3 patients had
deep vein thrombosis and 1 had pulmonary embolism. All 4 women had
cesarean deliveries (Tables 1, 2, and 3). There was no significant relation
between the use of AMCA and the occurrence of thromboembolism.

Conclusion.—No evidence of any thrombogenic effect of AMCA was
found. Therefore, there appears to be no need to alter indications for
AMCA treatment or the recommended dosages.

▶ Data concerning the use of antifibrinolytic agents during status gravida-
rum are very few. These include comments with respect to effects on the
mother as well as the fetus. This study with AMCA suggests that it can be

TABLE 3.—The Relationship Between the Occurrence of
Thromboembolism (TE) and the Use of AMCA in Patients Delivered
by Cesarean Section

| | Number of cases | | | |
	AMCA	controls	O. R.	95% C. L.
TE	1	4	0.65	0.1–5.8
No TE	168	439		

Abbreviations: O.R., odds ratio; C.L., confidence limits.
(Courtesy of Lindoff C, Rybo G, Åstedt B: *Thromb Haemost* 70:238–240, 1993.)

used during pregnancy to treat various bleeding disorders and, perhaps, thrombocytopenia associated with pregnancy. This agent can be helpful in the prevention of bleeding and does not appear to carry any adverse risks for the mother, and no undesirable side effects have been reported in the fetus. Logically, this information may also be applied to ε-aminocaproic acid, but before any firm statements can be made, data with that agent are needed.—W.R. Bell, M.D.

Long-Term Results of a Single Protocol for Thrombolysis in Acute Lower-Limb Ischaemia

Giddings AEB, Quraishy MS, Walker WJ (Royal Surrey County Hosp, Guildford, England)

Br J Surg 80:1262–1265, 1993

116-95-3-83

Introduction.—Acute ischemia of the lower limb is a common problem with an early mortality rate greater than 15% and an amputation rate of as much as 30%. Early reports have suggested that thrombolytic therapy is becoming more effective and safer in these patients. Long-term follow-up of a protocol for the treatment of acute ischemia of the lower extremity with intra-arterial streptokinase and surgery was reported.

Methods.—At a single hospital, 157 patients were studied prospectively from 1982 to 1988. The 15% of patients with acute white leg were managed with immediate balloon catheter embolectomy. Another 36% with subacute arterial thrombosis were managed with heparin, medical support, and elective investigation. This left 78 patients (50%) for treatment with thrombolysis. Fifty-two were managed after the development of a single protocol. Follow-up of all survivors was at least 4 years (mean, 45 months).

Outcome.—Lysis was deemed effective in removing all or most of the obstruction in 73% of patients and to have conferred a unique benefit in 67%. Thirty-five percent of patients died during follow-up, 13% of them in the first month. However, only 3 of these deaths were directly attributed to unrelieved limb ischemia. Thirty-four patients were still alive at 4 years, 23 of them with limb salvage. The benefit of treatment was sustained for this long in 58% of patients. Of the 11 amputations, 6 were done within 30 days. More delayed amputation followed persistent distal occlusion or progression of distal disease. Thrombolysis carried no complications leading to death or amputation.

Conclusion.—For properly selected patients with acute ischemia of the lower limb, personal supervision and an established protocol can maintain the risks of thrombolysis at an acceptable level. For patients who survive the initial event, thrombolytic therapy can allow sustained limb salvage for at least 4 years. Randomized clinical trials are needed to establish the ultimate role of this therapy.

▶ This study points out the long-term benefits of successful thrombolysis. In many instances, the long-term patency was better than with the use of surgical techniques. This is critically important and indicates that the conservative role of thrombolysis may represent a significant advance in the treatment of peripheral arterial vascular occlusive disease.—W.R. Bell, M.D.

A Prospective, Randomized, Blinded, and Placebo-Controlled Trial of Intraoperative Intra-Arterial Urokinase Infusion During Lower Extremity Revascularization: Regional and Systemic Effects

Comerota AJ, Rao AK, Throm RC, Skibinski CI, Beck GJ, Ghosh S, Sun L, Curl GR, Ricotta JJ, Graor RA, Flinn WC, Roedersheimer RL, Alexander JB (Temple Univ, Philadelphia; Cleveland Clinic, Ohio; Buffalo VA Hosp and Millard Fillmore Hosp, Buffalo, NY; et al)

Ann Surg 218:534–543, 1993   116-95-3–84

Background.—Intraoperative fibrinolytic therapy delivers a high concentration of plasminogen activator to a thrombus to establish regional fibrinolysis without increasing the risk of bleeding. The safety and dose-related regional and systemic effects of intraoperative intra-arterial urokinase infusion on serum fibrinogen and the fibrinolytic system were investigated.

Methods.—A total of 134 patients undergoing lower-limb extremity bypass for chronic limb ischemia received preoperative urokinase in a distal bolus infusion of 125,000 units (UK125), 250,000 units (UK250), or 500,000 units (UK500), or placebo. Blood samples were obtained from the femoral vein and arm before drug infusion, prereperfusion, and postreperfusion; systemic blood samples were obtained 2 hours after perfusion. Plasma fibrinogen, fibrin(ogen) degradation products (FDPs), fibrin breakdown products D-dimer and fragment B-β 15-42, and plasminogen were assayed.

Results.—A dose-dependent decline in plasminogen activity that was significant vs. placebo was produced by urokinase only at the highest dose, although all mean values were normal. Neither regional nor systemic plasma fibrinogen levels declined significantly. Increases in plasma FDPs were dose related. Both UK250 and UK500 significantly increased FDPs compared with placebo in regional circulation; UK500 increased FDPs in the systemic circulation as well. Urokinase increased D-dimer in a dose-response fashion; systemic D-dimer elevations were significant with UK250 and UK500. Fragment B-β 15-42 increased with higher urokinase doses, but the elevations were significant only with UK500 at prereperfusion in systemic circulation. Operative blood loss, blood replacement needs, and wound hematomas were not increased by urokinase.

Conclusion.—Intraoperative bolus urokinase infusion promoted distal fibrinolysis without causing bleeding complications and may be useful in patients undergoing surgery to revascularize chronic limb ischemia. Detailed randomized research is needed to clarify the clinical benefit.

▶ This article makes 2 very important points: first, that thrombolytic therapy with urokinase can be safely employed intraoperatively, second, and that this agent can greatly augment the benefits of a surgical procedure by bringing about thrombose resolution in microvasculature that is not amenable to surgical technique.—W.R. Bell, M.D.

The Effects of Different Anesthetic Regimens on Fibrinolysis and the Development of Postoperative Arterial Thrombosis

Rosenfeld BA, for the Perioperative Ischemia Randomized Anesthesia Trial Study Group (Johns Hopkins Hosp, Baltimore, Md)
Anesthesiology 79:435–443, 1993

116-95-3–85

Background.—Regional anesthesia (RA) has been associated with a lower incidence of postoperative thrombotic complications than general anesthesia (GA). The difference may result from reduced inhibition of fibrinolysis and smaller coagulation factor elevations. However, previous research comparing RA and GA was not controlled for important hemostatic and pharmacologic variables. The effects of RA and GA on hemostatic function and postoperative thrombotic complications were compared in a study that controlled for blood pressure, heart rate, and perioperative pain relief.

Methods.—Fifty-two patients undergoing elective lower-extremity vascular reconstruction received GA and then intravenous morphine; 43 received RA and then epidural fentanyl. Data collection involved serial physical examinations, ECG, and cardiac isoenzymes to detect arterial thrombosis. Fibrinogen, plasminogen activator inhibitor-1 (PAI-1), and D-dimer levels were measured preoperatively and 24 and 72 hours after surgery.

Results.—Twenty-four arterial thrombotic events occurred in 22 patients, including 4 nonfatal myocardial infarctions; 2 cases of unstable angina; 12 subsequent thrombectomies or revascularization procedures, or both; and 6 amputations. Based on multiple logistic regression analysis, the type of anesthesia and preoperative PAI-1 concentrations were the only variables predictive of postoperative arterial thrombosis. Of the patients who had thrombosis, 77% received GA. Preoperative PAI-1 levels were significantly increased in patients who had thrombosis to a mean of 20.5 AU/mL, vs. 11.2 AU/mL for those who did not have the complication.

Conclusion.—Impaired fibrinolysis may be causally correlated with postoperative arterial thrombosis. Combined with fentanyl analgesia, RA preserves postoperative fibrinolysis; perioperative use of this regimen may decrease the risk of arterial thrombotic complications in patients undergoing lower-extremity revascularization.

▶ This topical area has been thoroughly investigated by the authors of this report. It does appear that it is important to consider at the time of a surgical procedure all ingredients that occur that may be responsible for the increased frequency of arterial thrombosis. These authors point out that a RA combined with epidural fentanyl analgesia does not inhibit the activity of the fibrinolytic system, in contrast to other anesthetic regimens. Attention paid to such details may be important in the final outcome of the frequency of the thrombosis associated with surgical techniques.—W.R. Bell, M.D.

Dusart Syndrome: A New Concept of the Relationship Between Fibrin Clot Architecture and Fibrin Clot Degradability: Hypofibrinolysis Related to an Abnormal Clot Structure
Collet J-P, Soria J, Mirshahi M, Hirsch M, Dagonnet FB, Caen J, Soria C (Geffacs, Laboratoire Sainte-Marie, Paris; Hôpital de l'Hotel Dieu, Paris; Hôpital Lariboisière, Paris; et al)
Blood 82:2462–2469, 1993   116-95-3–86

Background.—Fibrinogen Dusart is a congenital dysfibrinogenemia that brings severe thrombotic disorder, embolism, and abnormal fibrin polymerization. The disorder has been associated with abnormal polymerization that decreases the availability of the plasminogen at the fibrin surface. It is unclear whether this anomaly is caused by an abnormal plasminogen-binding site or a decrease in availability of binding sites in the abnormal clot structure. Whether abnormal clot architecture could play a role in the thromboresistance of the fibrin Dusart and the high incidence of embolism was analyzed.

Methods.—Blood samples were obtained from normal individuals and a patient with fibrinogen Dusart. The viscoelastic properties of the clot were examined using permeation analysis of the fibrin gel and the compaction technique. Clot lysis was analyzed by the generation of fibrin degradation product as the clot was degraded by fibrinolytic enzymes.

Results.—Examination of the viscoelastic properties of the fibrin Dusart clot revealed its anomalous character: extreme rigidity and tight configuration of the fibrin network. Under permeation analysis, the Dusart clot was 175 times less permeable to flow than the control. The tight-network configuration of the Dusart clot was seen by its dramatic decrease of gel porosity, fiber diameter, and fiber mass-length ratio. All of these parameters were greatly decreased compared with the control. The abnormal features of the Dusart fibrin clot were corrected in a dose-dependent manner by adding dextran 40 (30 mg/mL) before coagulation, which restored the Dusart clot permeability to virtually the same value as the normal control clot.

Conclusion.—Evidence was provided of the abnormality of fibrin Dusart, which is an extremely rigid and tight fibrin gel structure composed of very thin, short, and highly branched fibers. Such modifications in clot architecture render the clot more susceptible to fragmentation under circulatory stress and account for the high incidence of pulmonary embolism observed in patients with this syndrome.

▶ The authors provide considerable evidence that if there is a dysfunctional fibrinolytic system, this can result in structural fibrinogen arrangement that predisposes to additional thrombus formation. These observations must be considered when other congenital dysfibrinogenemias are identified.—W.R. Bell, M.D.

Ultrasound-Assisted Thrombolysis
Sehgal CM, Leveen RF, Shlansky-Goldberg,RD (Hosp of the Univ of Pennsylvania, Philadelphia; VA Med Ctr, Omaha, Neb)
Invest Radiol 28:939–943, 1993   116-95-3–87

Background.—The use of thrombolytic agents to lyse thrombus has been adopted as a major treatment option for vascular disease. However, the procedures are limited in their effectiveness, whereas the complication rate, cost, and length of treatment time are high. The use of ultrasound for recanalization has been suggested as an alternative. It has significant benefits, yet brings side effects associated with high-energy acoustics. A further option of using low-intensity ultrasound in conjunction with thrombolytic agents to increase the rate of thrombolysis was investigated.

Method.—Blood samples were obtained from 5 volunteers and prepared in vitro to obtain stable clots. The clots from each donor were divided into control and experimental groups and were treated with and without urokinase by using a continuous-wave, 20-KHz ultrasound at power levels of 1–2 W. Clot lysis was calculated by the percentage weight change before and after treatments.

Results.—As expected, both urokinase and ultrasound, when used alone, produced clot lysis. However, when the 2 methods were combined, a significant increase in lysis was seen. Within 7 minutes of sonication, almost complete thrombus lysis occurred in the presence of urokinase. At different power levels of insonation, 1 W and 1.5 W, the combination of urokinase and ultrasound produced more than twice the lysis observed by either method alone.

Conclusion.—These preliminary results show that a single low dose of urokinase combined with ultrasound at the modest power level of 1.5 W brings a substantial increase in in vitro thrombolysis compared with clots treated with urokinase only. Although the mechanism by which this occurs is unclear, it suggests that ultrasound synergistically enhances thrombolysis. The clinical implications of these findings may allow for the future reduction of dose and time of fibrolytic administration.

▶ The idea to use ultrasound to assist the plasminogen system to bring about resolution of thrombus is excellent. The strategy may be particularly helpful if a catheter can be passed immediately adjacent to or even into the substance of the thrombus and ultrasound waves can be emitted to disrupt the thrombus. Once these occur, then the activity of the plasminogen system may be more efficacious in bringing about the dissolution of preformed thrombi. Further studies on this matter are obviously in order.—W.R. Bell, M.D.

4 Hematologic Malignancies

Introduction

The pages that follow demonstrate further progress in the management of hematologic malignancies since the publication of the last YEAR BOOK OF HEMATOLOGY. Progress is never as rapid as we all would wish, but it is gratifying to me to be able to report steady progress year after year in what we can offer patients who suffer from life-threatening diseases such as the hematologic malignancies. It will be interesting to see what effect the reorganization of medicine and the stoking of the furnaces of regulation will have on what has been steady achievement to date. Let us hope that the accomplishments recorded in the next YEAR BOOK OF HEMATOLOGY will be at least as gratifying as those abstracted in this volume.

Hodgkin's Disease

Associations between the Epstein-Barr virus (EBV) and Hodgkin's disease continue to be reported, although no proof that that virus causes Hodgkin's disease has been offered to date. Lin et al. (1) from the National Cancer Institute published an American Society of Clinical Oncology abstract in which no association between EBV and familial Hodgkin's disease was found. Familial Hodgkin's disease is being observed more frequently, although it is rare. However, families with Hodgkin's disease and other hematologic malignancies are more common, which suggests to me that Hodgkin's disease may be more closely related to other hematologic malignancies than previously appreciated. Therefore, it would seem that many hematologic malignancies may have causal factors in common and EBV might simply be an infective organism to which Hodgkin's patients are more susceptible. It will be interesting to follow future clarification of the EBV-Hodgkin's story.

The most important therapeutic advance in Hodgkin's disease recorded in this chapter is bone marrow transplantation (BMT). There is no doubt that lives that would have been lost have been saved across the world by this procedure. I am unsure about the role of allogeneic BMT in this disease, but I am convinced that any Hodgkin's disease patient who has relapsed with other than local disease should be considered for autologous BMT or peripheral blood stem cell support during aggressive high-dose chemotherapy. The latter is, in the minds of many experts, preferable to the former. It is likely, however, that this type of aggressive therapy is, for now, an interim solution until more effective drugs for Hodgkin's disease are discovered.

Non-Hodgkin's Lymphoma

The international index devised by the International Non-Hodgkin's Lymphoma Prognostic Factor Project appears to be a very useful guide to treatment selection for patients with aggressive lymphoma. All future study designs for aggressive lymphoma treatment should incorporate this index. It is now time to revise the International Working Formulation in an effort to simplify the pathologic diagnosis of these diseases and to take into account many important European contributions that have been given little attention in the current formulation. An example of what needs to be considered in future systems is primary cutaneous CD30-positive large-cell lymphoma, a T-cell lymphoma with a very favorable prognosis.

Treatment of HIV-related lymphoma has progressed surprisingly well recently. Several successful aggressive regimens have been developed, and experience with them has already taught us that lymphoma is not a rate-limiting illness in HIV infection. The lymphoma can be controlled, sometimes eradicated, and otherwise healthy patients with HIV can be returned to a healthy state. The paper by Gisselbrecht et al. (Abstract 116-95-4-29) is particularly noteworthy here, as is the paper by Sparano et al. (2).

An extremely important study conducted by the Southwest Oncology Group (Abstract 116-95-4-30) demonstrated that cyclosphosphamide, doxorubicin, vincristine, and prednisone (CHOP); methotrexate with leucovorin rescue, doxorubicin, cyclophosphamide, vincristine, prednisone, and bleomycin (MACOP-B); methotrexate in a low dose with leucovorin rescue, bleomycin, doxorubicin, cyclophosphamide, vincristine, and dexamethasone (m-BACOD); and prednisone, doxorubicin, cyclophosphamide, and etoposide and then cytarabine, bleomycin, vincristine, and methotrexate with leucovorin rescue (ProMACE-CytaBOM) are all essentially equally effective as therapy for advanced non-Hodgkin's lymphoma. They found that CHOP was less toxic than the other regimens. Some of us are not surprised by this result (3). This disappointment does not mean that we should give up trying to build a better lymphoma trap. However, it does mean that comparative studies should be done earlier in the development of a new regimen.

Multiple Myeloma

Initial enthusiasm for autologous BMT in myeloma has dwindled quite a bit, as evidenced by the report by Alexanian et al. (Abstract 116-95-4-42). It is time to prospectively compare this approach with others in a multi-institutional effort. The answer from such a study would be important in developing standards of care for this neoplasm.

New drugs for myeloma are needed, and phase II studies should be a priority in this disease.

Chronic Leukemias

The development of fludarabine for treatment of chronic lymphocytic leukemia (CLL) has progressed to studying it in previously untreated patients, and an early indication is that it is likely to replace oral alkylating agents as standard therapy in that setting. It is clear that complete responses in patients with CLL can be obtained with fludarabine, but the impact of the drug on survival cannot be determined for years. The role of newer antimetabolites such as 2-chlorodeoxyadenosine in fludarabine failures is unclear at the moment because conflicting reports have appeared.

There are no new treatments for chronic myelogenous leukemia (CML). Interferon has not been as useful as might be expected from previous reports in all hands as evidenced by the Cancer and Leukemia Group B study (Abstract 116-95-4–52). Long-term follow-up of CML patients treated with allogeneic BMT in 1 study reported by Gratwohl et al. (4) suggested that the procedure may not result in cure as often as initially thought. That being the case, unrelated-donor marrow transplants, which are associated with a 50% mortality rate even in young patients, should be considered extremely carefully.

Acute Myeloid Leukemia

Further progress has been made in the treatment of acute promyelocytic leukemia (APL) with all-*trans* retinoic acid (ATRA). Castaigne et al. (Abstract 116-95-4–70) point out that lower doses of the agent may be optimal, and Fenaux et al. (Abstract 116-95-4–71) demonstrated that ATRA combined with standard induction chemotherapy may give results superior to either approach alone. It seems clear from this work that the ATRA-chemotherapy combination will become standard therapy for APL. Diverio et al. (Abstract 116-95-4–69) reported on the usefulness of a reverse transcription–polymerase chain reaction assay to detect minimal residual disease in APL. The absence of disease detectable by this method correlated well with long-term disease-free survival. These clinical and laboratory results taken together suggest that APL may become the first adult acute leukemia to be routinely cured.

Acute Lymphocytic Leukemia

Evidence is mounting that magnetic fields may play a role in the etiology or pathogenesis of childhood acute lymphocytic leukemia (ALL). The evidence is all derived from retrospective epidemiologic surveys, but some reports, such as that of Feychting et al. (Abstract 116-95-4–73), are compelling. The issue deserves further study.

Major improvement in the therapy of poor-prognosis childhood ALL has been made, as reported by the Childrens Cancer Group (Abstract 116-95-4–81). Their work confirms and extends the important work initiated by the Berlin-Frankfurt-Münster group in 1976 (5). Results in poor-prognosis patients now approach those obtained in patients with a favorable prognosis. Unfortunately, results in adult ALL still lag far behind those obtained in children, as observed by Weiss et al. (Abstract 116-95-4-82).

I hope the reader will find this brief summary of the year useful and that the papers abstracted in this chapter will kindle ideas that will result in abstracts in future volumes of the YEAR BOOK OF HEMATOLOGY.

Peter H. Wiernik, M.D.

References

1. Lin: *Proc Am Soc Clin Oncol* 13:185, 1994.
2. Sparano JA, et al: *Blood* 81:2810, 1993.
3. Roth JA, et al (eds): *Thoracic Oncology*. Philadelphia, WB Saunders, 1989, p 458.
4. Gratwohl A, et al: *Bone Marrow Transplant* 12:509–516, 1993.
5. Henze G, et al: *Klin Padiatr* 193:145, 1983.

Hodgkin's Disease

Presence of Epstein-Barr Virus Harbouring Small and Intermediate-Sized Cells in Hodgkin's Disease: Is There a Relationship With Reed-Sternberg Cells?

Jiwa NM, Kanavaros P, De Bruin PC, Van Der Valk P, Horstman A, Vos W, Mullink H, Walboomers JMM, Meijer CJLM (Free Univ Hosp, Amsterdam)
J Pathol 170:129–136, 1993   116-95-4-1

Background.—Several investigators have recently shown a relationship between Epstein-Barr virus (EBV) and Hodgkin's disease by using several methods for detecting EBV. The relative values of these methods—polymerase chain reaction (PCR), DNA and RNA in situ hybridization, and immunohistochemistry—were determined in a study of the lymph nodes of patients with Hodgkin's disease.

Methods.—Forty-four patients with Hodgkin's disease (primarily the nodular sclerosing type) were investigated for EBV. In situ hybridization and immunohistochemistry were combined to correlate the presence and activity of the virus at the cellular level.

Findings.—In 18 of the patients (53%), EBV-DNA sequences were detected with PCR. In 12 of these 18, DNA and RNA in situ hybridization were also positive. Of the remaining 6 patients with positive results, 2 were also positive with RNA in situ hybridization and immunohistochemistry for the detection of latent membrane protein-1. No positive signal was obtained with DNA in situ hybridization. All studies positive by DNA or RNA in situ hybridization, or both, were also positive for latent membrane protein-1. With RNA in situ hybridization, the Reed-

Sternberg cells and their mononuclear variants stained positive, and small and intermediate cells often reacted with the EBV-specific probes (EBERs). Double staining with cellular markers showed that most smaller EBER-positive cells often did not express T, B, or histiocytic markers but that they, along with Reed-Sternberg cells, demonstrated cytoplasmic and membranous staining with the lectin PNA. The smaller EBER-positive cells were not detected in EBV-PCR–negative Hodgkin's disease. Reed-Sternberg cells that were EBER-positive and a high proportion of the intermediate-sized cells were almost always positive for latent membrane protein-1, whereas most small EBER-positive cells remained negative for latent membrane protein-1. Only a few EBER-1– and EBER-2–positive cells were observed in EBV-PCR–positive nonmalignant lymph nodes.

Conclusion.—Most of the smaller EBV-positive cells in Hodgkin's disease belonged to reactive EBV-infected lymphocytes. However, these findings support the hypothesis that at least some smaller cells may belong to the reservoir of neoplastic cells in Hodgkin's disease.

---

bcl-2 Expression in Hodgkin's Disease: Correlation With the t(14;18) Translocation and Epstein-Barr Virus

Bhagat SKM, Medeiros LJ, Weiss LM, Wang J, Raffeld M, Stetler-Stevenson M (Natl Cancer Inst, Bethesda, Md; City of Hope Natl Med Ctr, Duarte, Calif)
Am J Clin Pathol 99:604–608, 1993   116-95-4-2

Background.—The pathogenesis of Hodgkin's disease is not well understood. There is cytogenetic evidence in some cases of a translocation that fuses the *bcl*-2 oncogene to a constitutively expressed immunoglobulin gene, t(14;18). The cells containing this translocation in Hodgkin's disease have not been identified. To understand the role of the *bcl*-2 oncogene in Hodgkin's disease, a group of 13 patients with and without the translocation was selected for analysis with a monoclonal anti–*bcl*-2 antibody. These patients were also analyzed for Epstein-Barr virus (EBV) expression, which has been reported to increase *bcl*-2 expression.

Results.—Immunohistologic staining revealed *bcl*-2 protein in the Reed-Sternberg and Hodgkin's cells in 8 of the 13 patients, 3 with the translocation and 5 with no detectable translocation. Epstein-Barr virus RNA was detected in the Reed-Sternberg and Hodgkin's cells of 4 patients: 2 also had *bcl*-2–positive Reed-Sternberg and Hodgkin's cells. The *bcl*-2–Positive Reed-Sternberg and Hodgkin's cells did not correlate with clinical features, histologic subtype, detectable translocation, or presence of EBV RNA.

Conclusion.—Although *bcl*-2 was expressed by Reed-Sternberg and Hodgkin's cells in most cases of Hodgkin's disease, this expression was not correlated with the presence of the t(14;18) translocation or EBV RNA. Therefore, the t(14;18) translocation may not be important in the pathogenesis of Hodgkin's disease. Further studies are necessary to examine the possible roles of this translocation and of EBV in the pathogenesis of Hodgkin's disease.

▶ It is still not clear what role, if any, EBV plays in the etiology or pathogenesis of Hodgkin's disease. The fact that EBV is not associated with familial Hodgkin's disease suggests that other factors are more important in the genesis of the disease or that familial and random Hodgkin's disease are different entities (1).—P.H. Wiernik, M.D.

Reference

1. Lin A, et al: *Proc Am Soc Clin Oncol* 13:185, 1994.

Prognostic Role of Serum β_2-Microglobulin in Hodgkin's Disease
Dimopoulos MA, Cabanillas F, Lee JJ, Swan F, Fuller L, Allen PK, Hagemeister FB (MD Anderson Cancer Ctr, Houston)
J Clin Oncol 11:1108–1111, 1993   116-95-4–3

Introduction.—Serum levels of β_2-microglobulin (β_2M) are increased in a wide range of malignant and nonmalignant diseases. In patients with several lymphoid malignancies, elevated serum levels of $\beta2M$ are associated with a poor prognosis. The role of serum $\beta2M$ in the prognosis of patients with Hodgkin's disease was assessed.

Methods.—The cohort analyzed consisted of 160 previously untreated patients with Hodgkin's disease. Serum levels of $\beta2M$ were determined before the initiation of treatment and tested for their correlation with known prognostic factors for the disease. These variables, together with $\beta2M$, were evaluated for their role in predicting the probability of complete remission and time to treatment failure.

Results.—Mean and median serum $\beta2M$ levels in these patients were 2.1 mg/L and 1.9 mg/L, respectively. A cutoff value of 2.5 mg/L was used to separate patients into low- and high-serum $\beta2M$ groups. Forty-seven patients (29%) were in the high-value group. Elevated serum $\beta2M$ values were more common in older patients, those with B symptoms, those with more advanced Ann Arbor stage, and male patients with lower hemoglobin values. Most patients (89%) achieved complete remission, but the rate of complete remission was lower in patients with elevated $\beta2m$ levels (79%) than in those with low $\beta2M$ levels (93%). Relapse had occurred in 16% of patients after a median follow-up of 30 months. Variables predictive of shorter time to treatment failure were high serum $\beta2M$ level, low hemoglobin, and advanced Ann Arbor stage.

Conclusion.—Patients with Hodgkin's disease and low serum levels of the polypeptide $\beta2M$ had a significantly better prognosis than patients with high levels of $\beta2M$. The impact of elevated $\beta2m$ appeared to be

Moving?

I'd like to receive my *Year Book of Hematology* without interruption.
Please note the following change of address, effective:

Name: _____

New Address: _____

_____

City: _____ State: _____ Zip: _____

Old Address: _____

_____

City: _____ State: _____ Zip: _____

Reservation Card

Yes, I would like my own copy of *Year Book of Hematology*. Please begin my subscription with the current edition according to the terms described below.* I understand that I will have 30 days to examine each annual edition. If satisfied, I will pay just $69.95 plus sales tax, postage and handling (price subject to change without notice).

Name: _____

Address: _____

City: _____ State: _____ Zip: _____

Method of Payment
O Visa   O Mastercard   O AmEx   O Bill me   O Check (in US dollars, payable to Mosby, Inc.)

Card number: _____ Exp date: _____

Signature: _____

LS-0909

*Your *Year Book* Service Guarantee:

When you subscribe to the *Year Book*, we'll send you an advance notice of future volumes about two months before they publish. This automatic notice system is designed to take up as little of your time as possible. If you do not want the *Year Book*, the advance notice makes it quick and easy for you to let us know your decision, and you will always have at least 20 days to decide. If we don't hear from you, we'll send you the new volume as soon as it's available. And, of course, the *Year Book* is yours to examine free of charge for 30 days (postage, handling and applicable sales tax are added to each shipment.).

BUSINESS REPLY MAIL

FIRST CLASS MAIL   PERMIT No. 762   CHICAGO, IL

POSTAGE WILL BE PAID BY ADDRESSEE

Chris Hughes
Mosby-Year Book, Inc.
200 N. LaSalle Street
Suite 2600
Chicago, IL 60601-9981

NO POSTAGE
NECESSARY
IF MAILED
IN THE
UNITED STATES

BUSINESS REPLY MAIL

FIRST CLASS MAIL   PERMIT No. 762   CHICAGO, IL

POSTAGE WILL BE PAID BY ADDRESSEE

Chris Hughes
Mosby-Year Book, Inc.
200 N. LaSalle Street
Suite 2600
Chicago, IL 60601-9981

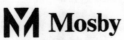

Dedicated to publishing excellence

more significant in patients with advanced disease. It is possible that $\beta2M$ serves as a tumor marker and reflects tumor burden in patients with Hodgkin's disease.

▶ This is a very useful clinical discovery. Because patients with Hodgkin's disease are rarely seen with impaired renal function or treated with interferon, $\beta2M$ determinations may turn out to be more useful in Hodgkin's disease than in myeloma.—P.H. Wiernik, M.D.

Serum Interleukin 6 Levels Are Elevated in Lymphoma Patients and Correlate With Survival in Advanced Hodgkin's Disease and With B Symptoms

Kurzrock R, Redman J, Cabanillas F, Jones D, Rothberg J, Talpaz M (Univ of Texas, Houston)

Cancer Res 53:2118–2122, 1993   116-95-4-4

Background.—B symptoms, such as fever, night sweats, and weight loss, are common among patients with lymphoma. These symptoms are also associated with poor prognosis. Aberrant production of pyrogenic cytokines could be responsible for these disease manifestations. Therefore, the relationship between these disease features and serum levels of tumor necrosis factor-α (TNF-α), IL-1β, γ-interferon (INF-γ), and IL-6 was examined in a group of patients with lymphoma.

Methods.—Within a 2-year period, serum samples from 28 patients with Hodgkin's lymphoma, 32 patients with non-Hodgkin's lymphoma, and 20 normal volunteers were collected and stored at $-70°C$. The samples were assayed for INF-γ by a specific and sensitive radioimmunoassay. The samples were assayed for the other cytokines by sensitive enzyme-linked immunosorbent assay techniques.

Results.—There were no statistically significant differences in the serum levels of INF-γ, TNF-α, or IL-1β. However, 35% of patients with lymphoma had detectable serum levels of IL-6, whereas none of the normal volunteers had detectable levels. Among the patients with B symptoms, 59% had detectable levels, whereas only 11% of the patients with lymphoma and no B symptoms had detectable levels. This was true among both groups of patients with lymphoma. The IL-6 levels were not significantly correlated with time from diagnosis, β_2-microglobulin, or lactate dehydrogenase levels. The median survival of patients with Hodgkin's disease who had detectable IL-6 levels was only 10 months, whereas those with undetectable serum levels have not reached median survival after 37.5 months of follow-up.

Conclusion.—Elevation of serum IL-6 levels is fairly common in patients with lymphoma and is associated with the presence of B symptoms. Elevated serum IL-6 levels are also associated with shorter survival in patients with Hodgkin's disease.

▶ This paper may explain why cyclosporin A was useful in the treatment of B symptoms of Hodgkin's disease, because the agent has been shown to inhibit IL-6 secretion. That may also account for the antimyeloma activity of cyclosporin A (1, 2).—P.H. Wiernik, M.D.

References

1. Zwitter M, et al: *Ann Intern Med* 106:843, 1987.
2. Wiernik PH, et al: *Leuk Lymphoma* 1994 (In press).

Comparison of CT and MRI in the Evaluation of Therapeutic Response in Thoracic Hodgkin Disease

Elkowitz SS, Leonidas JC, Lopez M, Cherick I, Schiff RG, Karayalcin G, Lanzkowsky P (Schneider Children's Hosp, New York)
Pediatr Radiol 23:301–304, 1993   116-95-4–5

Background.—The diagnosis and staging of Hodgkin's disease are usually based on a combination of imaging studies and histologic tests. Computed tomography is particularly useful in assessing the extent of disease in the chest. However, this technique does not allow for easy differentiation between residual neoplastic activity and scar tissue after treatment, nor does it allow for the identification of early recurrence. Magnetic resonance imaging could be a potential alternative because of its ability to discern tissue characteristics such as increased cellularity and edema by their higher water content as opposed to mature fibrous tissue. The clinical usefulness of MRI was compared with that of CT in evaluating the response to therapy in a group of patients with thoracic Hodgkin's lymphoma.

Methods.—Twenty-three patients with histologically verified Hodgkin's disease underwent 47 matched CT and MRI examinations of the chest within 1 week of each other. Five patients entered the study at the time of diagnosis; the other 18 had already been treated and were in remission. Disease activity was based on history, clinical examination, and laboratory values. Because none of these methods is infallible, disease activity was assigned only after a follow-up of at least 6 months to verify disease status. When the imaging study indicated no active disease and the patient was in clinical remission, the imaging examination was considered true negative. If it indicated active disease and the patient was at the onset of disease or in relapse, it was considered true positive. False negative or false positive status was assigned to imaging studies negative for disease activity in the presence of active new disease or relapse or to imaging studies that were positive in the presence of clinical remission.

Results.—On all 47 occasions, CT and MRI correctly identified active disease. The sensitivity of CT was high, but its specificity was very low (27%) because of residual masses. The positive predictive value of CT was therefore low, but the negative predictive value was high. Better results were seen with MRI. The follow-up examination indicated signal intensity consistent with complete fibrous replacement in 5 patients in clinical remission, which was confirmed by follow-up studies. In 10 additional patients with MRI showing persistently high signal on T2-weighted images despite verified early clinical remission, subsequent MRI examinations indicated fibrosis within 3–5 months. In the remaining patients, a persistently high signal intensity on T2-weighted images was seen for as long as 13 months of follow-up, despite continuous remission.

Conclusion.—The value of MRI in assessing the response to treatment of Hodgkin's lymphoma is limited. Nevertheless, MRI does characterize tissue somewhat better than CT, being more specific in excluding neoplastic activity when residual masses of uniformly low signal appear on T2-weighted images. However, in areas of persistently high signal on T2, the findings are inconclusive, and MRI is no better than CT.

▶ A useful observation compatible with findings in adults.—P.H. Wiernik, M.D.

Beguiled by the Gallium: Thymic Rebound in an Adult After Chemotherapy for Hodgkin's Disease
Burns DE, Schiffman FJ (Brown Univ, Providence, RI)
Chest 104:1916–1919, 1993   116-95-4-6

Background.—Gallium scanning has been found useful in diagnosing, staging, and differentiating between residual active disease or relapse and benign mediastinal enlargement after chemotherapy in patients with Hodgkin's and non-Hodgkin's lymphomas. However, in adult patients, gallium uptake in the mediastinum after chemotherapy may be indicative of benign thymic hyperplasia rather than tumor recurrence.

Case Report.—Woman, 18, reported general malaise, back pain, and persistent cough of 6 weeks' duration after an upper respiratory tract infection. Cervical lymphadenopathy was found during physical examination, and a chest radiograph showed mediastinal enlargement. After a staging workup, the patient was diagnosed as having Hodgkin's disease involving the mediastinal lymph nodes and lung parenchyma. A pretreatment gallium-67 scan revealed increased uptake in the mediastinum. Treatment included 6 monthly cycles of chemotherapy. After this treatment, the chest radiograph and chest CT revealed resolution of disease and a repeat gallium scan yielded normal results. A surveillance gallium scan performed 4 months later showed increased activity in the mediastinal and hilar regions. Corresponding chest CT and MRI revealed a retrosternal mass. Before

initiating aggressive treatment for presumed disease recurrence, a biopsy specimen of the mass was taken, and it revealed normal thymus tissue. This mediastinal mass, now considered as thymus, remained evident on both MRI and chest
CT. However, a gallium scan done 10 weeks after the biopsy specimen was
taken did not show abnormal radionuclide uptake in the mediastinum despite
the persistent mass. The patient has remained disease-free for more than 3 years
after the initial treatment. The most recent examinations, including a normal gallium scan and stable CT and MRI, have verified the absence of disease recurrence.

Conclusion.—After chemotherapy, thymus enlargement can occur in
adults with Hodgkin's disease. This fact should be considered when interpreting imaging studies, including gallium scans.

▶ The point about thymic enlargement in young patients is very important. I
have seen several patients who were thought to require further therapy because the possibility of thymic enlargement was not considered.—P.H. Wiernik, M.D.

**Cardiac Disease Following Treatment of Hodgkin's Disease in Chil-
dren and Adolescents**
Hancock SL, Donaldson SS, Hoppe RT (Stanford Univ, Calif)
J Clin Oncol 11:1208–1215, 1993   116-95-4-7

Study Population.—Because heart disease is such a frequent cause of
death in patients treated for Hodgkin's disease, the risks of cardiac disease were evaluated in 635 patients who were treated for this cancer before age 21 years in the past 3 decades. The patients had a mean age at
treatment of 15½ years. The mean follow-up was 10.3 years (representing 6,564 person-years of observation). Mortality rates were compared
with those in the age-, sex-, and race-matched general population.

Treatment.—A large majority of patients received mediastinal irradiation either primarily or later, using mantle fields. Total lymphoid irradiation was administered to 244 patients. In 71% of patients, the mediastinal dose was 40 Gy or greater. Subcarinal blocking was routinely used
after 1970 to limit the dose to much of the heart to 30–35 Gy. A 4.8-MV
or 6-MV linear accelerator was used for all treatments.

Findings.—Twelve patients have died of heart disease. Seven deaths
resulted from acute myocardial infarction, 3 resulted from valvular or
congenital heart disease, and 2 resulted from radiation-induced pericar-
ditis or pancarditis. All these patients had received a mediastinal radiation dose of 42–45 Gy between the ages of 9 and 20 years. The relative
risk of death from any cardiac disease was 29.6, and for fatal acute myocardial infarction, the risk was 41.5. None of the patients receiving lower
mediastinal radiation doses or no mediastinal radiation therapy have
died.

Implications.—At a minimum, cardiac abnormalities must be carefully sought in children and adolescents receiving mediastinal irradiation for Hodgkin's disease. The risk may be minimized by delivering a lower dose and less extensive radiation therapy and by using chemotherapy.

Factors Affecting Late Mortality From Heart Disease After Treatment of Hodgkin's Disease
Hancock SL, Tucker MA, Hoppe RT (Stanford Univ, Calif; Natl Cancer Inst, Rockville, Md)
JAMA 270:1949–1955, 1993

116-95-4-8

Purpose.—Although most patients with Hodgkin's disease can achieve long-term, relapse-free survival with treatment, intercurrent or treatment-induced disease may affect overall survival. The many radiation-induced or radiation-associated heart diseases may be particularly important causes of death. The risk of death from radiation-associated cardiac disease in a large sample of patients with Hodgkin's disease was examined retrospectively.

Methods.—The study sample comprised 2,232 patients with Hodgkin's disease treated in a 30-year period. Their risk of cardiac death was compared with that of a matched general population. In the first 11 years of the experience, radiation was administered in daily fractions of 2.2 to 2.75 Gy, with little cardiac blocking. Thereafter, subcarinal blocking was used routinely, limiting the radiation dose to the heart. In the last 15 years, fraction sizes were limited to 1.5 to 1.8 Gy, and most patients younger than 17 years of age were treated with combination chemotherapy and low-dose, limited-field radiation. Follow-up averaged 9.5 years.

Findings.—A total of 327 patients died of Hodgkin's disease and 290 died of other causes. Overall, 4% died of cardiac causes. The patients' relative risk of cardiac death was 3.1 times that of the general population, and the absolute risk was 28 excess deaths per 10,000 person-years of observation. The absolute risk was higher in men because of the baseline increased cardiac risk among men in the general population. The routine use of cardiac blocking decreased the relative risk of cardiac-related death from 4.3 to 2.6. The relative risk of death from acute myocardial infarction decreased significantly with age at mediastinal irradiation, from 45 for those treated before 19 years of age to 1.8 (nonsignificant) for those treated after 50 years of age. The risk also increased with time since treatment.

Conclusion.—The risk of death from cardiac causes is about 3 times higher in patients with Hodgkin's disease treated with mediastinal irradiation than in the general population. Risk is elevated in patients treated at younger ages and in those with longer time since treatment. The routine use of cardiac blocking has decreased the risk of death from cardiac causes other than myocardial infarction. Advances in treatment may bring further reductions in the cardiac risk.

▶ Concern for late cardiac complications of radiation therapy was one of the major factors that led to the study of chemotherapy as initial therapy for early-stage Hodgkin's disease. The same concern must be expressed for the use of doxorubicin in young patients (1).—P.H. Wiernik, M.D.

Reference

1. Lipshultz SE, et al: N Engl J Med 324:808, 1991.

Hodgkin's Disease: The Protective Effect of Childbearing
Kravdal Ø, Hansen S (Central Bureau of Statistics, Oslo, Norway; Cancer Registry, Oslo, Norway)
Int J Cancer 55:909–914, 1993   116-95-4–9

Objective.—The influence of reproductive factors on the occurrence of Hodgkin's disease was examined by reviewing register and census data for cohorts of 1.3 million Norwegian men and the same number of women born between 1935 and 1974.

Findings.—There were 695 cases of Hodgkin's disease in men and 441 in women during the review. Hazard model estimates indicated that for a given age and a given birth cohort, the incidence of Hodgkin's disease in women was inversely related to current parity. Higher parity explained part of the downward incidence trend observed after the middle 20s (Fig 4–1). A clear relationship was noted only for nodular sclerosing Hodgkin's disease. The risk of Hodgkin's disease developing in men exceeded that in childless women. The lower risk of Hodgkin's disease in women of high parity could not be attribued to lower social status.

Conclusion.—An inverse relationship between the number of children a woman delivers and her risk of development of Hodgkin's disease was supported.

▶ A very interesting observation that needs to be confirmed.—P.H. Wiernik, M.D.

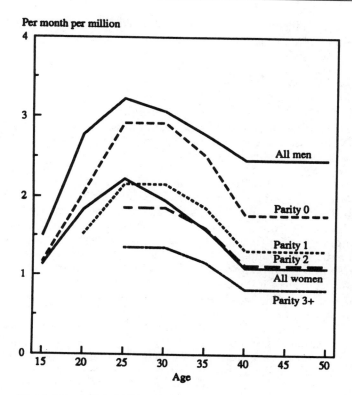

Per month per million

Model: Cohort+Age+Parity or Cohort+Age

Fig 4–1.—Incidence of Hodgkin's disease, by parity, predicted for women and men born in 1945. (Courtesy of Kravdal Ø, Hansen S: *Int J Cancer* 55:909–914, 1993.)

Hodgkin's Disease in the Very Young

Cleary SF, Link MP, Donaldson SS (Stanford Univ, Calif)
Int J Radiat Oncol Biol Phys 28:77–83, 1993   116-95-4–10

Background.—Although early studies suggested a worse prognosis for the youngest patients with Hodgkin's disease, more recent studies have shown no difference in the natural history and response to treatment of pediatric vs. adult patients. There are few data regarding the treatment response and survival of preadolescent patients with Hodgkin's disease, who constitute only a small percentage of patients with this disease.

Patients.—This retrospective study analyzed the outcome of 91 children, aged 10 years or younger with Hodgkin's disease. The patients were treated within a 30-year period, during which they represented only 4% of all patients with Hodgkin's disease. Eighty percent were boys.

Findings.—Histologic examination showed mixed cellularity in 33% and lymphocyte predominance in 13%, more common than in adolescent or adult patients. The 5-year survival was 94%, and the 10-year survival was 92%, compared with 93% and 86% for adolescents and 84% and 73% for adults. Freedom from relapse was also better in young children: 88% at 5 and 85% at 10 years. The 25-year actuarial survival was 78%, compared with 67% for adolescents and 41% for adults.

Young children were more likely to have stage I and less likely to have stage IV disease. The course of disease was at least similar to that of adolescents and somewhat better than that of adults for young children at all stages of disease. The actuarial 25-year survival was 73% for young children with stage I or II disease and 89% for those with stage III or IV disease. Corresponding figures were 79% and 28% for adolescents and 45% and 41% for adults. About two thirds of the young children were treated with the combination of low-dose radiation and chemotherapy, and one third were treated by primary external-beam radiation therapy. At a median follow-up of 11 years, the radiation therapy group had a 64% freedom from relapse and a 75% survival, compared with 97% and 93%, respectively, for the combined-modality group.

Conclusion.—This retrospective study demonstrates an excellent response to treatment in preadolescent children with Hodgkin's disease, with a freedom from relapse and survival significantly better than those of older patients. Prognostic advantages in the youngest patients may include the different histologic and stage distribution and the more frequent use of combined-modality therapy for even early-stage disease. Age is a significant prognostic factor of multivariate analysis.

Treatment of Pediatric Hodgkin Disease Tailored to Stage, Mediastinal Mass, and Age: An Italian (AIEOP) Multicenter Study on 215 Patients

Vecchi V, Pileri S, Burnelli R, Bontempi N, Comelli A, Testi AM, Carli M, Sotti G, Rosati D, Di Tullio MT, Grazia G, Massolo F, Aricó M, Colella R, Pession A, Rondelli R, Paolucci G (Bologna Univ, Italy; G Gaslini Inst, Genova, Italy; "La Sapienza" Univ, Roma; et al)
Cancer 72:2049–2057, 1993   116-95-4–11

Background.—The use of combination chemotherapy and radiation therapy has greatly improved the survival rates of children with Hodgkin's disease. However, some patients have had serious complications as a result of these treatments. A treatment protocol that would optimize treatment results and minimize serious side effects was sought in a multicenter study.

Methods.—Between November of 1983 and December of 1989, 215 consecutive children younger than age 15 years with Hodgkin's disease diagnosed were included in the study. All patients were given a diagnosis with clinical staging, histologic classification, and radiologic studies. They were divided into 3 groups. Group 1 included patients in the early stages of disease who received 3 courses of Adriamycin, bleomycin, vinblastine, and imidazole carboxamide (ABVD). Group 2 included patients in intermediate stages who were treated for 6 months with alternating cycles of ABVD and nitrogen mustard, vincristine, procarbazine, and prednisone (MOPP). Group 3 included patients in advanced stages who received alternating courses of MOPP and ABVD for 6 months. All groups then received low-dose radiation therapy, with the doses being determined by age and the response to initial chemotherapy. Group 3 patients then received an additional 4 courses of MOPP-ABVD.

Results.—Complete remission or good partial remission was achieved by 87% of the patients after initial chemotherapy. In group 1, 91.6% had a good response; in groups 2 and 3, 85% had a good response. After radiation therapy, all group 1 patients achieved complete remission. Radiation therapy brought a slight increase in response in group 2 but brought no improvement in group 3 patients. The most significant factors in predicting a poor prognosis were a large mediastinal mass, systemic symptoms, and nodular sclerosing histologic subtype (as opposed to the mixed-cellularity subtype). Age was also a prognostic factor, with children younger than age 7 years achieving significantly better freedom from progression.

Discussion.—A more conservative treatment regimen is sufficient in patients with less aggressive disease. However, further research must be done on chemotherapeutic protocols for higher-risk patients, because this 8-drug regimen did not yield improved survival compared with other regimens. Patients with large mediastinal mass may benefit from the earlier use of radiation therapy between chemotherapy courses. Children younger than age 7 years also have fewer unfavorable prognostic factors, suggesting that Hodgkin's disease has a less aggressive expression in younger children.

Pediatric Stage IV Hodgkin Disease: Long-Term Survival
Bader SB, Weinstein H, Mauch P, Silver B, Tarbell NJ (Harvard Med School, Boston)
Cancer 72:249–255, 1993   116-95-4–12

Background.—The optimal treatment for stage IV Hodgkin's disease in children is uncertain, partly because of the small number of published reports. The use of chemotherapy alone and in combination with low-dose radiation therapy in pediatric patients with stage IV Hodgkin's disease was evaluated.

Methods.—Forty-two children aged 18 years or younger with stage IV Hodgkin's disease were treated with combination chemotherapy consisting of mechlorethamine, vincristine, procarbazine, and prednisone with or without doxorubicin, bleomycin, vinblastine, and dacarbazine; 20 of these patients received adjunctive radiation therapy.

Results.—During a median follow-up of 83 months the 7-year actuarial freedom from progression of Hodgkin's disease was 69%, and the overall survival was 78%. Only 1 recurrence developed after 2 years. Twenty-six patients had a complete response to initial chemotherapy, 11 had a partial response, 1 had no response, and 4 had progressive disease. The 7-year freedom from progression rate was 73% for patients with a complete response to chemotherapy and 90% for those with a partial response. The actuarial overall 7-year survival was 88% among patients with a complete response and 80% among those with a partial response. Neither the 7-year freedom from progression nor overall survival rates differed significantly between those with a complete response and those with a partial response. However, the prognosis was significantly worse in patients who did not respond or had progressive disease after chemotherapy; their 7-year actuarial survival was 40%. Nine patients who responded completely to induction chemotherapy received adjunctive radiation. Although crude relapse rates were comparable among those receiving radiation therapy and those who did not, 4 of 5 patients who had relapses after chemotherapy alone had "B" symptoms and recurrences at initial disease sites. Adjuvant radiation therapy improved progression-free survival for patients with B symptoms.

Conclusion.—The risk of relapse is high in children with stage IV-B Hodgkin's disease who are treated with chemotherapy alone. These patients may benefit from combined treatment with chemotherapy and then radiation therapy.

▶ The excellent results obtained in children with Hodgkin's disease in these state-of-the-art studies (Abstracts 116-95-4–10 through 116-95-4–12) are obviously satisfying. It should be noted that no advantage for the use of doxorubicin can be found in these series.—P.H. Wiernik, M.D.

Hodgkin Disease in Patients 60 Years of Age or Older: Histologic and Clinical Features of Advanced-Stage Disease
Mir R, Anderson J, Strauchen J, Nissen NI, Cooper MR, Rafla S, Canellos GP, Bloomfield CD, Gottlieb AJ, Peterson B, Barcos M, Cancer and Leukemia Group B (Long Island Jewish Med Ctr, New Hyde Park, NY; Univ of Nebraska, Omaha; Mount Sinai Hosp, New York; et al)
Cancer 71:1857–1866, 1993   116-95-4–13

Objective.—The clinical and pathologic features of disease were reviewed in 171 patients aged 60 and older who received 4 different Hodgkin's disease treatment protocols between 1969 and 1988.

Histologic Findings.—Hodgkin's disease was diagnosed in 114 patients, two thirds of the total. Another 52 patients (30%) had a diagnosis of non-Hodgkin's lymphoma, and 5 patients had miscellaneous disorders. Of the 114 patients with a diagnosis of Hodgkin's disease, 51% were classified as having nodular sclerosing Hodgkin's disease, and 39.5%, mixed cellularity disease. Most patients with non-Hodgkin's lymphoma had either diffuse mixed small cleaved and large-cell lymphoma or diffuse large-cell lymphoma.

Clinical Features.—Males predominated in a ratio of 1.6 to 1. Only 7 patients were older than 74 years of age. Nearly 90% of patients had stage IIIB or stage IVB disease when first seen. In patients with either Hodgkin's disease or non-Hodgkin's lymphoma the most common sites of involvement were the para-aortic and the iliac–inguinal–femoral lymph nodes.

Outcome.—Patients with nodular sclerosing Hodgkin's disease and those with mixed cellularity disease had median survival times of 1.7 and 1.4 years, respectively, which was not a significant difference. There also was no significant difference in the overall survival between the patients with Hodgkin's disease (1.5 years) and those with non-Hodgkin's lymphoma (1.3 years). In the most recent treatment protocol, the patients with Hodgkin's disease had lower 5-year survival than those aged 40–59 years or those younger than 40 years of age. In addition, the older patients had more frequent involvement of the gastrointestinal tract and less frequent involvement of the cervical and mediastinal-hilar node groups than did younger patients.

Wide-Field Radiation Therapy With or Without Chemotherapy for Patients With Hodgkin Disease in Relapse After Initial Combination Chemotherapy

Uematsu M, Tarbell NJ, Silver B, Coleman CN, Rosenthal DS, Shulman LN, Canellos G, Weinstein H, Mauch P (Harvard Med School, Boston)
Cancer 72:207–212, 1993   116-95-4–14

Introduction.—Patients with Hodgkin's disease who relapse after initial chemotherapy appear to have a poor outlook, particularly if the first complete remission is brief. Frequently disease recurs at sites of initial node involvement, and in some patients this may be the only form of recurrence. The course of disease was examined in patients whose relapse after combination chemotherapy was limited to nodal sites and who were treated with wide-field, high-dose radiation therapy with or without further chemotherapy.

Patients and Treatment.—The 28 patients (median age, 26 years) relapsed after initial treatment with combination chemotherapy only and had disease limited to the nodes at this time. Nodular sclerosing disease was the most frequent type. Most often treatment with mechlorethamine, vincristine, prednisone, and procarbazine (MOPP) was delivered at the outset. Eleven patients were seen with stage IV disease. Six patients were in second relapse at the time that wide-field radiation therapy was recommended. All but 4 patients received radiation therapy doses comparable to those usually recommended for patients having early-stage disease who receive no other form of treatment. Half of the 28 patients, all in initial relapse, received further combination chemotherapy before radiation therapy.

Results.—The actuarial rate of freedom from relapse 7 years after salvage treatment was 93% for patients receiving both chemotherapy and radiation therapy and 36% for those receiving radiation therapy alone. The respective 7-year survival rates were 85% and 36%. Only 1 of the 14 patients given combined treatment for nodal relapse had a further relapse, and 12 of these patients were alive without progressive disease a median of 5.5 years after retreatment. All but 5 of the 14 patients had persistent or progressive disease or relapsed within about 1 year of initial chemotherapy.

Conclusion.—A combination of further combination chemotherapy and high-dose, wide-field radiation therapy should be considered for patients in nodal relapse of Hodgkin's disease after initial chemotherapy.

Effect of Filgrastim (G-CSF) in Hodgkin's Disease Patients Treated With Radiation Therapy

Knox SJ, Fowler S, Marquez C, Hoppe RT (Stanford Univ, Calif)
Int J Radiat Oncol Biol Phys 28:445–450, 1994   116-95-4–15

Background.—Myelosuppression is a frequent sequel of radiation therapy and may necessitate a considerable delay in treatment. As a result, cancer cure rates may decline. Filgrastim (recombinant human G-CSF) significantly hastens the recovery of neutrophils after chemotherapy and marrow transplantation. It has also been found to have a radioprotective effect on progenitor cells of human bone marrow in vitro.

Objective.—The value of filgastrim in preventing neutropenia was examined in 7 patients with Hodgkin's disease who were to receive large-

Mean ($\pm$ Standard Deviation) of Nadir Counts in Historical Series and in Filgrastim Patients During Second Treatment Course			
	Historical series	Filgrastin	p value*
WBC $\times 10^3/mm^3$	3.32 $\pm$ 1.06	5.98 $\pm$ 1.24	0.0014
ANC $\times 10^3/mm^3$	2.39 $\pm$ 0.97	4.71 $\pm$ 1.07	0.0015
Platelets $\times 10^3/mm^3$	239.1 $\pm$ 91.9	219.3 $\pm$ 42.2	0.3082

Abbreviation: ANC, absolute neutrophil count.
*Calculated with a 1-tailed student *t*-test assuming unequal variance.
(Courtesy of Knox SJ, Fowler S, Marquez C, et al: *Int J Radiat Oncol Biol Phys* 28:445–450, 1994.)

field subdiaphragmatic radiation therapy after thoracic "mantle" treatment. Five of the patients had nodular sclerosing Hodgkin's disease.

Methods.—Filgrastim was begun on the first day of subdiaphragmatic radiation therapy. Patients gave themselves subcutaneous injections throughout the 5- to 6-week treatment, starting with a dose of 3 $\mu g/kg/$ day. The total dose of subdiaphragmatic therapy ranged from 3,550 to 4,320 centigray. The results were compared with those in a historical series of 100 consecutive patients who underwent only radiation therapy.

Results.—Filgrastim treatment significantly increased the total white cell and absolute neutrophil counts in patients who underwent large-field irradiation. Counts remained significantly higher than in the historical series at all intervals (table). Neutrophilia with increased proportions of bands and immature myeloid forms developed in all filgrastim-treated patients. Two of the 7 patients had a WBC count less than 3,000/mm³ 1 week after the end of filgrastim therapy. The only side effect was mild musculoskeletal pain that responded to nonsteroidal anti-inflammatory drugs or acetaminophen.

Conclusion.—Filgrastim effectively prevents the severe leukopenia and neutropenia that may result from large-field subdiaphragmatic irradiation in patients with Hodgkin's disease.

▶ The main question remains unresolved. Are patients who receive G-CSF significantly more likely to have uninterrupted, full-dose radiation therapy than patients who do not receive the growth factor?—P.H. Wiernik, M.D.

Sex Differences in Risk of Second Malignant Tumours After Hodgkin's Disease in Childhood
Tarbell NJ, Gelber RD, Weinstein HJ, Mauch P (Joint Ctr for Radiation Therapy, Boston; Harvard School of Public Health, Boston; Harvard Med School, Boston)
Lancet 341:1428–1432, 1993   116-95-4–16

Background.—Some investigators have reported a high incidence of second malignancies in survivors of Hodgkin's disease. The risk of a second tumor was investigated in a large series of children treated during the past 20 years with wide-field irradiation or combination chemotherapy, or both.

Methods.—Included were 191 patients aged 16 years or younger at the time of diagnosis. All were treated between 1969 and 1988 at 1 center. The median follow-up from diagnosis was 11 years. Initially, 109 children were treated with radiation therapy alone, 21 received chemotherapy alone, and 61 received both treatments.

Findings.—The actuarial survival rate at 10 years was 89%. Fifteen patients had second tumors 6–20 years after the diagnosis of Hodgkin's disease. Overall, the estimated cumulative incidence of second malignancies at 15 years was 12%. Ten second tumors arose among 66 girls, compared with 5 in 125 boys, for cumulative incidences of 24% and 5%, respectively. Compared with boys, girls had a relative risk of 4.5 for second tumors. The incidence of second tumors among boys was 18 times that expected for the normal population. In girls, it was 57 times the expected incidence. Thirteen second malignancies were solid tumors, including 4 breast cancers.

Conclusion.—Continued surveillance in survivors of Hodgkin's disease is very important. Girls have a greater risk of having a second tumor than boys. The cumulative incidence of second cancer increases from 10 years after therapy.

▶ Why the difference?—P.H. Wiernik, M.D.

Acute Hypersensitivity Reactions to Etoposide in a VEPA Regimen for Hodgkin's Disease

Hudson MM, Weinstein HJ, Donaldson SS, Greenwald C, Kun L, Tarbell NJ, Humphrey WA, Rupp C, Marina NM, Wilimas J, Link MP (St Jude Children's Research Hosp, Memphis, Tenn; Univ of Tennessee, Memphis; Stanford Univ, Calif; et al)
J Clin Oncol 11:1080–1084, 1993   116-95-4-17

Background.—Etoposide, a semisynthetic derivative of podophyllotoxin, is known to be effective in treating many malignancies. Its major known side effect is dose-limiting myelosuppression; however, hypersensitivity reactions have also been reported. The high incidence of hypersensitivity reactions to etoposide seen in patients with Hodgkin's disease was examined, and methods of successful management were investigated.

Method.—A total of 45 children with Hodgkin's disease were enrolled in a combined-modality treatment protocol. The treatment plan included 6 cycles of vinblastine, etoposide, prednisone, and doxorubicin (VEPA) chemotherapy and low-dose involved-field radiation therapy.

Results.—Of the 45 patients treated with VEPA, 23 had 1 or more acute hypersensitivity reactions at a median of 5 minutes after administration of VEPA. The median age of these 23 patients at diagnosis was 15 years; 12 were boys. One patient had stage I disease, 5 had stage II, 6 had stage III, and 11 had stage IV. Signs and symptoms of hypersensitivity were flushing, respiratory problems, changes in blood pressure, and abdominal pain with or without nausea and vomiting. Respiratory problems included dyspnea, chest pain and tightness, bronchospasm, and cyanosis. The symptoms were relieved by withdrawing the etoposide infusion and administering diphenhydramine or hydrocortisone, or both. In 3 patients, epinephrine was required to treat bronchospasm. All patients made a complete recovery and were rechallenged with etoposide. Fifteen tolerated subsequent slower infusion of etoposide at a lower concentration with antihistamine or corticosteroid premedication, or both. The other 5 experienced a recurrence of hypersensitivity. Three of these patients had similar symptoms when etoposide was replaced with teniposide. Three patients who had isolated hypotensive episodes at the end of the etoposide infusion received subsequent infusions without incident.

Conclusion.—A surprisingly high incidence of hypersensitivity to etoposide was seen in this study of patients with Hodgkin's disease treated with VEPA chemotherapy. However, rechallenge with the drug was successful in 78% of patients.

Non-Hodgkin's Lymphoma

p53 Mutations Are Associated With Histologic Transformation of Follicular Lymphoma

Lo Coco F, Gaidano G, Louie DC, Offit K, Chaganti RSK, Dalla-Favera R (Columbia Univ, New York; Mem Sloan-Kettering Cancer Ctr, New York)
Blood 82:2289–2295, 1993   116-95-4-18

Purpose.—Most low-grade non-Hodgkin's lymphomas progress toward intermediate- and high-grade lymphomas. In the course of this progression, the tumor may transform from a follicular to a diffuse type. The mechanisms of this histologic progression are unknown. The possible pathogenetic role of relevant genetic abnormalities affecting proto-oncogenes and tumor suppressor genes was investigated.

Methods.—Sequential biopsy specimens were obtained from 21 patients with non-Hodgkin's lymphoma with clinical progression. Five had histologic transformation of their lymphoma from the follicular to the diffuse type, and 16 did not. Southern blot analysis was used to find evidence of karyotypic changes, c-*myc* rearrangements, and deletions affecting 6q27. The p53 mutations were sought by single-strand conformation polymorphism analysis and direct sequencing of polymerase chain reaction–amplified products.

Results.—Tumor progression was not associated with any apparent new cytogenetic abnormality. The c-*myc* gene was normal in all specimens. Of 5 patients with histologic transformation, 4 had a p53 gene mutation, compared with none of the patients without histologic transformation. One patient had the same mutation in a biopsy specimen taken before transformation occurred, which correlated with the presence of diffuse-type areas within a predominant follicular pattern. One patient with a p53 mutation also had a deletion of 6q27 in the post-transformation biopsy specimen.

Conclusion.—An association between the mutation of the p53 tumor suppressor gene and the histologic transformation of follicular lymphoma was documented. If confirmed in a larger number of patients, this finding could have important clinical implications for the early diagnosis of transformation.

▶ This important paper offers a molecular explanation for a common clinical observation.—P.H. Wiernik, M.D.

Long-Term Reduction in Sperm Count After Chemotherapy With and Without Radiation Therapy for Non-Hodgkin's Lymphomas
Pryzant RM, Meistrich ML, Wilson G, Brown B, McLaughlin P (Univ of Texas, Houston)
J Clin Oncol 11:239–247, 1993   116-95-4–19

Background.—A cancer chemotherapy regimen of cyclophosphamide, doxorubicin, vincristine, prednisone, and bleomycin (CHOP-Bleo) plus radiation therapy has produced long-term remission in patients with stage I through III low-grade lymphoma. Post-treatment fertility is frequently a concern because these patients tend to be young. Gonadal toxicity of CHOP-Bleo chemotherapy with or without radiation therapy was evaluated.

Methods.—Seventy-one patients with non-Hodgkin's lymphoma received CHOP-Bleo chemotherapy. Some patients were treated with other drugs; 33 underwent radiation therapy. Standard evaluation of semen volume, sperm motility, and sperm count were performed before treatment in 26 patients, during treatment in 9, and after treatment in 58. Semen analysis data were compared with those of 141 historical controls.

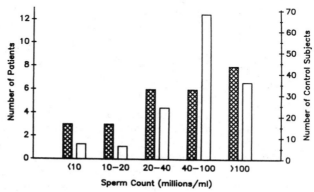

Fig 4–2.—Comparison of sperm count distributions from 26 patients with lymphoma before treatment (*hatched column*) and from control populations (*open column*). When multiple pretreatment counts were obtained, averages were taken using a cube-root transformation. Control data are from 141 nonexposed chemical plant workers and medical students. (Courtesy of Pryzant RM, Meistrich ML, Wilson G, et al: *J Clin Oncol* 11:239–247, 1993).

Results.—The median pretreatment sperm counts for patients and controls were almost identical (Fig 4–2). There was a trend toward an increased percentage of patients with sperm counts of less than 20 × 10^6/mL. Constitutional symptoms were the only variable that significantly correlated with a decreased sperm count. A significantly greater percentage of patients with stage B symptoms had sperm counts of less than 20 × 10^6/mL compared with those of controls. After treatment, 72% of the patients' sperm counts recovered to minimally fertile levels; 67% of all patients reached normal sperm levels. A Kaplan-Meier estimate of time-course recovery to sperm counts of .1 × 10^6/mL indicated that post-treatment sperm counts increase gradually, plateauing at approximately 5 years.

Conclusion.—A trend toward subfertility in male patients with lymphoma and constitutional stage B symptoms is suggested. However, pretreatment sperm counts are similar to controls in many men with lymphoma, including some with B symptoms. These patients may be candidates for sperm banking.

▶ The most significant finding here is that with time, sperm counts recover in most patients. This is also true for patients with Hodgkin's disease (1). —P.H. Wiernik, M.D.

Reference

1. Aisner J, et al: *J Clin Oncol* 11:507, 1993.

Large-Cell and Immunoblastic Lymphoma of the Mediastinum: Prognostic Features and Treatment Outcome in 57 Patients

Kirn D, Mauch P, Shaffer K, Pinkus G, Shipp MA, Kaplan WD, Tung N, Wheeler C, Beard CJ, Canellos GP, Shulman LN (Brigham and Women's Hosp, Boston; Dana-Farber Cancer Inst, Boston; Beth Israel Hosp, Boston; et al)

J Clin Oncol 11:1336–1343, 1993   116-95-4-20

Background.—The prognosis of patients with large-cell lymphoma of the mediastinum after chemotherapy and radiation therapy is not well defined. The value of radiation therapy remains unclear. Furthermore, prognostic factors have not been documented. A retrospective study was performed to determine the clinical characteristics and treatment outcomes of patients with large-cell and immunoblastic lymphoma of the mediastinum.

Methods.—Fifty-seven patients seen with primary, mediastinal large-cell and immunoblastic lymphoma between 1979 and 1991 were included. Initial sites of disease, radiologic features, treatment, outcomes, and prognostic factors were noted.

Findings.—Almost all patients had disease confined to sites above the diaphragm. In these patients, bulky disease and extensive intrathoracic infiltration were common. All patients underwent intensive chemotherapy. Forty-four percent underwent chest irradiation. The overall survival at 5 years was estimated to be 50%, with a freedom-from-relapse rate of 45%. Factors predicting disease relapse after chemotherapy were pleural effusion, a number of involved extranodal sites, a lactic dehydrogenase ratio of more than 3 and an incomplete treatment response as evidenced by residual mass on chest radiograph or persistent gallium-67 (^{67}Ga) avidity after chemotherapy. Factors predicting decreased survival rate included a pleural effusion, a number of involved extranodal sites, and a positive ^{67}Ga scan after therapy.

Conclusion.—After the initial treatment, patients with large-cell lymphoma of the mediastinum have about a 50% chance of surviving without disease. A pleural effusion on initial assessment was associated with a very poor outcome. Bulk disease in itself was a negative predictive factor only in patients without pleural effusions compared with patients without bulk disease. All patients with involvement of 2 or more extranodal sites had relapses after standard chemotherapy.

Primary Mediastinal B-Cell Lymphoma With Sclerosis: An Aggressive Tumor With Distinctive Clinical and Pathologic Features
Lazzarino M, Orlandi E, Paulli M, Boveri E, Morra E, Brusamolino E, Kindl S, Rosso R, Astori C, Buonanno MC, Magrini U, Bernasconi C (Univ of Pavia, Italy)
J Clin Oncol 11:2306–2313, 1993   116-95-4–21

Purpose.—Primary mediastinal B-cell lymphoma with sclerosis is a recently documented non-Hodgkin's lymphoma subtype. The clinical and pathologic features of this non-Hodgkin's lymphoma variant were reviewed.

Patients.—Between 1982 and 1992, 30 patients (median age, 26 years) were seen with nonlymphoblastic non-Hodgkin's lymphoma localized in the mediastinum. The median interval between symptom onset and definitive diagnosis was 30 days. Twenty-eight patients initially had chest symptoms attributable to an enlarging anterior mediastinal mass. Histologic confirmation was obtained via thoracotomy or mediastinoscopy in 20 patients and from lymph nodes in the lower supraclavicular site in 10 patients.

Results.—The tumor was bulky in 22 patients (73%), and 17 patients (57%) had superior vena cava syndrome (SVCS). However, SVCS did not always correlate with bulkiness because 2 patients with obvious SVCS had a nonbulky mediastinum. In addition, patients without symptoms of SVCS showed subclinical vena caval compression at CT scanning. Overall, 24 patients (80%) had vena caval obstruction. Fourteen patients

(47%) had infiltration of contiguous thoracic structures, and 4 patients (13%) had extrathoracic spread at diagnosis. All patients had extensive sclerosis. Of 29 evaluable patients, 16 (55%) achieved a complete response with chemotherapy, and 14 of the 16 underwent consolidation radiation therapy to the mediastinum. None of the 13 patients who did not have a complete remission responded to various salvage treatments, and all died within 12 months. Four patients with a complete remission relapsed within a year, and none survived. The 3-year actuarial survival rate was 38% for all patients and 72% for remitters.

Conclusion.—Primary mediastinal B-cell lymphoma with sclerosis is a highly aggressive variant of non-Hodgkin's lymphoma with unique clinical and histomorphologic features; therefore, it merits separate consideration among the non-Hodgkin's lymphomas.

▶ Combined-modality therapy does not seem to solve this problem in non-Hodgkin's lymphoma as readily as it does in Hodgkin's disease. Non-Hodgkin's lymphoma with a large mediastinal mass has a poor prognosis with or without sclerosis, irrespective of treatment specifics.—P.H. Wiernik, M.D.

A Predictive Model for Aggressive Non-Hodgkin's Lymphoma
The International Non-Hodgkin's Lymphoma Prognostic Factors Project (Dana-Farber Cancer Inst, Boston; Nebraska Lymphoma Study Group, Omaha; Istituto Nazionale Tumori, Milan, Italy; et al)
N Engl J Med 329:987–994, 1993   116-95-4–22

Background.—Many patients with intermediate- or high-grade non-Hodgkin's lymphoma are cured by combination chemotherapy, but those who are not ultimately die of the disease. The Ann Arbor staging system does not always accurately predict the long-term outcome.

Objective and Methods.—In an attempt to develop a model with which to predict the outcome of aggressive non-Hodgkin's lymphoma, clinical predictors were sought in adult patients receiving combination chemotherapy at 16 centers in the United States, Europe, and Canada between 1982 and 1987. All the patients received regimens containing doxorubicin. Clinical features that remained independently predictive of survival in step-down regression analyses were incorporated into models identifying groups of patients of all ages and groups of patients aged 60 years and younger with differing mortality risks.

Findings.—The 3,273 patients with tumors in Ann Arbor stages I through IV had a complete response rate of 66%. The 5-year relapse-free survival rate was 59% in patients who responded completely and 52% overall (table). In 2,031 patients of all ages, a model based on age, tumor stage, serum concentration of lactate dehydrogenase (LDH), performance status, and number of extranodal disease sites identified 4 risk groups with predicted 5-year survival rates of 73%, 51%, 43%, and 26%.

Outcome According to the Patients' Characteristics

CHARACTERISTIC	COMPLETE RESPONSE		RELAPSE-FREE SURVIVAL		OVERALL SURVIVAL	
	RATE (%)	P VALUE	5-yr rate (%)	P value	5-YR RATE (%)	P VALUE
All patients	66		59		52	
Sex						
Male	66	0.849	60	0.112	52	0.455
Female	66		57		53	
Age						
≤60 yr	68	<0.001	67	<0.001	60	<0.001
>60 yr	62		49		41	
Ann Arbor stage						
I	94		75		79	
II, tumor <10 cm	85		68		68	
II, tumor ≥10 cm	77	<0.001	69	<0.001	64	<0.001
II, tumor size unknown	65		69		62	
III	67		56		52	
IV	52		48		40	
I or II	83	<0.001	70	<0.001	69	<0.001
III or IV	57		51		44	
Site of involvement						
Bone marrow						
Absent	69	<0.001	62	<0.001	56	<0.001
Present	55		40		37	
Gastrointestinal tract						
Absent	69	0.004	59	0.023	54	0.009
Present	62		68		51	
Liver						
Absent	68	<0.001	60	<0.001	55	<0.001
Present	49		46		34	
Lung						
Absent	68	<0.001	60	0.022	54	<0.001
Present	50		46		39	
Central nervous system						
Absent	67	0.001	59	0.046	53	<0.001
Present	46		20		29	
Spleen						
Absent	67	<0.001	62	<0.001	55	<0.001
Present	54		39		40	
Extranodal site						
None	75		61		61	
1 site	69	<0.001	62	<0.001	56	<0.001
>1 site	53		52		40	
≤1 site	72	<0.001	61	<0.001	58	<0.001
>1 site	53		52		40	
Dimension of largest tumor						
<10 cm	72	<0.001	58	0.005	55	0.005
≥10 cm	60		68		51	
Performance status						
Ambulatory (0 or 1)	70	<0.001	58	0.019	55	<0.001
Not ambulatory (2–4)	45		54		35	
B symptoms						
Absent	75	<0.001	62	<0.001	61	<0.001
Present	52		52		40	

(continued)

Table *(continued)*

Serum LDH level							
≤1× normal	81	<0.001	65	<0.001	67	<0.001
>1× normal	60		53		44	
Serum albumin level							
≥1× normal	76	<0.001	64	0.393	60	<0.001
<1× normal	55		51		37	
Serum β_2-microglobulin level							
≤1× normal	75	0.004	59	0.739	65	<0.001
>1× normal	55		75		39	

(Courtesy of The International Non-Hodgkin's Lymphoma Prognostic Factors Project: *N Engl J Med* 329:987–994, 1993.)

In 1,274 patients aged 60 years or younger, an age-adjusted model based on tumor stage, level of LDH, and performance status identified 4 risk groups with predicted 5-year survival rates of 83%, 69%, 46%, and 32%. In both models, an increased risk of death reflected both a lower complete response rate and more frequent relapse from complete response.

Conclusion.—Both of these models, the international index and the age-adjusted international index, are significantly more accurate than the Ann Arbor classification in predicting long-term survival in patients with intermediate- and high-grade non-Hodgkin's lymphoma who receive combination chemotherapy.

▶ The international index should be used in the design of future clinical trials for this disease.—P.H. Wiernik, M.D.

Primary Cutaneous CD30-Positive Large Cell Lymphoma: Definition of a New Type of Cutaneous Lymphoma With a Favorable Prognosis: A European Multicenter Study of 47 Patients
Beljaards RC, Kaudewitz P, Berti E, Gianotti R, Neumann C, Rosso R, Paulli M, Meijer CJLM, Willemze R (Free Univ Hosp, Amsterdam; Univ Hosp, Munich; Univ of Milano, Italy; et al)
Cancer 71:2097–2104, 1993   116-95-4-23

Background.—Large-cell lymphoma appears in extremely varied clinical, histologic, and immunophenotypical expressions. Recent studies have described patients with large-cell lymphoma confined to the skin, which expresses CD30 (Ki-1/Ber-H2) antigen and has a favorable prognosis. However, there has been disagreement about the definition of this condition and whether to use morphologic or immunophenotypic criteria.

Methods.—Clinical records and histologic and immunohistochemical data were gathered from 5 centers on patients with large-cell lymphoma who were CD30-positive and had no extracutaneous disease or history of any other lymphoma. Patients were treated with a variety of therapies, including polychemotherapy, radiation therapy, surgical excision, or excision followed by radiation therapy.

Results.—Of the 47 patients, 46 had complete remission after the initial treatment, with a disease-free interval of 2–59 months. Spontaneous remissions occurred in 11 patients who had both small nodular and large tumorous cutaneous lesions. Twenty-seven patients relapsed; 15 had cutaneous relapses and 12 had extracutaneous relapses. Four of the latter group died of systemic lymphoma. In 40 patients, the CD30-positive tumor cells had anaplastic cytomorphology; 7 had nonanaplastic CD30-positive cells. There was no relationship between the cytomorphology of the tumor cells and clinical presentation or outcome.

Discussion.—Expression of the CD30 antigen seems to be the defining feature of this large-cell lymphoma subgroup, and differentiation between morphologic features appears to be irrelevant. Other studies describing the unfavorable clinical course of patients with CD30–large-cell lymphoma and localized cutaneous disease have suggested that the CD30 expression is also a more important predictor than the extent of the disease. These CD30-positive lymphomas are seen with solitary or localized skin lesions and are characterized by frequent cutaneous relapses, the possibility of spontaneous remission, and favorable prognosis. The 25% rate of spontaneous remission suggests that these CD30-positive lymphomas may lie further along on a continuum that includes lymphomatoid papulosis, another more benign self-healing cutaneous disease. Because systemic polychemotherapy was no more effective than other therapies, it is suggested that more conservative treatment be used for small or localized disease.

▶ This is a real entity that deserves special attention in the design of clinical trials.—P.H. Wiernik, M.D.

Clinical Aspects of Primary Thyroid Lymphoma: Diagnosis and Treatment Based on Our Experience of 119 Cases
Matsuzuka F, Miyauchi A, Katayama S, Narabayashi I, Ikeda H, Kuma K, Sugawara M (Kuma Hosp, Kobe, Japan; Kagawa Med School, Japan; Kure Hosp, Japan; et al)
Thyroid 3:93–99, 1993   116-95-4–24

Introduction.—Primary thyroid lymphoma accounts for, at most, 5% of all thyroid cancers. It most often arises from B lymphocytes and only rarely from T cells. Nearly all cases are associated with Hashimoto's thyroiditis, with or without hypothyroidism. No definitive treatment has been established.

Series.—One hundred nineteen patients with thyroid lymphoma seen at 1 center in Japan in the period 1963–1990 were reviewed. Women were affected more than twice as often as men. The mean patient age was 60 years.

Clinical Features.—Some patients had evidence of Epstein-Barr virus infection. Antimicrosomal antibodies were identified in 68% of patients, and all 65 patients in whom peritumoral tissues were examined had histologic changes of Hashimoto's thyroiditis. In addition, 41% of patients were either overtly or subclinically hypothyroid. All the patients had a growing thyroid mass; most had noted a rapidly growing neck mass for 2–3 months. Only 6% of patients had distant metastasis at the time of diagnosis. Ultrasound studies showed a typical asymmetric pseudocystic pattern in 43 of the 46 patients examined. Cytologic studies demonstrated an abundant lymphoid cell infiltrate. Fine-needle aspiration biopsy specimens yielded the correct diagnosis in 78% of 83 patients.

Treatment and Outcome.—Before fine-needle aspiration biopsy and chemotherapy were available, 11 of 31 patients died of lymphoma. Subsequently, mortality from lymphoma declined to 5%. Patients with predominantly stage 2 lymphoma consistently survived when given radiation therapy and 6 courses of cyclophosphamide, Adriamycin, vincristine, and prednisolone (CHOP) chemotherapy. In contrast, radiation therapy plus 1 or 2 courses of CHOP or nitrogen mustard, vincristine, procarbazine, and prednisolone (MOPP) chemotherapy yielded a survival rate of 75%.

▶ Another special situation. Combined-modality therapy seems to be on solid ground here.—P.H. Wiernik, M.D.

Management of Lymphoproliferative Disorders After Cardiac Transplantation

Chen JM, Barr ML, Chadburn A, Frizzera G, Schenkel FA, Sciacca RR, Reison DS, Addonizio LJ, Rose EA, Knowles DM, Michler RE (Columbia Univ, New York; Armed Forces Inst of Pathology, Washington, DC)
Ann Thorac Surg 56:527–538, 1993   116-95-4-25

Background.—One serious complication commonly arising from immunosuppression after organ transplantation is the development of post-transplantation lymphoproliferative disorders (PTLDs). These PTLDs are heterogenous for clinical appearance, histopathologic features, and therapy regimens. A more accurate system for assessment and classification of these disorders was sought.

Methods.—In a 9-year, single-center study, 424 cardiac transplant recipients who had survived for more than 30 days were assessed for PTLD incidence; 19 had PTLD. The 2 control populations included 19 age- and sex-matched patients without PTLD and the remaining 405 members of the initial cohort. The PTLD cohort was assessed for the time of diagnosis after transplant, the PTLD involvement site, and histopathologic category. In addition, Epstein-Barr virus (EBV) serologic titers were measured and OKT3 treatment use was noted. Survival and rejection-free intervals were assessed.

Results.—There was a significantly higher incidence of PTLD among women and those with cardiomyopathy. Rejection-free intervals were twice as long for patients without PTLD. Of the 4 sites noted (lung, gastrointestinal tract, adenoids and lymph nodes, and other extranodal sites), patients with PTLD had a high incidence of gastrointestinal and lung involvement, and those patients had significantly better survival rates than patients with other sites of involvement. Histopathologic features had no prognostic significance. There was no correlation between the time of diagnosis after transplant and survival. There was no significant correlation between EBV titer levels or OKT3 use and disease progression.

Discussion.—The irrelevance of the interval between transplant and diagnosis suggests that the moment of transformation to malignancy does not occur at a predictable time after transplantation. The more favorable prognosis for patients with PTLD with lung or gastrointestinal involvement may reflect earlier detection of disease in these sites. The heterogeneity of PTLD dictates an individualized approach to therapy, although decreasing immunosuppression therapy may improve survival. The multifactorial process of disease transformation requires further study so that a better understanding of diagnosis and treatment can develop.

▶ This is probably the largest series of such patients. For a review of the literature prior to this paper, see the reference (1).—P.H. Wiernik, M.D.

Reference

1. Sklarin NT, et al: *Am J Hematol* 37:105, 1991.

Role of Magnetic Resonance Imaging in Predicting Relapse in Residual Masses After Treatment of Lymphoma

Hill M, Cunningham D, MacVicar D, Roldan A, Husband J, McCready R, Mansi J, Milan S, Hickish T (Royal Marsden Hosp, Sutton, Surrey, England; Inst of Cancer Research, Sutton, Surrey, England)
J Clin Oncol 11:2273–2278, 1993   116-95-4–26

Background.—After patients are treated for lymphoma, a residual mass is often detected radiologically. Some of these patients have active lymphoma remaining in this mass and will have a relapse unless treated. Therefore, a reliable, noninvasive method for discriminating between fibrosis and lymphoma in the context of a residual mass is required. Magnetic resonance imaging has the potential to fill this role, because malignant tissue has been reported to have different signal intensity from both normal and fibrotic tissue. Low signal intensity in the mass on T2-

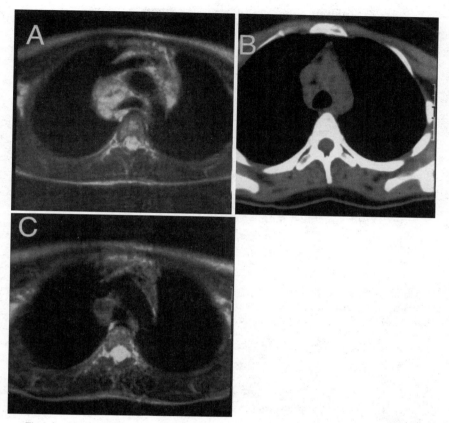

Fig 4–3.—A, pretreatment T2-weighted image shows abnormal high signal intensity in the paratracheal area and in the prevascular space (*arrows*). **B,** post-treatment CT scan shows abnormal attenuation within the prevascular space (*arrow*). **C,** post-treatment T2-weighted MRI shows low signal-intensity paratracheal mass (*arrow*). Low signal–intensity areas within the anterior mediastinal fat (*curved arrow*) are characteristic of inactive lymphoma. (Courtesy of Hill M, Cunningham D, MacVicar D, et al: J Clin Oncol 11:2273–2278, 1993.)

weighted sequences is the most important parameter (Fig 4–3). The efficacy of MRI, gallium-67 single-photon emission CT (SPECT), and erythrocyte sedimentation rate (ESR) in predicting early relapse at the site of a residual mass in patients who had been treated for lymphoma was evaluated.

Methods.—Thirty-four patients who had residual masses after treatment for lymphoma were examined by means of MRI, SPECT, and ESR within 3 months of the end of therapy. Patients were monitored for relapse for 1 year. The sensitivity, specificity, negative predictive value, and positive predictive value were calculated for each method of investigation. The time-to-relapse curves were derived, and the log-rank test was used to determine whether patients with a positive result on investigation were more likely to have a relapse than were those with negative results.

Results.—Of the 34 patients with lymphoma and residual masses, 14 had relapses. Eleven of these relapses were within the residual mass area. Magnetic resonance imaging had a 90% specificity, 71% positive predictive value, and 75% negative predictive value, but only a sensitivity of 45%. The results for SPECT were similar, with an even lower sensitivity of 33%. The ESR was inferior in predicting relapses when compared with the other 2 investigation methods. Magnetic resonance imaging was the only investigation that had statistical significance in predicting relapse, which was more evident in patients with Hodgkin's lymphoma. The combination of SPECT and MRI results was no better at predicting relapse than MRI alone.

Conclusion.—The MRI is a useful tool in the prediction of relapse in the context of a residual mass after treatment for lymphoma. The development of more sensitive investigation techniques would further enhance the prediction of relapse.

The Significance of Isolated Gallium-67 Uptake in the Hilar Lymph Nodes of an Untreated Lymphoma Patient

Larcos G, Farlow DC, Antico VF, Gruenewald SM (Westmead Hosp, Australia)
Clin Nucl Med 18:1039–1041, 1993　　　　　　　　116-95-4–27

Introduction.—Although single-photon emission CT (SPECT) examination of the thorax using radiogallium citrate is a sensitive means of detecting lymphoma, it may increase the number of false positive results obtained.

Case Report.—Woman, 69, had enlarged lymph nodes in her right inguinal region, and an excisional biopsy specimen revealed follicular small-cell non-Hodgkin's lymphoma. Thorough investigation failed to demonstrate disease elsewhere in the body. Planar imaging after administration of gallium-67 demonstrated uptake in the right ilioinguinal region, and, in addition, SPECT imaging showed moderately intense uptake in both hila. A radiation dose of 46 Gy was delivered to the right ilioinguinal region. The adenopathy resolved, but another SPECT study done 6 months later showed persistent hilar activity. Thoracic CT scanning remained negative. The patient was monitored without treatment and had a relapse 28 months later, with enlarged nodes in the left inguinal region, both axillas, and the right supraclavicular fossa. A radiogallium study showed abnormality at these sites and persistent low-grade hilar uptake, but the thoracic CT scan did not demonstrate disease.

Implications.—In some patients with untreated non-Hodgkin's lymphoma, isolated uptake of radiogallium in the pulmonary hila on thoracic SPECT imaging may not indicate the presence of disease. Nevertheless, careful clinical and CT studies are required to rule out indolent disease.

▶ These papers (Abstracts 116-95-4–26 and 116-95-4–27) illustrate the superiority of MRI over gallium-67 SPECT in this situation.—P.H. Wiernik, M.D.

Novel Oral Combination Chemotherapy in the Treatment of Intermediate-Grade and High-Grade AIDS-Related Non-Hodgkin's Lymphoma
Remick SC, McSharry JJ, Wolf BC, Blanchard CG, Eastman AY, Wagner H, Portuese E, Wighton T, Powell D, Pearce T, Horton J, Ruckdeschel JC (Albany Med College, NY; St Clare's Hosp and Health Ctr, New York; Univ of South Florida, Tampa; et al)
J Clin Oncol 11:1691–1702, 1993   116-95-4–28

Objective.—A novel 4-agent oral chemotherapy regimen was evaluated for efficacy and safety in 18 patients with biopsy specimen–proven, AIDS-related, non-Hodgkin's lymphoma. All patients had intermediate- or high-grade disease, and all but 1 had diffuse large-cell or large-cell immunoblastic lymphomas.

Treatment.—The regimen consisted of lomustine, 100 mg/m², on day 1; etoposide, 200 mg/m², on days 1–3; cyclophosphamide, 100 mg/m², on days 22 through 31; and procarbazine, 100 mg/m², on days 22 through 31. Treatment cycles were repeated at 6-week intervals.

Assessment.—The quality of life was evaluated prospectively using both the Functional Living Index-Cancer and the Brief Symptom Inventory. Levels of cell-associated p24 antigen were measured by indirect immunofluorescence and flow cytometry.

Results.—Of the 47 treatment cycles initiated, 38 were completed; the median number per patient was 2.5. The rate of objective treatment response was 61%. Patients had a median survival of 7 months, but the 7 who had a complete response had a median survival of 15 months. Myelosuppression was the most common and the most severe form of toxicity, but the regimen was, in general, tolerable. There were 2 treatment-related deaths (11%). The overall cost of treatment was about half that of the cyclophosphamide, doxorubicin, vincristine, and prednisone (CHOP) regimen and less than one third that of the modified combination of methotrexate, bleomycin, doxorubicin, cyclosphosphamide, vincristine, and dexamethasone with intrathecal cytarabine (M-BACOD) regimen.

Advantages.—The oral regimen of combination chemotherapy used is easily administered and is well received by patients. The medical risk to personnel is eliminated, and the treatment is substantially less expensive than intravenous regimens. Such convenient regimens will become increasingly attractive as the HIV epidemic continues.

Human Immunodeficiency Virus-Related Lymphoma Treatment With Intensive Combination Chemotherapy

Gisselbrecht C, for the French-Italian Cooperative Group (Hôpital Saint Louis, Paris)

Am J Med 95:188–196, 1993   116-95-4-29

Background.—Patients who are seropositive for HIV have an increased risk of high-grade non-Hodgkin's lymphoma. Treatment is complicated by underlying AIDS. However, patients without severe AIDS may benefit from intensive strategies used in non–HIV-related lymphoma.

Methods.—One hundred forty-one patients with lymphoma who were HIV-seropositive were treated with aggressive chemotherapy in a prospective, multicenter trial. All patients had a performance status of less than 3 and no active opportunistic infections. Treatment consisted of 3 cycles of doxorubicin (Adriamycin), 75 mg/m²; cyclophosphamide, 1,200 mg/m²; vindesine, 2 mg/m², for 2 days; bleomycin, 10 mg, for 2 days; and prednisone, 60 mg/m², for 5 days (ACVB). A consolidation phase of high-dose methotrexate plus leucovorin, ifosfamide, etoposide, asparaginase, and cytarabine (LNH84) was then administered. Central nervous system prophylaxis was routinely done with intrathecal methotrexate. After chemotherapy, azidothymidine maintenance was begun. The median follow-up was 28 months.

Findings.—Sixty-three percent of the patients had complete remissions, and 13% had partial remissions. Thirteen patients did not respond. Twenty patients (14%) died during administration of ACVB, 8 from progressive disease. The median and disease-free survival times were 9 and 16 months, respectively. The median survival for nonresponders was 5 months. Twenty-three patients died of opportunistic infections while in persistent complete remission. Factors strongly associated with shorter survival were a CD4-positive lymphocyte count of less than 100×10^6/L, performance status greater than 1, immunoblastic lymphoma, and previous AIDS. Patients with none of these risk factors had a 50% probability of survival at 2 years.

Conclusion.—Intensive chemotherapy is feasible and effective in certain patients with HIV-related lymphomas. A subgroup of patients without adverse prognostic factors achieved long-term remission.

▶ The complete response rate and median survival of the patients in the study by Remick et al. (Abstract 116-95-4-28) are inferior to those in the Gisselbrecht et al. study (Abstract 116-95-4-29). The latter are more comparable with our own results (1). Furthermore, an oral regimen may be more difficult for some AIDS patients to tolerate than a parenteral one.—P.H. Wiernik, M.D.

Reference

1. Sparano JA, et al: *Blood* 81:2810, 1993.

Comparison of a Standard Regimen (CHOP) With Three Intensive Chemotherapy Regimens for Advanced Non-Hodgkin's Lymphoma

Fisher RI, Gaynor ER, Dahlberg S, Oken MM, Grogan TM, Mize EM, Glick JH, Coltman CA Jr, Miller TP (Loyola Univ, Maywood, Ill; Southwest Oncology Group Statistical Ctr, Seattle; Abbott Northwestern Hosp, Minneapolis; et al)
N Engl J Med 328:1002–1006, 1993   116-95-4–30

Background.—National trials have shown that the cyclophosphamide, doxorubicin, vincristine, prednisone (CHOP) regimen, a first-generation treatment for non-Hodgkin's lymphoma, has cured about 30% of patients with advanced-stage intermediate-grade disease or high-grade disease. Studies have indicated that as many as 65% of these patients might be cured by third-generation regimens such as low-dose methotrexate with leucovorin rescue, bleomycin, doxorubicin, cyclophosphamide, vincristine, and dexamethasone (m-BACOD); prednisone, doxorubicin, cyclophosphamide, and etoposide, followed next by cytarabine, bleomycin, vincristine, and methotrexate with leucovorin rescue (ProMACE-CytaBOM); and methotrexate with leucovorin rescue, doxorubicin, cyclophosphamide, vincristine, prednisone, and bleomycin (MACOP-B).

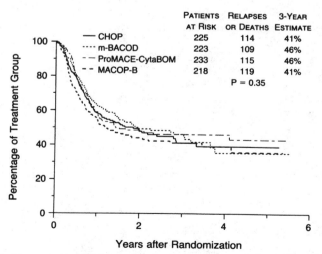

	PATIENTS AT RISK	RELAPSES OR DEATHS	3-YEAR ESTIMATE
CHOP	225	114	41%
m-BACOD	223	109	46%
ProMACE-CytaBOM	233	115	46%
MACOP-B	218	119	41%
		P = 0.35	

Fig 4–4.—Time to treatment failure in the treatment groups. The 3-year estimate is of survival without disease. (Courtesy of Fisher RI, Gaynor ER, Dahlberg S, et al: *N Engl J Med* 328:1002–1006, 1993.)

Objective.—The Southwest Oncology Group and the Eastern Cooperative Oncology Group combined to initiate a prospective, randomized, phase III trial evaluating these regimens in 899 patients with biopsy specimen–confirmed non-Hodgkin's lymphoma. Patients with bulky stage II, stage III, or stage IV disease of intermediate and high grade (other than lymphoblastic lymphoma) were eligible for the trial. Randomization was based on marrow infiltration, bulky disease, age, and lactate dehydrogenase concentration.

Results.—Complete responses were achieved in 44% of patients receiving CHOP therapy, 48% receiving the m-BACOD regimen, 56% receiving ProMACE-CytaBOM, and 51% receiving MACOP-B. After 3 years, 44% of patients were alive without disease. Differences in disease-free survival between the various treatment groups were not significant (Fig 4–4), nor were differences in the overall survival at 3 years. Toxicity was similar to that reported in phase II trials of the same regimens and did not differ significantly in the various treatment groups.

Conclusion.—The CHOP regimen still is the best available treatment for patients with advanced-stage intermediate-grade non-Hodgkin's lymphoma or high-grade disease. Significant improvement will require innovative approaches rather than merely different combinations of existing drugs.

▶ This is probably the most important advanced lymphoma paper in several years from a clinical care point of view. I am not at all surprised by the results.—P.H. Wiernik, M.D.

Combination Chemotherapy for Intermediate and High Grade Non-Hodgkin's Lymphoma

Dhaliwal HS, Rohatiner AZS, Gregory W, Richards MA, Johnson PWM, Whelan JS, Gallagher CJ, Matthews J, Ganesan TS, Barnett MJ, Waxman JH, Stansfeld AG, Wrigley PFM, Slevin ML, Malpas JS, Lister TA (St Bartholomew's Hosp, London)
Br J Cancer 68:767–774, 1993　　　　　　　　116-95-4–31

Introduction.—The newer, more intensive chemotherapeutic regimens for advanced intermediate- and high-grade non-Hodgkin's lymphoma have produced higher remission rates and more durable remissions than cyclophosphamide, doxorubicin, vincristine, and prednisolone (CHOP) and other first-generation protocols. However, some of these results could be the result of improved patient selection. Whether a compromise between methotrexate with leucovorin rescue, doxorubicin, cyclophosphamide, vincristine, prednisone, and bleomycin (M-BACOD) and conventional CHOP chemotherapy could maintain efficacy while avoiding the complications of bleomycin and high-dose methotrexate was investigated.

Patients.—The study included 118 consecutive adults with newly diagnosed intermediate- and high-grade non-Hodgkin's lymphoma. All were treated with CHOP with mid-cycle methotrexate and leucovorin rescue (CHOP-M). During each cycle, patients received intrathecal methotrexate as CNS prophylaxis.

Outcome.—Sixty-four percent of patients achieved clinical remission, including complete remission in 41% and good partial remission in 23%. The remaining patients either died before completion of therapy or had persistent disease. Complete remission was less likely in patients with hyponatremia, advanced age, and hypoalbuminemia. After at least $4\frac{1}{2}$ years' follow-up, two thirds of patients with clinical remission were still well. The actuarial 8-year projected remission duration was 70%. Four patients died in complete remission, and 1 had an isolated CNS recurrence. Factors predicting remission duration on multivariate analysis were serum sodium and advanced age. At 8 years, 45% of the patients were alive, and the actuarial projected survival was 42%. Factors negatively affecting survival rates on multivariate analysis were hypoalbuminemia, advanced age, hyponatremia, male sex plus age older than 50 years, and diffuse large-cell or large-cell immunoblastic histology. Cutoff points of 32 g/L^{-1} for albumin and 136 mmol/L^{-1} for sodium were able to define categories of patients with different outcomes.

Conclusion.—The CHOP-M regimen appears to be at least as good as CHOP for patients with intermediate- or high-grade non-Hodgkin's lymphoma, but it is not as good as other second- or third-generation chemotherapy regimens. Treatment-related mortality is 20%, including some patients in apparent remission. The prognostic factors of serum albumin, serum sodium, and age identify patient subgroups with significantly different outcomes.

▶ Based on the Southwest Oncology Group study (Abstract 116-95-4–30), it is reasonable to conclude that methotrexate and leucovorin added nothing to the results in intermediate-grade lymphoma in this British study. However, those drugs may have improved outcome for the high-grade lymphoma patients. Why should serum sodium correlate with prognosis?—P.H. Wiernik, M.D.

Randomized, Double-Blind, Placebo-Controlled, Phase III Study of Recombinant Human Granulocyte-Macrophage Colony-Stimulating Factor as Adjunct to Induction Treatment of High-Grade Malignant Non-Hodgkin's Lymphomas

Gerhartz HH, Engelhard M, Meusers P, Brittinger G, Wilmanns W, Schlimok G, Mueller P, Huhn D, Musch R, Siegert W, Gerhartz D, Hartlapp JH, Thiel E, Huber C, Peschl C, Spann W, Emmerich B, Schadek C, Westerhausen M, Pees H-W, Radtke H, Engert A, Terhardt E, Schick H, Binder T, Fuchs R, Hasford J, Brandmaier R, Stern AC, Jones TC, Ehrlich HJ, Stein H, Parwaresch M, Tiemann M, Lennert K (Munich Univ; GSF, Munich; Essen Univ, Germany; et al)

Blood 82:2329–2339, 1993   116-95-4–32

Background.—Hematotoxicity is the major dose-limiting factor in cancer chemotherapy. Adjunct administration of recombinant human GM-CSF (rhGM-CSF) has been shown to significantly reduce neutropenia and infection rates in patients undergoing bone marrow transplantation. Because studies have shown the importance of high-dose chemotherapy in curing lymphomas, the use of rhGM-CSF may be helpful in limiting hematotoxicity in these patients.

Methods.—During a 2-year period, 182 patients with untreated high-grade malignant non-Hodgkin's lymphomas from 18 centers were entered into a randomized, double-blind, placebo-controlled study. One hundred twenty-five patients completed appropriate chemotherapy regimens and received either 6 cycles of rhGM-CSF injections or placebos during chemotherapy-free intervals. There was no prophylactic antibiotic use. Patients were divided into low- and high-risk prognostic groups to determine the effects of this combined therapy.

Results.—The only adverse reactions to the rhGM-CSF treatment were cutaneous reactions at the injection site, which necessitated discontinuance of medication in some patients. The patients treated with rhGM-CSF had higher mean leukocyte counts, quicker leukocyte recovery, and shorter leukopenic episodes through all 6 cycles than did controls. The incidence of infection, days of hospitalization, days with fever, and necessity for antibiotic treatment were all significantly decreased in the group treated with rhGM-CSF. Overall, tumor response was mildly improved with rhGM-CSF treatment. However, in the high-risk subset, the improvement in tumor response for patients receiving rhGM-CSF was highly significant. Survival rates were not significantly altered with rhGM-CSF treatment.

Discussion.—The use of rhGM-CSF has significant beneficial effects in controlling the hematotoxic effects of the intensive chemotherapy required in treating non-Hodgkin's lymphoma. Because these effects were maintained through all 6 cycles, rhGM-CSF use is recommended in all cycles to ensure the maximum benefit. In addition, rhGM-CSF should be administered during chemotherapy-free intervals to produce maximum treatment benefits.

▶ This study demonstrates the efficacy of GM-CSF (*Escherichia coli*–derived) in lymphoma patients treated with an aggressive regimen. The German oncology community deserves credit for pioneering growth factors in hematologic malignancies. We have begun to catch up, at least with respect to leukemia studies. A recent Eastern Cooperative Oncology Group study (1) demonstrated similar benefit in elderly leukemia patients undergoing induction therapy (yeast-derived GM-CSF); however, a Cancer and Leukemia Group B study (2) of similar design failed to show an advantage in elderly leukemia patients supported during induction with *E. coli*–derived GM-CSF, the preparation used by Gerhartz et al. in this lymphoma study. The doses of GM-CSF in the CALGB leukemia study and the German lymphoma study were similar. The real question concerning the German study is, based on the Southwest Oncology Group study results (Abstract 116-95-4–30), is it necessary to treat what was primarily a group of intermediate-grade lymphoma patients so intensively that they *need* growth factor support?—P.H. Wiernik, M.D.

References

1. Rowe JM, et al: *Blood* 82(suppl 1):329a, 1993.
2. Stone R, et al: *Proc Am Soc Clin Oncol* 13:304, 1994.

P-VABEC: A Prospective Study of a New Weekly Chemotherapy Regimen for Elderly Aggressive Non-Hodgkin's Lymphoma
Martelli M, Guglielmi C, Coluzzi S, Avvisati G, Amadori S, Giovannini M, Torromeo C, Mandelli F (University "La Sapienza," Rome)
J Clin Oncol 11:2362–2369, 1993   116-95-4–33

Background.—In the past 20 years, the use the multiagent chemotherapy has dramatically changed the prognosis of aggressive non-Hodgkin's lymphoma. This treatment induces durable remission in a significant percentage of patients in advanced stages of the disease. However, the prognosis and cure rate for elderly patients with aggressive non-Hodgkin's lymphoma remain unknown. A prospective study was performed to assess a new combination chemotherapy designed specifically for elderly patients.

Methods.—During a 2-year period, 60 previously untreated patients with aggressive non-Hodgkin's lymphoma were treated with a new weekly alternating 6-drug chemotherapeutic regimen (P-VABEC). All patients were older than 60 years of age. Doxorubicin, etoposide, and cyclosphamide were alternated weekly with vincristine and bleomycin. Oral prednisone was given every day for the entire treatment. Twenty-six patients underwent 8 courses, and 34 underwent 12 courses.

Results.—Seventy-five percent of the patients had a complete response, 17% had a partial response, and 8% had no response. Of the 45 complete responders, 20 relapsed. Four of 10 partial responders had disease progression, and another 3 patients died while in complete remission. At a median of 25 months, 28 patients were still alive and responding. The projected 2-year overall survival, disease-free survival, and event-free survival rates were 64%, 57%, and 55%, respectively. Patients undergoing 8 treatment courses had complete remission rates and actuarial curves of overall, disease-free, and event-free survival similar to those of patients who received 12 courses.

Conclusion.—This regimen is one of the briefest first-line chemotherapy regimens reported in the treatment of elderly patients with aggressive non-Hodgkin's lymphoma. The regimen was active and well tolerated. Prospective randomized trials are now needed to determine the efficacy of this regimen compared with that of other standard regimens.

EPOCH Chemotherapy: Toxicity and Efficacy in Relapsed and Refractory Non-Hodgkin's Lymphoma

Wilson WH, Bryant G, Bates S, Fojo A, Wittes RE, Steinberg SM, Kohler DR, Jaffe ES, Herdt J, Cheson BD, Chabner BA (Natl Cancer Inst, Bethesda, Md)
J Clin Oncol 11:1573–1582, 1993   116-95-4-34

Background.—There is evidence that expression of the multidrug resistance gene, *mdr-1,* and its product, *p*-glycoprotein, is increased in cases of relapsed or refractory lymphoma. Cultured *mdr-1* tumor cells are less resistant when exposed to low concentrations of natural product drugs for a protracted period than when briefly exposed to higher concentrations.

Objective.—A regimen of etoposide, vincristine, doxorubicin, cyclophosphamide, and prednisone (EPOCH) chemotherapy was designed for use in patients with relapsed or refractory non-Hodgkin's lymphoma of varying grade. The natural product component was infused for 96 hours.

Patients.—Seventy-four consecutive patients who had relapse after or failed to respond to standard combination chemotherapy were included in the trial. Seventy were assessable for response to EPOCH treatment. The median age was 50 years. Three fourths of patients had intermediate- or high-grade histologic disease. Diffuse large-cell and large-cell immunoblastic types were most frequent, accounting for 61% of cases. Seventy-seven percent of patients had stage IV disease.

Treatment.—Initially etoposide was administered for 72 hours in a dose of 150 mg/m², but subsequently a total dose of 200 mg/m² was administered in 96 hours. Prednisone was administered for 2 weeks at first but later was administered for 6 days. Currently, etoposide, vincristine, and doxorubicin are administered by continuous infusion for 96 hours, cyclophosphamide as an intravenous bolus on day 6, and prednisone orally on days 1–6. Each cycle of treatment lasts 3 weeks. Patients who fail to tolerate full drug doses after the initial cycle are eligible to receive G-CSF.

Results.—The overall response rate was 87%, and the rate of complete response was 27%. Patients received a median of 4.5 treatment cycles; the optimal response occurred after 4 cycles. All patients with low-grade lymphoma responded, although only 1 had a complete response. Complete responses were most frequent (42%) in patients with de novo aggressive lymphoma. There were no significant differences in event-free survival according to histologic subgroup. A complete response to the last chemotherapy administered was the best single predictor for a complete response to EPOCH therapy. Brief neutropenia and minimal gastrointestinal toxicity were characteristic. Both treatment-related deaths were related to disseminated fungal infection.

Conclusion.—Chemotherapy with EPOCH is a relatively safe and highly effective means of partially reversing drug resistance in patients with non-Hodgkin's lymphoma who are resistant to or have relapsed from the same drugs administered on a bolus schedule.

▶ For another infusional regimen with excellent results in the same setting, see Sparano JA, et al. (1).—P.H. Wiernik, M.D.

Reference

1. Sparano JA, et al: *J Clin Oncol* 11:1071, 1993.

Effective Therapy for Poor-Prognosis Non-Hodgkin's Lymphoma With 8 Weeks of High–Dose-Intensity Combination Chemotherapy
Waits TM, Greco FA, Greer JP, Johnson DH, Wolff SN, Stein RS, McMaster ML, Hainsworth JD (Vanderbilt Univ, Nashville, Tenn)
J Clin Oncol 11:943–949, 1993   116-95-4–35

Background.—Despite marked advances in the treatment of aggressive non-Hodgkin's lymphoma, the outcomes of conventional regimens remain poor in some patients. The results of an 8-week, multidrug, high-dose–intensity chemotherapy regimen were reported.

Methods.—Seventy patients with advanced intermediate- or high-grade non-Hodgkin's lymphoma were treated between April of 1986 and April of 1991. The patients ranged in age from 18 to 69 years (median, 41 years). Seventy-three percent had stage IV disease. Fifty-three percent had Shipp's category 3 disease. Twenty-four percent had small non-cleaved-cell lymphoma. In half the patients, the Eastern Cooperative Oncology Group performance status was 2 or higher. In 34%, 2 or more extranodal sites were involved. Twenty-four percent had bone marrow

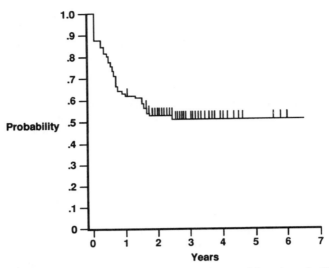

Fig 4–5.—Failure-free survival for the entire group is 52% (95% confidence interval, 40% to 64%) after a median follow-up of 35 months. Patients who remain failure-free are represented by the *tick marks*. (Courtesy of Waits TM, Greco FA, Greer JP, et al: *J Clin Oncol* 11:943–949, 1993.)

involvement. The chemotherapeutic regimen included cyclophospha-mide, etoposide, doxorubicin, vincristine, bleomycin, methotrexate with leucovorin rescue, and prednisone.

Findings.—Sixty-two patients completed the planned treatment. Eighty-one percent achieved complete remission. The actuarial 5-year failure-free survival rate was 52% (Fig 4–5). At a median follow-up of 35 months, 37 patients were still alive and free of disease. Factors associated with an adverse prognosis were age older than 50 years, bone marrow involvement, and a serum lactic dehydrogenase level of more than 500 IU/L. Most treatment-related toxicity resulted from myelosuppression. All patients had severe leukopenia, which lasted for a median of 9 days. Seven patients (10%) died of myelosuppression-associated complications. Five were older than 60 years of age.

Conclusion.—This brief, intensive treatment was effective in patients with non-Hodgkin's lymphoma with a poor prognosis. The treatment outcomes in patients with small noncleaved-cell lymphoma or Shipp's category 3 disease were similar to those of the overall group. Patients older than 60 years of age did not tolerate the treatment well and should not receive it.

Central Lymphatic Irradiation for Stage III Nodular Malignant Lymphoma: Long-Term Results

Jacobs JP, Murray KJ, Schultz CJ, Wilson JF, Goswitz MS, Stevens CW, Cox

JD (Med College of Wisconsin, Milwaukee; Univ of Texas, Houston; Walter Reed Army Med Ctr, Washington, DC; et al)
J Clin Oncol 11:233–238, 1993

116-95-4-36

Background.—The clinical course of nodular malignant lymphomas is typically indolent. The median survival of patients with this lymphoma is about 7 years. Various treatment strategies have been tried in patients with stage III disease. The long-term outcomes of central lymphatic irradiation for stage III nodular malignant lymphoma were reported.

Methods.—Thirty-four patients were treated between 1969 and 1985. Twenty-six had nodular poorly differentiated lymphoma, 4 had nodular mixed lymphocytic/histiocytic lymphoma, and 4 had nodular histiocytic lymphoma. Patients ranged in age from 30 to 73 years. Nineteen of the patients were women. In all patients, lymphatic irradiation encompassed cervical, supraclavicular, axillary, mediastinal, para-aortic, mesenteric, pelvic, and femoral lymphatics to total doses of 20–30 Gy in fractions of 1–1.8 Gy. In 17 patients, Waldeyer's ring was treated initially. The median follow-up was 9 years, 8 months.

Findings.—The life-table actuarial 15-year overall survival was 28%, disease-free survival was 40%, and cause-specific survival was 46%. There was only 1 relapse after 9 years. Patients with 5 or fewer sites of involvement had a significantly improved disease-free survival rate. Twenty patients had salvage therapy, including further irradiation or chemotherapy, or both. Ten percent of this group are alive and well with no evidence of disease. Radiation Therapy Oncology Group acute hematologic, gastrointestinal, and salivary toxicity scores were 2 or less in 83% of the patients treated at 1 center. Ninety-six percent had late toxicity scores of 2 or less. Twenty-three percent of the patients receiving initial treatment to Waldeyer's ring had persistent xerostomia.

Conclusion.—Given the long natural history of stage III modular malignant lymphoma, the best treatment for this disease is controversial. Initial comprehensive central lymphatic irradiation may be the preferred approach to obtaining a durable, relapse-free interval for these patients.

Cyclosporine Treatment of Refractory T-Cell Lymphomas

Cooper DL, Braverman IM, Sarris AH, Durivage HJ, Saidman BH, Davis CA, Hait WN (Yale Univ, New Haven, Conn)
Cancer 71:2335–2341, 1993

116-95-4-37

Objective.—In organ transplant recipients, cyclosporine prolongs graft survival via reduced transcription of cytokines believed to mediate T-cell expansion and subsequent graft rejection, especially IL-2. This mechanism of action could make cyclosporine effective against T-cell neoplasms. A phase II trial of cyclosporine in patients with refractory T-cell lymphomas was conducted.

Methods.—Participants included 16 patients with peripheral or cutaneous T-cell lymphoma (PTCL or CTCL, respectively) that progressed after at least 1 previous course of therapy. Most had multiple courses of chemotherapy or radiation therapy, or both. A group of 11 had CTCL, and a group of 5 had PTCL. All were treated with cyclosporine, which was administered orally at a starting dosage of 7.5 mg/kg twice daily.

Results.—Two patients responded in the CTCL group and none responded in the PTCL group. In both of the responders, disease recurred to almost baseline levels within 1 week of discontinuation of cyclosporine. When therapy was restarted, the patients responded again. Only 3 patients continued therapy for more than 3 weeks, with most stopping because of disease progression. Renal toxicity was significant.

Conclusion.—This phase II study documents a poor response rate to cyclosporine in patients with refractory T-cell lymphomas. Either these tumors are not dependent on IL-2, or the cyclosporine did not reach its intracellular target. The responses that do occur suggest that cyclosporine is cytostatic rather than cytocidal; alternatively, responses may result from the anti-inflammatory effects of cyclosporine.

▶ The occasional response to cyclosporine by patients with lymphoma, immune thrombocytopenia purpura, myeloma, agranulocytosis, and post-treatment thrombocytopenia deserves further evaluation.—P.H. Wiernik, M.D.

Radioimmunotherapy of B-Cell Lymphoma With [131I]Anti-B1 (Anti-CD20) Antibody

Kaminski MS, Zasadny KR, Francis IR, Milik AW, Ross CW, Moon SC, Crawford SM, Burgess JM, Petry NA, Butchko GM, Glenn SD, Wahl RL (Univ of Michigan, Ann Arbor; Coulter Corp, Hialeah, Fla)
N Engl J Med 329:459–465, 1993   116-95-4-38

Background.—Almost 50% of all patients with advanced-stage intermediate- and high-grade lymphomas do not achieve complete remission or experience disease recurrence after remission, despite treatment with various combined chemotherapeutic regimens. As part of an ongoing phase I trial, the effect of radioimmunotherapy with iodine-131(^{131}I)–labeled B-cell–specific anti-CD20 monoclonal antibody (MoAb) was evaluated in patients with CD20-positive B-cell lymphomas refractory to primary chemotherapy.

Patients and Methods.—Ten patients aged 36–74 years were included. All had tumor tissue that was reactive to either anti-B1 or L26 antibodies, and all had experienced a relapse or were unresponsive to chemotherapy. No other treatment had been undertaken for at least 4 weeks before initiation of the study. Anti-B1 (anti-CD20) mouse MoAb trace labeled with ^{131}I (15 mg containing 5 mCi) was administered intravenously at approximately 1-week intervals. Therapy was first administered

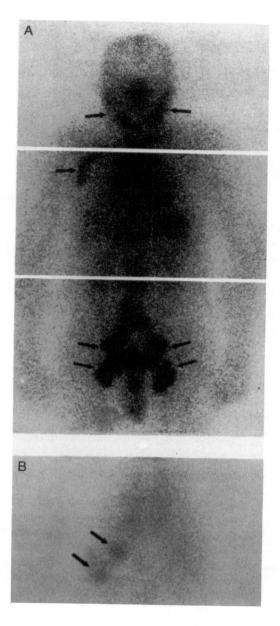

Fig 4–6.—Gamma camera images of patients with B-cell lymphomas after injection of ^{131}I-labeled anti-B1 antibody. **A,** anterior view of 1 patient obtained 120 hours after trace-labeled antibody injection. There are multiple tumors (*arrows*) 2–6 cm in diameter involving the neck, the right axilla, and the iliac, inguinal, and femoral regions. **B,** posterior view of another patient obtained 235 hours after antibody injection. There is distinct focal uptake (*arrows*) within the spleen consistent with intrasplenic tumor targeting. A CT scan of this patient also demonstrated low-attenuation lesions in the spleen consistent with involvement by lymphoma. (Courtesy of Kaminski MS, Zasadny KR, Francis IR, et al: *N Engl J Med* 329:459–465, 1993.)

to all 10 without pretreatment with unlabeled anti-B1 antibody. To assess the effect of administering unlabeled antibody on the distribution of radiolabeled antibody and tumor targeting, a second trace-labeled dose was administered to 8 patients immediately after pretreatment with 135 mg of unlabeled antibody. Between 1 and 2 weeks later, 2 patients received a third trace-labeled dose after infusion of 685 mg of unlabeled antibody. At least 1 week later, the pretreatment dose of unlabeled antibody that produced the highest ratio of the tumor dose to the whole-body dose in the tracer studies was used to deliver higher doses of radioactivity for radioimmunotherapy to 9 patients. Three patients, 2 of whom were treated twice 6–8 weeks apart, received doses designed to deliver 25 centigray (cGy) to the whole body. Four patients, 1 of whom was treated twice, received 35 cGy, and 2 patients, 1 of whom was treated twice, received 45 cGy. Each dose contained 34–66 mCi of activity. After each tracer dose, serial quantitative γ-camera images and whole body radioactivity measurements were obtained.

Results.—Images were obtained for all known disease sites larger than 2 cm (Fig 4–6). A variable effect of pretreatment doses of unlabeled anti-B1 antibody on tumor targeting with the radiolabeled antibody was noted. Tumor responses were found for 6 of the 9 treated patients, including those with bulky or chemotherapy-resistant disease. Of those, 4 patients experienced complete remission, and 2 had partial remissions. Objective responses to tracer infusions were observed in 3 patients before radioimmunotherapeutic doses were administered. Of those with complete remission, 1 remained in remission for 8 months, and the other 3 have had no disease progression for 11, 9, and 8 months. Mild or no myelosuppression was noted.

Conclusion.—Treatment with radioimmunotherapy with ^{131}I-labeled anti-B1 antibody is promising.

Radiolabeled-Antibody Therapy of B-Cell Lymphoma With Autologous Bone Marrow Support

Press OW, Eary JF, Appelbaum FR, Martin PJ, Badger CC, Nelp WB, Glenn S, Butchko G, Fisher D, Porter B, Matthews DC, Fisher LD, Bernstein ID (Univ of Washington, Seattle; Fred Hutchinson Cancer Research Ctr, Seattle; Coulter Corp, Miami, Fla; et al)
N Engl J Med 329:1219–1224, 1993   116-95-4-39

Introduction.—In lymphoma patients, larger doses of cytotoxic therapy could be used if selectively targeted to tumor sites. Specifically, radiolabeled monoclonal antibodies recognizing B-lymphocyte surface antigens may represent an effective new therapeutic technique. A phase I dose-escalation trial of anti-CD20 and anti-CD37 antibodies labeled with iodine-131 (^{131}I) was conducted in patients with relapsed B-cell lymphoma.

Methods.—Forty-three patients with B-cell lymphoma in relapse underwent sequential biodistribution studies with escalating doses of antibody—.5, 2.5, and 10 mg/kg—trace-labeled with ^{131}I, 5–10 mCi. γ-Camera imaging and tumor biopsy specimens were performed to evaluate the radiation dose to the tumor as well as to normal organs. Patients with a favorable biodistribution, that is, those whose tumors took up more radiation than did their liver, lungs, or kidneys, were eligible for therapeutic infusion of ^{131}I-labeled antibodies according to the dose-escalation protocol.

Results.—Biodistribution was favorable in 24 patients. Nineteen received therapeutic infusion of ^{131}I-labeled antibodies, 234–777 mCi, and then received autologous marrow reinfusion. This treatment resulted in complete remission for 16 patients, a partial response in 2, and a minor response in 1. Complete remission persisted for as long as 53 months in 9 patients. For patients who received doses of less than 27.25 Gy to normal organs, the toxic effects, including myelosuppression, nausea, infection, and cardiopulmonary toxicity, were moderate.

Conclusion.—The response rate to high-dose radioimmunotherapy in patients with relapsed B-cell lymphoma with a favorable antibody biodistribution was high. Doses delivering more than 27.25 Gy to the lungs cause cardiopulmonary toxicity. Antibody biodistribution is more likely to be favorable in patients without splenomegaly and with tumor burdens of less than 500 mL.

▶ Radiolabeled antibody therapy of lymphoma is a promising new approach to therapy that may ultimately be most useful as a means of eradicating minimal residual disease.—P.H. Wiernik, M.D.

Multiple Myeloma

The Bone Marrow of Multiple Myeloma Patients Contains B Cell Populations at Different Stages of Differentiation That Are Clonally Related to the Malignant Plasma Cell

Billadeau D, Ahmann G, Greipp P, Van Ness B (Univ of Minnesota, Minneapolis; Mayo Clinic, Rochester, Minn)
J Exp Med 178:1023–1031, 1993   116-95-4–40

Background.—Multiple myeloma is characterized by the proliferation of a clonal plasma cell population in the bone marrow. Myeloma cells apparently are limited to this microenvironment and are rarely detected peripherally. Nevertheless, the disease disseminates widely throughout the axial skeleton. It has proved difficult to isolate multiple myeloma tumor cell lines because of their slow rate of growth.

Objective and Methods.—An attempt was made to identify earlier cells in the B-cell lineage that are clonally related to plasma cell tumor and that may represent the growth fraction of the tumor. Isotypes clonally related to plasma cell tumor were sought by using allele-specific oligonucleotides (ASOs) derived from the third complementarity determining the region of the rearranged tumor immunoglobulin heavy-chain gene. The RNA from the bone marrow was reverse-transcribed with a panel of constant region primers, and ASO–polymerase chain reaction amplification was then carried out.

Results.—Preswitch isotype species that are clonally related to myeloma were demonstrated. Separation of the marrow cells into CD45+ and CD38+ cell populations resulted in a lineage-specific expression of the clonally related RNA molecules. The Cμ and Cδ molecules were found in the CD45+ cell population, and the Cγ in the CD38+ population.

Conclusion.—The presence of B-cell populations that are clonally related to the plasma-cell tumor was demonstrated, supporting the concept of myeloma precursors. It appears important to characterize clonally related cells because they may influence the outcome of treatment.

▶ This discovery, aside from its scientific importance, may facilitate the establishment of cell lines representing precursor myeloma cells from patients with myeloma.—P.H. Wiernik, M.D.

Low-Dose Gallium Nitrate for Prevention of Osteolysis in Myeloma: Results of a Pilot Randomized Study
Warrell RP Jr, Lovett D, Dilmanian FA, Schneider R, Heelan RT (Mem Sloan-Kettering Cancer Ctr, New York; Hosp for Special Surgery, New York; Brookhaven Natl Lab, Upton, NY)
J Clin Oncol 11:2443–2450, 1993   116-95-4–41

Background.—Osteolysis produces considerable morbidity in patients with myeloma, but few studies have attempted to document the natural course of bone loss or its reversal during cytotoxic drug treatment. Gallium nitrate has proved to be a very effective and safe means of treating cancer-related hypercalcemia. The drug strongly inhibits bone resorption, and it also blocks the resorptive effects of IL-1, tumor necrosis factor, and parathyroid hormone in vitro. Gallium nitrate also stimulates the synthesis of bone collagen and promotes the incorporation of calcium into bone mineral.

Study Plan.—Thirteen patients with multiple myeloma whose disease had been stabilized with cytotoxic drug therapy were randomized to receive gallium nitrate for 6 months or to observation only for 6 months and then gallium treatment for the next 6 months. The drug was administered subcutaneously in a dose of 30 mg/m²/day for 2 weeks of every month. In addition, a dose of 100 mg/m² was administered by intravenous infusion for 5 days every other month. Paired comparisons were available for 13 active treatment periods and 7 observation periods.

Results.—Total body calcium, determined by delayed γ-neutron activation, declined during 4 of 7 observation periods but increased during 9 of 13 treatment periods. A mean group difference of 3% was evident at 6 months. Regional bone density, as determined by dual-photon absorptiometry, declined 1.4% during observation but did not change during gallium treatment. The mean vertebral fracture index declined 27% during observation but only 2% during active treatment. The mean body height decreased less in patients receiving gallium (.06 vs. .57 in.). Seven of 12 gallium-treated patients reported a major reduction in bone pain, whereas none of 7 patients who were observed had such a response. One gallium recipient had an episode of renal insufficiency, but treatment was in general very well tolerated.

Conclusion.—The adjuvant administration of a remineralizing drug such as gallium nitrate is able to slow or possibly even reverse osteolysis in patients receiving cytotoxic treatment for myeloma.

▶ For 18 years, these authors and others have been trying to find a situation for which gallium nitrate is the treatment of choice. These preliminary results suggest that they may have found one. However, conclusive data on the use of this agent in this setting will most likely come from prospective, randomized studies that compare gallium nitrate with other agents thought to prevent osteolysis in myeloma.—P.H. Wiernik, M.D.

Limited Value of Myeloablative Therapy for Late Multiple Myeloma
Alexanian R, Dimopoulos M, Smith T, Delasalle K, Barlogie B, Champlin R (Univ of Texas, Houston)
Blood 83:512–516, 1994   116-95-4–42

Introduction.—Myeloablative therapy, supported by autologous bone marrow or blood stem cell transplantation, has been tried in many patients with resistant multiple myeloma. Although the results in patients with primary resistant disease and in those who have responded to initial chemotherapy have been encouraging, myeloablative treatment may be less effective in patients with later phases of multiple myeloma.

Patients and Mehods.—The use of myeloablative therapy, supported by autologous bone marrow or blood progenitor cells, was examined in 49 patients with multiple myeloma who had received at least 1 year of previous chemotherapy. The median age was 52 years. Twenty-three had resistant relapse despite treatment with vincristine-doxorubicin by continuous infusion with pulse dexamethasone. Fifteen had primary resistance lasting longer than 1 year, and 11 had consolidated disease during remission after successful vincristine-doxorubicin by continuous infusion with pulse dexamethasone treatment of resistant disease. For most patients, myeloablative therapy consisted of melphalan and total body irradiation. The results of treatment were compared with those of clinically similar patients who did not receive intensive therapy, most because they refused it or their insurance company would not cover it.

Results.—The resistant relapse group had a 61% response rate, with a median remission of 5 months. In the prolonged primary resistance group, 6 of 15 patients responded. However, the overall survival in this group was comparable to that of controls. The late remission group had a remission time similar to that of the control.

Conclusion.—Myeloablative treatment with autologous bone marrow or blood stem cell support is not useful for most patients with multiple myeloma after the first year of chemotherapy. This treatment reduces myeloma but makes no important difference in remission or survival time. Intensive therapy is potentially useful only early in the course of multiple myeloma.

▶ If autologous bone marrow transplantation is to be effective in a given myeloma patient, it must be done early in the disease. Randomized studies comparing early autologous bone marrow transplantation with other treatments are urgently required in myeloma.—P.H. Wiernik, M.D.

Chronic Leukemia

HAIRY-CELL LEUKEMIA

Marrow Mast Cell Hyperplasia in Hairy Cell Leukemia
Macon WR, Kinney MC, Glick AD, Collins RD (Vanderbilt Univ, Nashville, Tenn)
Mod Pathol 6:695–698, 1993   116-95-4-43

Background.—Random cases of hairy-cell leukemia (HCL) were found to be associated with large numbers of marrow mast cells, comparable to levels in other B-cell neoplasms. Increases in marrow mast cells in HCL have not previously been reported.

Methods.—Marrow mast cells were counted per high magnification field (HMF) on toluidine-blue–stained marrow biopsy specimens from 34 patients with HCL. In 9 cases, counts were also made on splenic sections. Biopsy specimens from 28 normal marrow transplant donors and 10 normal spleens were used for comparison.

Findings.—Mast cells were distributed irregularly throughout normal and HCL marrows. They tended to be more concentrated about the hairy cells in patients focally involved by HCL. The mean number of mast cells per HMF was 12.7 in HCL marrow and 1.1 in controls. Eighty-six percent of normal marrows averaged less than 2 mast cells per HMF, whereas 88% of patients with HCL averaged 2 or more mast cells per HMF. In patients with HCL and controls, splenic mast cells averaged less than 1 per HMF. At electron microscopic evaluation, marrow mast cells in patients with HCL showed normal substructure with many granules. Mast cell surfaces showed filopodia that frequently came in contact with those of hairy cells.

Conclusion.—Varying degrees of mast cell hyperplasia are found in most HCL marrows but not spleens. There appears to be a biological interaction between mast cells and hairy cells. Although the significance of marrow mast cell hyperplasia in HCL is not known, these mast cells may contribute to the increased reticulin fiber network seen in HCL marrows.

The Bone Marrow Fibrosis of Hairy-Cell Leukemia Is Caused by the Synthesis and Assembly of a Fibronectin Matrix by the Hairy Cells
Burthem J, Cawley JC (Univ of Liverpool, England)
Blood 83:497–504, 1994

116-95-4-44

Background.—Hairy-cell leukemia (HCL), a proliferation of clonal B lymphocytes with features of activation, is characterized by fine reticulin fibrosis in the bone marrow. However, fibroblast infiltration has never been observed in the marrow, and the origin of the fibrosis remains unclear. In previous research on hairy-cell (HC)–adhesive protein interactions, homotypic aggregates of HCs contained large amounts of fibronectin, suggesting that HCs can form as fibronectin matrix. This possibility was investigated.

Methods and Findings.—Hairy-cells of HCL produced an insoluble matrix of fibronectin in vitro. Fibronectin synthesis was demonstrated by the appearance of cellular fibronectin on the surface of cells cultured in serum-free medium and by immunoprecipitation of the metabolically labeled protein from HC aggregates. In addition, HCs assembled fibronectin into disulfide-bonded multimers. A 70-kD amino-terminal fragment of the molecule that blocks fibronectin multimer formation by fibroblasts blocked this assembly. Hairy cells expressed abundant fibronectin receptor VLA-5, which is not seen on normal circulating B lymphocytes but is important in matrix formation. Hairy cells also adhered to fibronectin fragment containing the VLA-5 binding site. In vivo, fibronectin was demonstrated in association with infiltrating HCs in bone marrow sections from patients with HCL.

Conclusion.—The VLA-5 of HCs may be implicated in their assembly of fibronectin matrix. The HC synthesis and assembly of fibronectin matrix appear to be partially responsible for the bone marrow fibrosis that characterizes HCL.

▶ Marrow mast cell hyperplasia in HCL is an interesting finding of unknown significance. Macon et al. (Abstract 116-95-4-43) suggest that it may contribute to the fibrosis observed in marrows of patients with HCL. However, it should be noted that marrow mast cells are frequently found in increased numbers in other chronic B-lymphoproliferative disorders in which marrow fibrosis is not a feature. Burthem and Cawley (Abstract 116-95-4–44) offer a better explanation for the fibrosis.—P.H. Wiernik, M.D.

CHRONIC LYMPHOCYTIC LEUKEMIA

Activity of P-Glycoprotein in B-Cell Chronic Lymphocytic Leukemia Determined by a Flow Cytometric Assay

Ludescher C, Hilbe W, Eisterer W, Preuss E, Huber C, Gotwald M, Hofmann J, Thaler J (Univ of Innsbruck, Austria)

J Natl Cancer Inst 85:1751–1758, 1993   116-95-4–45

Purpose.—Some patients with chemoresistant hematologic malignancies have overexpression of P-glycoprotein, which is encoded by the *MDR1*, or PGY1, gene. Better techniques of detecting P-glycoprotein expression are needed, as reflected by the inconsistent data regarding the frequency and clinical relevance of multidrug resistance in B-cell chronic lymphocytic leukemia (B-CLL). Peripheral blood cell P-glycoprotein activity was measured in patients with B-CLL, with special attention to possible clinical correlations.

Methods.—Forty-two consecutive patients with B-CLL were studied, 22 treated and 20 untreated. Peripheral blood cell P-glycoprotein activity was assessed by dual fluorescence in a flow cytometric assay that detects efflux of the fluorescent dye rhodamine 123, which the P-glycoprotein pump transports from the cell. The monoclonal antibody Leu12/CD19 was used to co-stain leukemic cells. In 26 patients, expression of *MDR1* and *MDR3* messenger RNA was measured by polymerase chain reaction.

Findings.—Eighty-one percent of patients showed marked rhodamine-123 efflux, which was abolished when multidrug resistance inhibitors were used. There was no correlation between rhodamine-123 efflux and Rai stage, lymphocyte count, or disease duration or progression. The untreated patients had a lower percentage of cells with rhodamine-123 efflux than patients who had received at least 1 multidrug resistance–associated drug. Both *MDR1* and *MDR3* mRNA were detected in all patients but 1. A significant correlation was noted between rhodamine-123 reflux and *MDR1* but not *MDR3* messenger RNA expression.

Conclusion.—Patients with B-CLL appear to have intrinsic rather than acquired P-glycoprotein overexpression. This activity is enhanced after treatment with multidrug resistance–associated drugs but does not appear to be related to more aggressive disease. Clinical screening for multidrug resistance may be possible with the combination of polymerase chain reaction and an assay of P-glycoprotein function, although further analysis is needed to determine whether the rhodamine-123 assay is directly related to drug resistance.

▶ P-glycoprotein has been measured by a variety of techniques, and the data have been analyzed by assuming a variety of arbitrary cutoff points for defining P-glycoprotein positivity. This paper takes the most informative approach to determining the significance of P-glycoprotein by reporting on *functional* P-glycoprotein. Standardization of techniques is needed for the measurement of P-glycoprotein and for the interpretation of its levels of expression. Hopefully, in the future, arbitrary definitions of positive and negative cell populations will give way to more appropriate, biologically relevant definitions.—P.H. Wiernik, M.D.

Pentostatin in Prolymphocytic Leukemia: Phase II Trial of the European Organization for Research and Treatment of Cancer Leukemia Cooperative Study Group

Döhner H, Ho AD, Thaler J, Stryckmans P, Sonneveld P, de Witte T, Lechner K, Lauria F, Bödewadt-Radzun S, Suciu S, Solbu G, Witt B, Hunstein W, Zittoun R (Univ of Heidelberg, Germany; Univ of California, San Diego; Universitätsklinik für Innere Medizin, Innsbruck, Austria; et al)
J Natl Cancer Inst 85:658–662, 1993   116-95-4–46

Background.—B- and T-cell prolymphocytic leukemias are aggressive variants of chronic lymphoid leukemia, with shorter survival duration and less responsiveness to therapy than chronic lymphocytic leukemia. Pentostatin (2′-deoxycoformycin [DCF]) is a purine analog that has demonstrated activity in the treatment of chronic lymphoid malignancies. Therefore, a prospective phase II trial was conducted by the Leukemia Cooperative Group of the European Organization for Research and Treatment of Cancer to examine the activity and toxicity of DCF in the treatment of prolymphocytic leukemia.

Methods.—Twenty patients with prolymphocytic leukemia were administered DCF, 4 mg/m², intravenously once a week for 3 weeks and then every other week for 3 doses. Responsive patients received maintenance therapy once a month for as long as 6 months.

Patients.—Of the 20 patients included in this study, 14 had B-cell and 6 had T-cell prolymphocytic leukemia. Three patients had received no previous treatment, 8 had received 1 or 2 treatment rounds, and 9 had received more than 2 previous chemotherapeutic treatments.

Results.—One patient died during the first 6 weeks of treatment of unknown cause. One patient died of disseminated toxoplasmosis during maintenance therapy after achieving partial remission. Of the 20 patients, 9 achieved partial remission. The median duration of response to therapy was 9 months. No complete remissions occurred. Toxic effects included nausea and vomiting, infections, and transient increases in liver enzymes and creatinine levels. Thrombocytopenia developed in 8 patients.

Conclusion.—Pentostatin has activity as a therapy for previously untreated and salvage cases of prolymphocytic leukemia. Trials with DCF alone or in combination with other agents should be done to improve the poor prognosis of patients with prolymphocytic leukemia.

▶ Prolymphocytic leukemia is uncommon, if it exists at all. I think it is better to consider this entity as simply far-advanced chronic lymphocytic leukemia. At any rate, it is noteworthy that DCF has activity in patients with immature forms of chronic lymphocytic leukemia, as does fludarabine.—P.H. Wiernik, M.D.

Results of Fludarabine and Prednisone Therapy in 264 Patients With Chronic Lymphocytic Leukemia With Multivariate Analysis-Derived Prognostic Model for Response to Treatment
O'Brien S, Kantarjian H, Beran M, Smith T, Koller C, Estey E, Robertson LE, Lerner S, Keating M (MD Anderson Cancer Ctr, Houston)
Blood 82:1695–1700, 1993   116-95-4–47

Background.—Prednisone is often used along with chlorambucil in the treatment of chronic lymphocytic leukemia (CLL). Prednisone and fludarabine were studied in an attempt to improve the remission rates and duration of remission in CLL.

Methods.—Two hundred sixty-four patients with CLL received fludarabine, 30 mg/m², intravenously for 30 minutes each day for 5 days and prednisone, 30 mg/m², orally each day for 5 days. This course was repeated every month.

Findings.—The overall response and complete response rates were 52% and 37%, respectively, in 169 previously treated patients. In this patient group, the respective overall and complete response rates were 74% and 63% in patients with Rai stage 0–II disease; and 64% and 46% in patients with Rai stage III–IV disease. Among previously untreated patients, overall and complete remission rates were 79% and 63%, respectively. Respective overall and complete remission rates in this group were 85% and 70% in patients with Rai 0–II disease and 64% and 46% in those with Rai III–IV disease. The incidence of minor infections or fever of unknown origin, occurring in 22% of the courses, was similar in all patient groups. The incidences of sepsis and pneumonia were significantly associated with the extent of previous treatment and Rai stage, ranging from 3% of courses in previously untreated patients with Rai stage 0–II disease to 13% in previously treated patients with Rai stage III–IV disease. *Listeria* sepsis or *Pneumocystis carinii* pneumonia developed in 14 patients. Response and infection rates were identical to those occurring in 110 patients treated with the same dose schedule of fludarabine alone. Factors significantly associated with poorer response were Rai stages III–IV, previous treatment, older age, and low albumin levels.

Conclusion.—The combination of fludarabine and prednisone is an effective regimen for treating patients with CLL. However, adding prednisone did not increase the response rate compared with that achieved with fludarabine alone.

Long-Term Follow-Up of Patients With Chronic Lymphocytic Leukemia Treated With Fludarabine As a Single Agent

Keating MJ, O'Brien S, Kantarjian H, Plunkett W, Estey E, Koller C, Beran M, Freireich EJ (Univ of Texas, Houston)
Blood 81:2878–2884, 1993

116-95-4-48

Background.—The traditional treatment of chronic lymphocytic leukemia (CLL) is based on alkylating agents and corticosteroids. No effective therapy was available for patients resistant to these agents until the recent discovery of the activity of nucleoside analog fludarabine and 2-chlorodeoxyadenosine, and the adenosine deaminase inhibitor 2-deoxycoformycin. The use of fludarabine, a fluorinated analog of ara-adenine that is relatively resistant to deamination by adenosine deaminase, in the management of CLL was investigated.

Methods.—A total of 113 patients with CLL participated; 78 had been treated previously. Treatment with fludarabine as a single agent was administered in blocks of 3 courses, after which patients were reevaluated. In patients who achieved a complete or partial response, progressive disease was considered to have occurred when the absolute lymphocyte count had increased to more than $10,000/\mu L$ on 2 occasions a month apart or when the percentage of bone marrow lymphocytes was increased to more than 50%. Reenlargement of nodes, liver, or spleen was considered evidence of progressive disease.

Results.—The response to therapy and survival after receiving fludarabine were strongly correlated with the extent of previous therapy, the stage of disease, and whether the patients were refractory to alkylating agents. Other influencing factors associated with survival were age and serum level of albumin when therapy began. The median to progression of responders who had not undergone previous treatment was 33 months, in contrast to 21 months for those who had undergone previous treatment. Survival after progression of disease was also closely linked to the degree of previous therapy. No successful salvage regimen after initial fludarabine therapy was seen in patients refractory to alkylating agents, although the drug did achieve further remissions in patients who had received fludarabine as their initial treatment or who were not refractory to alkylating agents. Patients in unmaintained remission had a low morbidity rate on discontinuation of fludarabine, with less than 1 episode of infection per patient-year at risk. The morbidity during this time was linked to clinical response and was influenced by whether the patients had received previous treatment.

Conclusion.—Long-term follow-up of patients treated with fludarabine indicates that the response rate, survival, and time to progression are closely correlated with the degree of previous therapy. The best responses were seen in previously untreated patients. It is recommended that patients who have received previous treatment who then receive fludarabine should undergo postremission therapy.

▶ An intergroup study in the United States is currently comparing fludarabine with chlorambucil and a combination of both drugs for untreated CLL. The authors of this paper from M.D. Anderson Cancer Center deserve most of the credit for bringing fludarabine to the clinic. It is the first significant advance for CLL therapy in decades.—P.H. Wiernik, M.D.

Lack of Effect of 2-Chlorodeoxyadenosine Therapy in Patients With Chronic Lymphocytic Leukemia Refractory to Fludarabine Therapy

O'Brien S, Kantarjian H, Estey E, Koller C, Robertson B, Beran M, Andreeff M, Pierce S, Keating M (Univ of Texas, Houston)

N Engl J Med 330:319–322, 1994   116-95-4–49

Background.—Fludarabine and 2-chlorodeoxyadenosine are nucleoside analogs that have been proved effective in treating patients with chronic lymphocytic leukemia (CLL). The drugs are believed to have similar mechanisms of action, but a small number of patients who fail to respond to fludarabine have responded to 2-chlorodeoxyadenosine.

Objective.—The efficacy of 2-chlorodeoxyadenosine was examined in 28 patients with CLL that had proved refractory to fludarabine treatment. The patients had a median age of 63 years. A large majority had advanced disease with anemia or thrombocytopenia, or both.

Treatment.—All the patients had received alkylating agents before fludarabine, and two thirds received other treatment after a trial of fludarabine, most often an anthracycline-based regimen or etoposide with or without mitoxantrone. The median interval between fludarabine treatment and the use of 2-chlorodeoxyadenosine was 1 month. A daily dose of 4 mg of 2-chlorodeoxyadenosine per m² was administered by continuous infusion for 1 week. Treatment could be repeated at monthly intervals.

Results.—Of the 28 patients, 2 had a partial response to 2-chlorodeoxyadenosine treatment. Minor antitumor activity was noted in some other patients who failed to meet criteria for remission. Only 1 patient with anemia or thrombocytopenia improved appreciably. Ten patients died during the first 2 monthly courses of 2-chlorodeoxyadenosine. Myelosuppression was frequent; most patients had neutropenia and thrombocytopenia. Nonhematologic toxicity was minimal.

Conclusion.—Patients with CLL who do not respond to fludarabine and who have poor marrow reserve are not likely to enter remission if they receive 2-chlorodeoxyadenosine, which itself induces substantial myelosuppression.

▶ Others have had better results with 2-chlorodeoxyadenosine in CLL patients who have not responded to fludarabine (1). The difference in these experiences is unexplained.—P.H. Wiernik, M.D.

Reference

1. Juliusson G, et al: N Engl J Med 327:1056, 1992.

CHRONIC MYELOCYTIC LEUKEMIA

Suppression of Chronic Myelogenous Leukemia Colony Growth by Interleukin-4
Estrov Z, Markowitz AB, Kurzrock R, Wetzler M, Kantarjian HM, Ferrajoli A, Gutterman JU, Talpaz M (Univ of Texas, Houston)
Leukemia 7:214–220, 1993   116-95-4–50

Introduction.—Interleukin-4, a cytokine with pleiotropic activities, suppresses GM-CFU granulocyte-macrophage (CFU-GM) proliferation in normal bone marrow cultured with either GM-CSF or IL-3. In the same cultures, it also enhances the colony-stimulating effect of G-CSF.

Methods.—The effect of IL-4 on bone marrow or peripheral blood cells from 30 patients with chronic myelogenous leukemia (CML) was examined. Repetitive experiments were performed using the CFU-granulocyte-erythrocyte-monocyte-megakaryocyte colony culture assay, as well as IL-1β, IL-6, and GM-CSF enzyme-linked immunosorbent assays.

Findings.—When cells were cultured in the presence of EPO—alone or with phytohemagglutinin-conditioned medium, GM-CSF, or IL-3—IL-4 inhibited GM-CFU colony replication by 24% to 65%. This inhibition occurred in a dose-dependent fashion at concentrations of .01–10 μg/mL and was partially reversed by the addition of IL-1β, 100 units/mL, to the CML cultures. When low-density peripheral blood cells from patients with CML were incubated with IL-4, 75% of samples showed down-regulation of IL-1β and IL-6 production. When IL-4 was added to CML cultures grown in the presence of G-CSF, there was suppression of CML GM-CFU in 2 samples, stimulation in 3, and no significant effect in 2.

Conclusion.—Interleukin-4 appears to suppress CML colony growth in culture. This suppressive effect may be mediated by inhibition of IL-1 as well as by other mechanisms, such as inhibition of IL-6 production. There may be a subgroup of patients with CML in whom IL-4 has an in vivo antiproliferative effect. Its potential to suppress CML progenitor replication in vivo may make IL-4 a useful therapeutic agent in patients with CML.

▶ We may not know enough about IL-4 to test it clinically in CML yet, but because of its inhibition of IL-6 secretion, it should be, and is, studied in myeloma.—P.H. Wiernik, M.D.

Hematologic Remission and Cytogenetic Improvement After Treatment of Stable-Phase Chronic Myelogenous Leukemia With Continuous Infusion of Low-Dose Cytarabine

Robertson MJ, Tantravahi R, Griffin JD, Canellos GP, Cannistra SA (Dana-Farber Cancer Inst, Boston; Harvard Med School, Boston)
Am J Hematol 43:95–102, 1993   116-95-4–51

Objective.—Because low concentrations of cytarabine selectively inhibit the growth of neoplastic myeloid progenitor cells from patients with chronic myelogenous leukemia (CML) in vitro, infusion therapy with low-dose cytarabine was evaluated in patients with stable-phase CML.

Study Plan.—The 5 patients enrolled in the study had more than 50% Philadelphia chromosome (Ph)–positive metaphases on cytogenetic analysis of the bone marrow. There were fewer than 3% blasts in the peripheral blood and fewer than 5% in the bone marrow. Cytarabine was administered by continuous subcutaneous infusion using a portable syringe pump. The initial dose of 15 mg/m^2/day was increased in increments of 5 mg/m^2/at 2-week intervals to 30 mg/m^2/day. Treatment was limited by a total leukocyte count of less than 2,500/μL or a platelet count as low as 75,000/μL.

Results.—Forty-three cycles of low-dose cytarabine were administered. The median treatment time per cycle was 29 days. All 5 patients had a complete hematologic response. In 1 patient, Ph-positive metaphases were eliminated from the bone marrow. The median time to the best cytogenetic response was approximately 5 months. Treatment was, in general, well tolerated, but 1 patient was withdrawn because of persistent liver enzyme elevations. No patient became febrile or required platelet transfusion, but most cycles were associated with symptomatic anemia that necessitated red cell transfusion.

Conclusion.—Prolonged infusion of low-dose cytarabine is a relatively safe means of achieving hematologic control and cytogenetic improvement in patients with stable-phase CML.

Prolonged Subcutaneous Administration of Recombinant α2b Interferon in Patients With Previously Untreated Philadelphia Chromosome-Positive Chronic-Phase Chronic Myelogenous Leukemia: Effect

on Remission Duration and Survival: Cancer and Leukemia Group B Study 8583

Ozer H, George SL, Schiffer CA, Rao K, Rao PN, Wurster-Hill DH, Arthur DD, Powell B, Gottlieb A, Peterson BA, Rai K, Testa JR, LeBeau M, Tantravahi R, Bloomfield CD (Univ of North Carolina, Chapel Hill; Duke Univ, Durham, NC; Univ of Maryland, Baltimore; et al)

Blood 82:2975–2984, 1993

116-95-4–52

Introduction.—Because earlier studies suggested a possible role for interferon (INF)-α in treating chronic myelogenous leukemia (CML), the Cancer and Leukemia Group B undertook a multicenter study to determine the value of recombinant INF-α2b in untreated patients with newly diagnosed, Philadelphia chromosome–positive, chronic-phase CML. A total of 107 such patients received daily subcutaneous treatment with recombinant INF-α2b at a dose of 5×10^6 IU/m².

Results.—Very severe toxicity was unusual, and most lesser toxic effects tended to lessen after several weeks of treatment. It was possible to continue treatment by modifying the dose. Fifty-nine percent of patients achieved at least partial remission and 22% entered complete remission. Another 17% of patients had progressive disease. Of 84 evaluable patients, 21 had blast crisis develop, only 2 of whom remain alive. The overall median response duration was 52 months (Fig 4–7). The rate of partial or complete cytogenetic response in 78 evaluable patients was 40%. There were no significant differences in the duration of remission or survival according to whether a cytogenetic response took place.

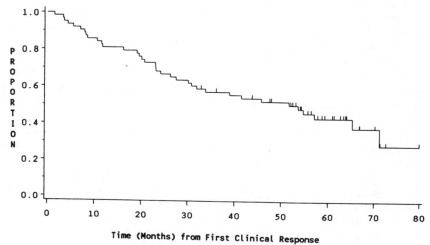

Time (Months) from First Clinical Response

Fig 4–7.—Proportion of patients still in remission as a function of time (Kaplan-Meier estimates) for the 63 patients with complete or partial response. At this point, 36 patients (57%) had not responded to treatment. The median length of response was 52 months. (Courtesy of Ozer H, George SL, Schiffer CA, et al: *Blood* 82:2975–2984, 1993.)

Conclusion.—Almost 60% of untreated patients with CML had at least a partial clinical response to treatment with recombinant INF-α.

Effect of Prior Interferon Alfa Therapy on the Outcome of Allogeneic Bone Marrow Transplantation for Chronic Myelogenous Leukemia
Giralt SA, Kantarjian HM, Talpaz M, Rios MB, Del Giglio A, Andersson BS, Przepiorka D, Deisseroth AB, Champlin RE (Univ of Texas, Houston)
J Clin Oncol 11:1055–1061, 1993   116-95-4-53

Background.—Treatment of chronic myelogenous leukemia (CML) has usually involved chemotherapy with busulfan or hydroxyurea, or both. These agents suppress leukocytosis but do not prevent progression of the disease. On the other hand, high-dose chemotherapy and then allogeneic bone marrow transplantation are capable of eradicating the malignancy. Interferon-α (INF-α) has also been shown to act against CML; however, it is unclear to what extent it affects engraftment, graft-vs.-host disease, regimen-related toxicity, and survival. Whether INF therapy affects the outcome of allogeneic bone marrow transplantation was investigated.

Methods.—A total of 77 patients with CML underwent allogeneic bone marrow transplantation between 1981 and 1991. The transplants were from HLA-identical related donors, after a total body irradiation–containing preparative regimen. Patients were classified into 2 groups on the basis of disease stage at the time of transplantation: first chronic phase or more advanced disease, as defined by clinical and hematologic findings. The 2 groups were further subdivided according to whether the patients had been previously treated with INF-α. The INF-α group in-cluded patients who had received doses of $3–5 \times 10^6$ units/m² 3 times a week or more for at least 4 weeks.

Results.—Forty-one patients underwent transplantation in chronic phase; 23 had previously received INF-α. No significant differences were observed between the patients treated with INF and those not treated with INF with respect to age, time of transplantation, preparative regi-men, or female donor–male recipient sex mismatches. Neither were any significant differences seen between those who had received INF and those who had not with regard to neutrophil recovery of more than 1×10^9/L, platelet recovery of more than 50×10^9/L, incidence of grade II–IV graft-vs.-host disease, incidence of chronic graft-vs.-host disease, disease-free survival, relapse, or 100-day transplant-related mortality. Similarly, in patients with more advanced disease at time of transplanta-tion, no significant differences in these outcomes were seen between pa-tients who had received INF and those who had not.

Conclusion.—Previous treatment with INF-α did not adversely affect transplant outcome. Further studies are required to investigate the complementary roles of INF-α and allogeneic bone marrow transplantation in the treatment of CML.

▶ The Robertson et al. study (Abstract 116-95-4–51) is provocative. More than a decade ago, the Cancer and Leukemia Group B (CALGB) conducted studies of cytosine arabinoside (Ara-C) in chronic-phase CML and found the agent not useful in that setting. However, Robertson et al. used a different schedule and dose, which appear to be effective. Perhaps the combination of low-dose continuous-infusion Ara-C plus INF-α should be tested, because others have reported greater benefit from INF than was observed by Ozer et al. (Abstract 116-95-4–52) in the CALGB trial and by Giralt et al. (Abstract 116-95-4–53).—P.H. Wiernik, M.D.

MYELODYSPLASIA

Therapy-Related Myelodysplasia and Acute Myeloid Leukemia. Cytogenetic Characteristics of 115 Consecutive Cases and Risk in Seven Cohorts of Patients Treated Intensively for Malignant Diseases in The Copenhagen Series

Pedersen-Bjergaard J, Philip P, Larsen SO, Andersson M, Daugaard G, Ersbøll J, Hansen SW, Hou-Jensen K, Nielsen D, Sigsgaard TC, Specht L, Østerlind K (Rigshospitalet, Copenhagen; Herlev County Hosp, Copenhagen; Serum Inst, Copenhagen)
Leukemia 7:1975–1986, 1993

116-95-4–54

Purpose.—Secondary or therapy-related acute myeloid leukemia (t-AML) often presents as myelodysplasia (t-MDS). It is the most serious complication of cancer treatment and offers a unique opportunity to study the development of chemically induced leukemia in humans. The findings of 115 consecutive patients with t-MDS or t-AML were studied.

Methods.—Cytogenetic studies of these patients were conducted during a 16-year period. These cytogenetic findings were correlated with the patients' general type of therapy and compared with the findings in de novo acute myeloid leukemia. Forty-five of the patients were identified by close follow-up of 7 Danish cohorts of patients treated for 6 different types of primary malignant lymphomas or solid tumors. These cohorts were compared to evaluate their risk for t-MDS and t-AML.

Results.—For patients receiving primary treatment with alkylating agents, the risk for therapy-related disease increased by about 1% per year from 2 to at least 8 years after the beginning of treatment. Most patients were seen with t-MDS, showing loss of an entire chromosome 5 or 7 or of various parts of the long arms. These leukemias fell into the M1, M2, or M4 subtypes. The leukemic risk increased much more sharply, beginning after only 1 year of therapy, in patients receiving drugs targeted at DNA-topoisomerase II (e.g., etoposide, doxorubicin, 4-epidoxorubicin, or mitoxantrone) in combination with drugs acting directly on DNA (e.g., cisplatin or alkylating agents). Cases of t-AML or t-MDS of early onset usually were seen as overt M4 or M5 leukemia with balanced translocations to chromosome bands 11q23 or 21q22. In contrast, the later-onset cases were often similar to those occurring in patients treated with alkylating agents alone.

Conclusion. —The t-AML may develop in patients with either alkylation of DNA or poisoning of DNA-topoisomerase II. The clinical and cytogenetic characteristics of these secondary leukemias appear to be different. The 2 classes of drugs may act synergistically in causing secondary leukemia. For patients with germ cell tumors treated with etoposide, cisplatin, and bleomycin, the risk for secondary leukemia may increase exponentially with increased doses of cisplatin and etoposide.

▶ There is, of course, no doubt that certain chemotherapeutic agents are associated with the development of so-called secondary leukemias. However, the agents may only play a role in leukemogenesis when leukemogenesis is an intrinsic feature of the primary disease. Alkylating agents are associated with an increased incidence of leukemia in myeloma, a disease observed to transform to an AML without treatment. Furthermore, the same agent that frequently causes myeloma in BALB/c mice, intraperitoneal mineral oil, less frequently causes acute myelomonocytic leukemia without myeloma in that model. Alkylating agents rarely, if ever, induce acute leukemia in chronic lymphocytic leukemia, which suggests that the underlying disease is as important as its treatment in the evolution of secondary leukemia.—P.H. Wiernik, M.D.

All-*Trans* Retinoic Acid in Patients With Myelodysplastic Syndromes: Results of a Pilot Study

Aul C, Runde V, Gattermann N (Heinrich Heine Univ, Düsseldorf, Germany)
Blood 82:2967–2974, 1993   116-95-4–55

Background. —Myelodysplastic syndromes (MDS) are common diseases in the elderly and are usually fatal. There is no standardized therapy; in some cases, only supportive treatment can be offered. All-*trans* retinoic acid (ATRA) induces remission in most patients with acute promyelocytic leukemia, prompting speculation on its possible use in treating other hematologic malignancies.

Methods. —A 3-month, dose-escalating trial of ATRA was performed in 15 patients with primary or secondary MDS. Four had refractory anemia, 2 had refractory anemia with ring sideroblasts, 7 had refractory anemia with excess blasts, and 2 had refractory anemia with excess blasts in transformation. To be included, patients had to have transfusion-dependent anemia, pronounced neutropenia or thrombocytopenia, or increasing numbers of blast cells in the peripheral blood or bone marrow. The ATRA therapy started at a dose of 30 mg/m²/day, administered orally in 2 equal doses every 12 hours. The dose was increased to 60 mg/m²/day at 4 weeks and to 90 mg/m²/day at 8 weeks. The treatment response was assessable in 14 patients.

Results.—There were no complete or partial remissions. A minor response was noted in 3 patients, including 2 patients with decreased transfusion requirements and 1 with increased neutrophil and platelet counts. Five patients progressed to more advanced MDS or overt leukemia; 3 with chromosomal abnormalities retained their cytogenetic marker after 10–12 weeks of ATRA treatment. All patients but 2 had at least low-grade dermatologic toxicity, and 2 patients had to stop treatment because of conjunctivitis or progressive neurologic symptoms.

Conclusion.—This pilot study reports disappointing results of ATRA treatment in patients with MDS. The reason for the lack of response in MDS compared with acute promyelocytic leukemia may have to do with the absence of the t(15;17) translocation. Future studies will assess the effects of combining ATRA with other differentiation-inducing agents, as well as the effects of other retinoids.

▶ This was an excellent idea that did not work out. The authors suggest that failure might have been expected because of the lack of t(15;17). However, other patients without this translocation have, on occasion, responded to ATRA (1).—P.H. Wiernik, M.D.

Reference

1. Wiernik PH, et al: *Leukemia* 5:504, 1991.

Acute Leukemias

ACUTE MYELOID LEUKEMIA

Radon Exposure and Leukaemia in Adulthood
Viel J-F (Faculty of Medicine, Besançon, France)
Int J Epidemiol 22:627–631, 1993   116-95-4–56

Background.—There are reported geographic correlations between indoor radon concentrations and the incidence of various types of leukemia. Studies from England, Scotland, Wales, and Canada have noted positive associations between leukemia and radon concentrations. The influence of radon exposure on adult leukemia rates in France was examined, adjusting for gamma-level and socioeconomic status.

Methods.—Detailed data were collected regarding indoor radon and gamma ray geometric means for 41 French administrative areas from 1984 to 1986. Data on leukemia deaths in adults aged 35–84 years were correlated with the mean radon exposure.

Findings.—In the 41 administrative areas, the indoor radon concentration averaged 12–147 Bq/m⁻³, whereas gamma-ray concentration was

28–142 nG/h^{-1}. Mortality from acute lymphoid leukemia was similar to the national level, but there was an excess of deaths from acute myeloid leukemia (AML). Poisson regression models and modified tests for partial correlation showed a significant and positive relation between AML mortality and indoor radon concentration. This association held regardless of adjustment for indoor gamma-ray dose, socioeconomic status, and linear gradient.

Conclusion.—Data from France support the hypothesis that indoor radon exposure is a leukemic environmental hazard. It is estimated that more than one fourth of deaths from AML may be caused by radon.

Risk of Leukemia After Treatment With Pituitary Growth Hormone
Fradkin JE, Mills JL, Schonberger LB, Wysowski DK, Thomson R, Durako SJ, Robison LL (Natl Inst of Diabetes and Digestive and Kidney Diseases, Bethesda, Md; Natl Inst of Child Health and Human Development, Bethesda, Md; Ctrs for Disease Control and Prevention, Atlanta, Ga; et al)
JAMA 270:2829–2832, 1993   116-95-4–57

Background.—The estimate of a twofold greater incidence of leukemia in recipients of growth hormone was based on incomplete data bases from Europe and North America. The incidence of leukemia and lymphoma was determined based on a study that evaluated the risk for Creutzfeldt-Jakob disease and other adverse effects of growth hormone among participants in the United States National Hormone and Pituitary Program.

Methods.—Eighty-four percent of 6,284 recipients of growth hormone or their proxies were contacted and interviewed; medical records or death certificates were reviewed for the deceased. Reported diagnoses of leukemia or lymphoma were confirmed by reviewing medical records. The person-years of risk for each subject were established from the date of first growth hormone treatment to the date of interview, death, or diagnosis of leukemia or lymphoma.

Results.—In 59,736 patient-years of follow-up, there were 3 cases of leukemia, which was not significantly higher than the 1.66 cases expected in an age-, race-, and gender-matched general population in the United States. However, extension of follow-up revealed 3 additional cases, yielding a minimum leukemia rate of 6, which is significantly higher than the expected 2.26. Leukemia was not associated with idiopathic growth hormone deficiency but was significantly correlated with craniopharyngioma. Five patients who had leukemia required growth hormone secondary to antecedent cranial tumor; 4 had undergone radiation therapy. Lymphoma was not excessive in this cohort.

Conclusion.—The overall incidence of leukemia is about 2.25 times higher among patients treated with pituitary growth hormone compared with that of the general population. This increase results from patients with antecedent tumors, primarily craniopharyngioma. Whether administration of growth hormone, underlying risk factors, or an interaction of the 2 components caused the heightened leukemia rate must be determined. Growth hormone–related malignancy should continue to be analyzed in patients receiving recombinant growth hormone.

▶ Six patients with leukemia and growth hormone deficiency who never received growth hormone therapy have been reported (1).—P.H. Wiernik, M.D.

Reference

1. Redmond GP, et al: *Pediatr Res* 31:83A, 1992.

Spontaneous Remission of Infantile Acute Nonlymphocytic Leukemia for 11 Years in a Child With Normal Karyotype
Penchansky L, Wollman MR, Gartner JC, Wenger SL (Univ of Pittsburgh, Pa; Children's Hosp of Pittsburgh)
Cancer 71:1928–1930, 1993   116-95-4-58

Background.—Leukemic-like hematologic abnormalities that spontaneously resolve rarely occur in karyotypically normal infants. One infant with self-limiting acute nonlymphocytic leukemia (ANLL) who later had karyotypically normal ANLL was described.

Case Report.—Male infant, 6 weeks, was first seen with fever and hepatosplenomegaly. A complete blood count indicated anemia and leukoerythroblastic leukocytosis. His bone marrow aspirate contained 20% blasts with a myeloid morphologic appearance. Cytochemical stains were weakly positive for Sudan black. Five percent of the blasts were positive for chloroacetate esterase, and all blasts were negative for nonspecific esterase. Acute leukemia (French-American-British M1) was the diagnosis, but chemotherapy was withheld because of his young age and the relatively low blast percentage in the bone marrow aspirate. Two weeks later, the fever resolved and hepatosplenomegaly diminished. However, the leukocyte count had increased and his marrow blast count was lower. The results of a bone marrow culture for granulocyte-monocyte colony formation in agar were normal. No treatment was initiated, and his hematologic parameters improved progressively and stabilized within 12 months. Eleven years later, the patient had prolonged fever, anemia, and neutropenia. Bone marrow aspiration revealed 33% blasts with myeloid morphology. Chemotherapy based on the Childrens Cancer Group Study Protocol 2891 for ANLL (French-American-British M1) resulted in remission after 3 months. The patient tolerated an allogeneic bone marrow transplant; however, leukemia recurred 5 months later. Six weeks after high-dose chemotherapy, bone marrow aspiration and a biopsy specimen revealed recovery marrow. The patient died of veno-occlusive disease after a second bone marrow transplant.

Conclusion.—The diagnosis and prognosis of karyotypically and phenotypically normal infants with an abnormal hematologic picture resembling that of ANLL are less straightforward compared with those of an older child or adult. Treatment should be withheld in these patients until the leukemic process is evident.

Transient Myeloproliferative Disorder in a Down's Neonate With Rearranged T-Cell Receptor β Gene and Evidence of *In Vivo* Maturation Demonstrated by Dual-Colour Flow Cytometric DNA Ploidy Analysis

Kwong YL, Cheng G, Tang TS, Robertson EP, Lee CP, Chan LC (Queen Mary Hosp, Hong Kong)

Leukemia 7:1667–1671, 1993   116-95-4–59

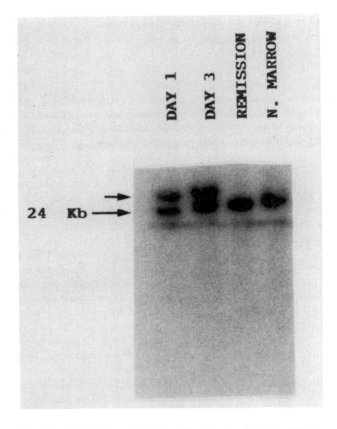

Fig 4–8.—Samples of DNA digested with *Bam*HI and analyzed with the TCR-β constant region probe. *Lane 1,* patient's day 1 peripheral blood sample; *lane 2,* patient's day 3 peripheral blood sample; *lane 3,* patient's day 30 bone marrow sample with disease in remission; *lane 4,* bone marrow sample from a normal donor. (Courtesy of Kwong YL, Cheng G, Tang TS, et al: *Leukemia* 7:1667–1671, 1993.)

Introduction.—The transient myeloproliferative disorder found in infants with Down syndrome is characterized by hepatosplenomegaly and markedly increased blasts in both the bone marrow and peripheral blood. Anemia and thrombocytopenia may or may not be seen. Spontaneous remission is the rule, but in approximately 20% of patients, acute leukemia develops.

Case Report.—Male infant, born at 34 weeks' gestation, had somatic features of Down syndrome. Mild respiratory distress was seen, and radiographs showed pulmonary congestion as well as marked enlargement of the liver and spleen. Leukocytosis was noted, with increased blasts in the circulation. Oliguria and bilirubinemia developed and responded to a double-volume exchange transfusion. The hepatosplenomegaly lessened gradually, but necrotizing enterocolitis developed, necessitating antibiotic treatment and total parenteral nutrition. Hematopoiesis appeared normal on marrow examination at 1 month of age.

Hematologic and Cytogenetic Findings.—Some of the circulating blast cells appeared undifferentiated, and others had features of megakaryoblasts. The blasts expressed myeloid, T-lymphoid, and megakaryocytic surface antigens but not B-lineage antigens. The T-cell receptor-β (TCR_β) gene was clonally rearranged; the immunoglobulin heavy-chain gene exhibited a germline configuration. Flow cytometric DNA ploidy analysis of blast cells showed that a 2N population predominated initially but that polyploidization occurred later as the number of circulating blasts declined. Eventually hematopoiesis returned to normal, as both blast cells and the clonally rearranged TCR_β gene disappeared (Fig 4-8).

Interpretation.—It appears that the abnormal clone eventually became mature in this case of transient myeloproliferative disorders. In neonates with Down syndrome and transient myeloproliferative disorder, trisomy 21 may lead to a transient state of enforced self-renewal, resulting in temporary clonal dominance of multilineate phenotype stem cells. An alternative explanation is that trisomy 21 confers a transformational potential that leads to either genetic misprogramming or a lineage switch but is not sufficient to produce the full picture of leukemia.

▶ Eventual development of acute leukemia in neonates who present with a spontaneously regressing leukemia-like disorder may be more common than was previously appreciated (1).—P.H. Wiernik, M.D.

Reference

1. Liang D-C, et al: *Leukemia* 7:1521, 1993.

Comparison of Acute Myeloid Leukemia Occurring De Novo or Preceded by a Myelodysplastic Stage: Differences in Cellular DNA Content

Widell S, Auer G, Hast R, Reizenstein P (Karolinska Inst, Stockholm)
Am J Hematol 42:293–298, 1993   116-95-4–60

Objective.—The DNA content of bone marrow cells from 11 patients with de novo acute myeloid leukemia (AML) was compared with that in cells from 10 patients whose acute leukemia was preceded by a phase of myelodysplasia (MDS-AML). Cells from 13 healthy controls were also examined.

Methods.—The DNA index, or mean amount of DNA per cell, was determined using a digital video-based image-analyzing system.

Findings.—Of 11 patients with de novo AML, 3 had DNA index values below the normal limit for both immature and mature bone marrow cells. Differences between this group of 3 patients and both patients with MDS-AML and controls were significant for blasts and promyelocytes, lymphocytes, and monocytes. Patients with MDS-AML had DNA index values comparable to those of controls.

Conclusion.—These findings, along with reports suggesting differences in granulocyte morphology, clonality, and HLA-DR expression, support the view that de novo AML and MDS-AML are biologically distinct disorders.

High Expression of bcl-2 Protein in Acute Myeloid Leukemia Cells Is Associated With Poor Response to Chemotherapy

Campos L, Rouault J-P, Sabido O, Oriol P, Roubi N, Vasselon C, Archimbaud E, Magaud J-P, Guyotat D (Centre de Transfusion Sanguine, Lyon, France; Hôpital Edouard Herriot, Lyon, France; Faculté de Médicine, St Etienne, France)
Blood 81:3091–3096, 1993   116-95-4–61

Background.—The proto-oncogene *bcl-2* encodes a mitochondrial protein that blocks programmed cell death, resulting in prolonged survival of lymphoid cells. Large amounts of the bcl-2 protein are found in lymphoid malignancies and also in normal tissues that undergo apoptotic cell death, such as the bone marrow. A monoclonal antibody to the bcl-2 protein was used to examine the expression of this gene product in 82 consecutive newly diagnosed cases of acute myeloid leukemia (AML).

Treatment.—The patients received intensive chemotherapy, starting with an anthracycline drug or mitoxantrone and cytosine arabinoside for induction of remission. Postinduction treatment included 2 intensive courses of treatment for patients aged 60 years and younger. Older patients received consolidation treatment with daunorubicin and cytosine arabinoside or low-dose cytosine arabinoside. Nine patients received al-

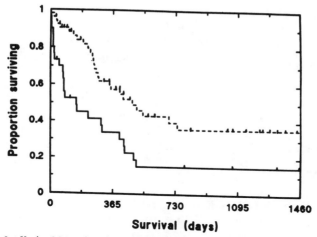

Survival (days)

Fig 4–9.—Kaplan-Meier plot of survival duration according to bcl-2 expression. *Solid curve,* cases with 20% or more bcl-2$^+$ cells; *dashed curve,* cases with less than 20% bcl-2$^+$ cells. Survival is significantly different (P < .005) by log-rank test. (Courtesy of Campos L, Rouault J-P, Sabido O, et al: *Blood* 81:3091–3096, 1993.)

logeneic bone marrow transplants, 6 of them at the time of first remission and 3 after relapse.

Findings.—The mean proportion of bcl-2$^+$ cells in marrow samples was 23%, but it ranged from zero to 95%. These cells were more numerous in French-American-British M4 and M5 cases and when the WBC count was high. In addition, the expression of the bcl-2 protein correlated with that of the stem cell marker CD34. The survival of blast cells in liquid culture correlated significantly with the percentage of bcl-2$^+$ cells. The overall complete response rate was 66%. Eighty-five percent of patients with fewer than 20% bcl-2$^+$ cells entered complete remission after chemotherapy, compared with only 29% who had 20% or more positive cells. In addition, a high level of expression of bcl-2 correlated with a significantly shortened survival (Fig 4–9).

Conclusion.—The proto-oncogene *bcl-2* is expressed on AML cells, and the level of its expression correlates with such biological aspects as hyperleukocytosis and blast cell behavior in liquid culture. In addition, a high level of expression correlates with compromised survival and, therefore, may mandate a modified approach to treatment.

▶ This is an interesting finding in AML. However, I think the same caution expressed in the article by Ludescher et al. (Abstract 116-95-4–45) about the methodology of measuring P-glycoprotein in leukemia cells needs to be expressed here. Rather than choosing an arbitrary point above which patients are labeled positive, other statistical analyses that choose the best breakpoint for predictor variables, such as the Classification and Regression Tree Analysis (CART), would be more useful.—P.H. Wiernik, M.D.

Autonomous Proliferation of Leukemic Cells in Vitro as a Determinant of Prognosis in Adult Acute Myeloid Leukemia

Löwenberg B, van Putten WLJ, Touw IP, Delwel R, Santini V (Dr Daniel den Hoed Cancer Ctr, Rotterdam, The Netherlands; Erasmus Univ, Rotterdam, The Netherlands)

N Engl J Med 328:614–619, 1993   116-95-4-62

Background.—In acute myeloid leukemia (AML), leukemic cells frequently sustain their own proliferation in vitro. In experimental leukemia models, autocrine mechanisms substantially transform the kinetics of cellular development, conferring a growth advantage. The spontaneous proliferation of AML was analyzed to determine its impact on clinical outcome.

Methods.—Tritiated thymidine uptake by leukemic cells from 114 patients with newly diagnosed AML and from 91 patients receiving chemotherapy was measured in serum-free and cytokine-free cultures. Cellular proliferation was quantified by the level of activity and related to overall survival and to treatment outcome.

Results.—The level of proliferation was low in cell samples from 37 patients, intermediate in 29, and high in 38. Proliferative activity correlated with disease stage; significantly greater levels of activity were observed in cells from patients with stage M4 or M5 AML compared with those from patients with stage M1 or M2 disease. The probability of 3-year survival was 36% among patients with low levels of proliferative activity, significantly higher than the 3% probability associated with high levels of proliferative activity. Chemotherapy patients with low proliferative activity had a 68% complete remission rate and a 49% probability of remaining relapse-free. In contrast, the remission rate of 39% and disease-free survival rate of 11% were significantly lower in those with a high level of proliferation. The 3-year disease-free survival among patients in complete remission after chemotherapy was 49% when proliferative activity was low and 9% with high activity. The overall survival was significantly higher among patients with low proliferative activity. Patients with intermediate levels of cell proliferation in vitro had intermediate rates of survival, relapse, and disease-free survival.

Conclusion.—The capacity of leukemic blasts for autonomous proliferation correlates with highly aggressive AML.

Clinical and Prognostic Significance of In Vivo Differentiation in Acute Myeloid Leukemia

Raza A, Preisler H, Lampkin B, Lykins J, Kukla C, Gartside P, Sheikh Y, Yousuf N, White M, Barcos M, Bennett J, Browman G, Goldberg J, Grunwald H, Larson R, Vardiman J, Vogler R (Roswell Park Mem Inst, Buffalo, NY; Univ of Rochester, NY; Health Science Ctr, Syracuse, NY; et al)
Am J Hematol 42:147–157, 1993

116-95-4-63

Background.—Neoplastic cell examination is possible in acute myelocytic leukemia (AML) before, during, and after chemotherapy. The leukemic cell proliferation and differentiation in serial bone marrow specimens obtained during standard chemotherapy for AML were investigated.

Methods.—Before initiation of remission induction therapy, 86 patients with standard-risk AML newly diagnosed received bromodeoxyuridine, and the labeling index, durations of S-phase, and myeloblast cell cycle were determined. Induction therapy consisted of cytosine arabinoside and daunomycin. A bone marrow biopsy specimen was taken on days 6 and 17 and at subsequent weekly intervals. Bone marrow aspirates were treated with monoclonal antibromodeoxyuridine antibody to determine the fate of bromodeoxyuridine-labeled cells.

Results.—In vivo differentiation was evident in 48 patients (Diff+). Bromodeoxyuridine-labeled granulocytes were apparent a week after induction therapy began. In contrast, the bromodeoxyuridine-labeled myeloblasts were prominent in biopsy specimens from patients without differentiation (Diff–). Serial marrow samples from Diff– patients contained neither labeled cells nor bromodeoxyuridine-labeled blasts, suggesting residual leukemia. Biopsy specimens from Diff+ patients revealed either substantial labeled cells or 3+ to 4+ differentiation, or they showed 1+ or 2+ differentiation. The durations of S-phase and myeloblast cell cycle were shortest for Diff– patients, slightly longer for 1–2+ Diff+, and longest for 3–4+ Diff+. Two thirds of Diff+ patients entered complete remission, which was comparable to the 73.6% remission rate of Diff–. However, the Diff+ group had a significantly longer duration of remission and a median has not been established; the median remission among Diff– cases was 220 days. The length of the S-phase correlated with longer remission: 7 patients with the longest S-phase remained in remission, whereas 24 with the shortest S-phase were in remission a median of 240 days.

Conclusion.—In vivo cell differentiation in patients with AML suggests a favorable long-term prognosis, either because of substantial normal residual hematopoiesis before induction therapy or leukemic cell differentiation.

Biological Characteristics of Newly Diagnosed Poor Prognosis Acute Myelogenous Leukemia

Raza A, Preisler HD, Li YQ, Larson RA, Goldberg J, Browman G, Bennett J, Grunwald H, Vogler R, Kukla C (Univ of Cincinnati, Ohio; Univ of Chicago; Cooper Hosp Univ, Camden, NJ; et al)

Am J Hematol 42:359–366, 1993   116-95-4–64

Background.—The prognosis for acute myelogenous leukemia (AML) that develops after exposure to hematopoietic toxins, after a preleukemia syndrome, or in patients older than age 70 years is generally poor. A combination of 2 or more of these characteristics significantly worsens the prognosis. The relationship between the expression of *fms, myc,* and IL-1β genes and treatment outcome in AML was investigated.

Methods.—Patients with at least 1 of the 3 poor-prognostic characteristics for AML were treated according to remission induction protocol INT 0059. Bone marrow aspirates and biopsy specimens were obtained before the start of chemotherapy and 12 hours after the last dose. Leukemic cell differentiation was assessed before and during induction therapy, and pretherapy leukemic cell expression of *fms, myc,* and IL-1β was assessed.

Results.—The expression of *fms* was studied in 23 pretherapy RNA specimens, and transcripts were detected in 5. The pretherapy leukemia cell mass did not correlate with the level of *fms* expression, although on day 6, the leukemia cell mass was significantly smaller in patients whose leukemia cells contained *fms* transcripts, compared with that of patients whose cells did not contain the gene. Furthermore, complete remission was more likely when leukemia cells contained *fms* transcripts. Bone marrow from patients with leukemia cells expressing *fms* had a higher percentage of cells that synthesized DNA. Relationships were not observed between *fms* expression and duration of remission or between *myc* expression and treatment outcome. Interleukin-1β transcripts were detected in pretherapy leukemia cells in 21 of 25 patients, and IL-1β expression correlated inversely with duration of remission.

Conclusion.—When compared with newly diagnosed standard-prognosis AML, the leukemia in patients with a poor prognosis is more likely to exhibit low levels of *fms* expression.

▶ These 2 papers (Abstracts 116-95-4-63 and 116-95-4-64), basically from 1 study, associate in vitro differentiation with favorable clinical outcome in AML.—P.H. Wiernik, M.D.

The 8;21 Chromosome Translocation in Acute Myeloid Leukemia Is Always Detectable by Molecular Analysis Using *AML1*

Maseki N, Miyoshi H, Shimizu K, Homma C, Ohki M, Sakurai M, Kaneko Y

(Saitama Cancer Ctr Hosp, Japan; Saitama Cancer Ctr Research Inst, Ina, Japan)
Blood 81:1573–1579, 1993

116-95-4-65

Background.—Specific chromosome translocations are associated with specific subtypes of acute myeloid leukemia (AML). The 8;21 translocation is associated with the M2 subtype of the French-American-British classification of AML. A novel gene (*AML1*) had previously been isolated on chromosome 21; the gene was rearranged by the t(8;21) translocation. Leukemic cell DNA from patients with AML was analyzed to determine whether *AML1* DNA rearrangement is detectable in all t(8;21) AML.

Patients and Methods.—Fifty-nine patients with AML, aged 6 months to 74 years, with leukemic cell samples available for both cytogenic and molecular analysis, were included. Karyotyping and Southern blot DNA analysis with an *AML1* probe were carried out on these samples.

Results.—The AML1 gene was rearranged in leukemic cells from 33 patients with AML with t(8;21)(q22;q22) or its variant, complex t(8;V;21). The *AML1* gene was also rearranged in 3 patients with AML and no t(8;21). The *AML1* gene rearrangement was not detected in leukemic cells from 23 patients with AML with normal diploidy or with non-t(8;21) cytogenic abnormalities.

Conclusion.—Juxtaposition of 5′ *AML1* to a gene located in the breakpoint region of 8q22 may be an essential step in the leukemogenesis of t(8;21) subtype AML. Southern hybridization with *AML1* probes may be sufficient to detect t(8;21), its variants, and masked t(8;21).

8;21 Translocation and Multilineage Involvement

Kwong YL, Ching LM, Liu HW, Lee CP, Pollock A, Chan LC (Queen Mary Hosp, Hong Kong)
Am J Hematol 43:212–216, 1993

116-95-4-66

Background.—One of the most common chromosomal aberrations in acute myeloid leukemia (AML) is translocation (8;21) (q22;q22). This aberration occurs in 7% to 12% of patients. One group of patients with t(8;21) was examined.

Methods and Findings.—The patients were 8 adults and 3 children. In 6, AML M2 was diagnosed according to strict French-American-British criteria. There was no peripheral blood monocytosis or marrow evidence of monocytic differentiation. However, 2 patients had significant fluoride-sensitive α-naphthol acetate esterase or increased serum lysozyme. In 3 patients, more than 20% of the cells in the marrow had monocytic features morphologically. More than 20% of the blasts had fluoride-sensitive α-naphthol acetate esterase. One patient had increased serum lysozyme as well; therefore, the diagnosis for this patient was AML M4. Gross granulocytic hyperplasia with 15% blasts was noted in 1 patient, along with a 4-cm splenomegaly. Chronic myeloid leukemia in acceleration was diagnosed in this patient. Another patient had trilineage myelodysplasia with 25% blasts and was given a diagnosis of refractory anemia with excessive blasts in transformation. Cytogenetic study revealed t(8;21) as the sole karyotypic aberration. The most common associated aberration was loss of a sex chromosome.

Conclusion.—Translocation (8;21) may occur in a wide range of hematologic abnormalities. It is therefore proposed that this translocation may involve different hemopoietic lineages.

▶ The paper by Maseki et al. (Abstract 116-95-4-65) elucidates some of the molecular mechanisms of leukemogenesis of AML associated with t(8;21). It is intriguing that the *AML1* gene in the chromosome 21 breakpoint region of that translocation has significant homology with 1 of the genes that controls morphogenesis in the fruit fly. The Kwong et al. paper (Abstract 116-95-4-66) reminds us that the t(8;21) may be associated with several different French-American-British types of AML.—P.H. Wiernik, M.D.

Management of Leukemic Hyperleukocytosis With Hydration, Urinary Alkalinization, and Allopurinol: Are Cranial Irradiation and Invasive Cytoreduction Necessary?
Nelson SC, Bruggers CS, Kurtzberg J, Friedman HS (Duke Univ, Durham, NC)
Am J Pediatr Hematol Oncol 15:351–355, 1993   116-95-4-67

Background.—Hyperleukocytosis, defined as a peripheral leukocyte count in excess of $100 \times 10^9/L$ secondary to acute leukemia, is a medical emergency that can lead to intracranial hemorrhage and death. Emergent cranial irradiation is used to prevent this complication, but this has serious associated morbidity when used in the young child. Exchange transfusion and leukapheresis are also used but are invasive and require an intensive care setting. Three young children with acute leukemia and hyperleukocytosis were successfully treated with intravenous hydration, alkalinization, and allopurinol therapy.

Results.—The average maximal decrease in the leukocyte count was 88% within 70 hours of the initiation of this conservative management regimen. A leukocyte count of less than $100 \times 10^9/L$ was observed an average of 15 hours after hospitalization. There were no complications.

Conclusion.—The pediatric patient with acute lymphocytic leukemia and hyperleukocytosis without evidence of leukostasis or life-threatening metabolic abnormalities can be managed by intravenous hydration, urinary alkalinization, and allopurinol. This method is safe, effective, and noninvasive.

▶ My impression of this report is that Nelson et al. were lucky. I agree that with a WBC count of 100,000/μL, hydration and measures to prevent urate nephropathy may suffice, but with a WBC count greater than 200,000/μL, I would advocate more aggressive measures. The authors quote Fritz RD, et al. (1), who pointed out the great likelihood of intracerebral hemorrhage in patients with blast counts greater than 300,000/μL. The mechanism is rupture of a capillary in the brain at the venous end where sludging of blast cells is most likely. The sludged blasts secrete uric acid, a vasodilator, which facilitates the capillary rupture. Hydration is not going to resolve a focal nidus of sludged leukemia cells at the venous end of a capillary. Low-dose cranial irradiation (200–300 centigray $\times$2) will. That, plus either immediate institution of induction therapy or hydroxyurea to prevent reformation of intracerebral foci of sludging, is the safest and least expensive way of preventing death from this complication.—P.H. Wiernik, M.D.

Reference

1. Fritz RD, et al: *N Engl J Med* 261:59, 1959.

Cyclosporin A and Cyclosporin SDZ PSC 833 Enhance Anti-CD5 Ricin A-Chain Immunotoxins in Human Leukemic T Cells

Jaffrézou J-P, Sikic BI, Laurent G (Centre National de la Recherche Scientifique, Toulouse, France; Centre Hospitalier Universitaire Purpan, Toulouse, France; Stanford Univ, Calif)
Blood 83:482–489, 1994   116-95-4-68

Objective.—Ricin A-chain immunotoxins (RTA-ITs) are among the most potent immunotoxins being investigated for possible use as anticancer drugs. Cyclosporin A may affect the efficacy or toxicity of RTA-IT therapy. The potential of cyclosporin A and its nonimmunosuppressive analog SDZ PSC 883 to enhance the effects of RTA-ITs was examined.

Observations.—At doses of 4 μmol/L, both cyclosporin A and SDZ PSC 833 enhanced the cytotoxicity of T101 RTA-ITs on the CEM III human lymphoblastic T-cell line by more than 100-fold. The 2 cyclosporines also significantly increased the cytotoxicity of T101 F(ab')$_2$, a more potent RTA-IT. Studies of plasma from patients receiving cyclosporin A showed a 31% to 60% increase in T101 RTA-IT–mediated cytotoxicity at plasma cyclosporin A levels of 3,090–4,860 ng/mL. Ricin A-chain immunotoxin binding, internalization, intracellular trafficking, and degradation were unaffected by cyclosporin A or SDZ PSC 883. The internalized T101 RTA-IT molecules studied were essentially intact.

Conclusion.—At clinically achievable concentrations, cyclosporin A and SDZ PSC 833 appear capable of in vivo enhancement of the effects of RTA-ITs. This enhancing effect may act only on a small population of RTA-ITs that cannot be detected by current techniques. Animal studies are now needed to confirm the results of this study.

Absence of Reverse Transcription-Polymerase Chain Reaction Detectable Residual Disease in Patients With Acute Promyelocytic Leukemia in Long-Term Remission

Diverio D, Pandolfi PP, Biondi A, Avvisati G, Petti MC, Mandelli F, Pelicci PG, Lo Coco F (Univ "La Sapienza," Rome; Univ of Perugia, Italy; Univ of Milano-Monza, Italy)

Blood 82:3556–3559, 1993   1 16-95-4–69

Background.—In several leukemic subtypes, hybrid fusion genes function as specific tumor markers. Amplifying chimeric complementary DNAs with reverse transcription–polymerase chain reaction (RT-PCR) permits sensitive detection of the neoplastic clone for diagnosis and monitoring studies in these leukemias. However, the clinical importance of minimal residual disease assessment with PCR has not been definitively established.

Methods and Findings.—Nine patients with acute promyelocytic leukemia in remission for 4–12 years were assessed for minimal residual disease by means of RT-PCR amplification of the specific PML/RAR-α fusion gene. Seven patients had been treated with conventional chemotherapy alone, 1 had undergone allogeneic bone marrow transplantation (BMT), and 1 had undergone autologous BMT as consolidation therapy after chemotherapy. The t(15;17) rearrangement was documented in 8 patients. None had detectable residual PML/RAR-α transcripts. All patients are currently in unmaintained complete remission 48–154 months after complete remission and 6–17 months after PCR assessment.

Conclusion.—Long-term survival in patients with acute promyelocytic leukemia appears to be associated with eradication of cells carrying the specific PML/RAR-α rearrangement. Thus, PCR negativity should be considered the treatment goal in such patients. These findings further support the clinical relevance of PCR monitoring in patients with acute promyelocytic leukemia. In other leukemic subtypes, the prognostic value of PCR assessment is still unclear.

▶ This study by Diverio et al. demonstrates a strong correlation between undetectable PML/RAR-α by RT-PCR and disease-free survival of patients with acute promyelocytic leukemia. However, their study does not provide information on patients who achieve clinical complete remission and remain RT-PCR–positive. They studied only patients in complete remission for years and did not study patients at the time complete remission was diagnosed.—P.H. Wiernik, M.D.

Effectiveness and Pharmacokinetics of Low-Dose All-*trans* Retinoic Acid (25 mg/m²) in Acute Promyelocytic Leukemia

Castaigne S, Lefebvre P, Chomienne C, Suc E, Rigal-Huguet F, Gardin C,

Delmer A, Archimbaud E, Tilly H, Janvier M, Isnard F, Travade P, Montfort L, Delannoy A, Rapp MJ, Christian B, Montastruc M, Weh H, Fenaux P, Dombret H, Gourmel B, Degos L (Hôpital Saint Louis, Paris; Hôpital Purpan, Toulouse, France; Hôpital Beaujor, Paris; et al)
Blood 82:3560–3563, 1993

Background.—All-*trans* retinoic acid (ATRA) has proved to be an effective treatment for patients with newly diagnosed acute promyelocytic leukemia and for those in first relapse. Doses of 45–100 mg/m²/day have induced complete remission through promoting differentiation, but dose-ranging studies are unavailable.

Objective and Methods.—An open multicenter study was begun in 1990 to evaluate ATRA therapy at an initial dose of 25 mg/m²/day until complete remission took place. Of the 30 patients, 12 had not been treated previously. Fourteen were in first relapse, and 4 had failed to respond to conventional first-induction chemotherapy.

Results.—Ten of 12 patients with recent diagnoses had complete remission after 1–3 months of treatment. Of the 14 patients treated when in first relapse, 10 entered complete remission, and another had a transient partial response. All 4 patients who did not respond to conventional chemotherapy entered complete remission. The median time to complete remission was 45 days. Hyperleukocytosis developed in 9 patients. All 5 patients receiving comprehensive consolidation treatment remained in continuous complete remission after 6–14 months, but 8 of 11 patients receiving mild consolidation courses have relapsed. Eight patients had complications possibly related to retinoic acid syndrome, and 3 of them died. Pharmacokinetic studies indicated that plasma drug levels were comparable to those achieved with a daily dose of 45 mg/m².

Conclusion.—Treatment of acute promyelocytic leukemia with ATRA seems promising. An initial dose of 25 mg/m²/day appears to be effective.

▶ The low-dose ATRA regimen has not been studied in the United States.—P.H. Wiernik, M.D.

Effect of All Transretinoic Acid in Newly Diagnosed Acute Promyelocytic Leukemia: Results of a Multicenter Randomized Trial
Fenaux P, Le Deley MC, Castaigne S, Archimbaud E, Chomienne C, Link H, Guerci A, Duarte M, Daniel MT, Bowen D, Huebner G, Bauters F, Fegueux N, Fey M, Sanz M, Lowenberg B, Maloisel F, Auzanneau G, Sadoun A, Gardin C, Bastion Y, Ganser A, Jacky E, Dombret H, Chastang C, Degos L, European APL 91 Group (Service Clinique des Maladies du Sang–Hôpital St Louis, Paris)
Blood 82:3241–3249, 1993

Background.—Investigators have shown that all-*trans* retinoic acid (ATRA) selectively differentiates abnormal promyelocytes into mature granulocytes in acute promyelocytic leukemia and induced a complete remission in 80% to 90% of patients with new diagnosis and those in first relapse. Treatment with ATRA rapidly improved coagulopathy without inducing aplasia, suggesting that it may decrease the incidence of fatal bleeding and sepsis in acute promyelocytic leukemia. However, ATRA was associated with a rapid increase in leukocytes and signs of "ATRA syndrome," with a potentially fatal outcome, in about one third of patients. Also, most patients who achieved complete remission and who were maintained with ATRA alone or with relatively mild chemotherapy rapidly relapsed. Therefore, the efficacy of ATRA combined with intensive chemotherapy was tested in patients with a new diagnosis of acute promyelocytic leukemia.

Methods and Findings.—Patients aged 65 years or younger received chemotherapy with daunorubicin–cytosine arabinoside alone or combined with ATRA in the multicenter, randomized trial. The event-free survival was the major end point. After the first interim analysis, the study was terminated early because the event-free survival was significantly greater in patients receiving combined treatment. One hundred one patients were enrolled at the time of study termination. Of 49 patients in the group receiving combined treatment, 91% achieved complete remission, and 9% died early. In the group receiving chemotherapy only, 81% achieved complete remission, 8% died early, and 10% had resistant leukemia. The difference in complete remission rates between groups was not significant. The duration of coagulopathy in the combined-treatment group was significantly decreased compared with that in the chemotherapy-only group. The estimated Kaplan-Meier event-free survival was 79% in the combined-treatment group and 50% in the chemotherapy-only group at 1 year. Estimated relapse rates were 19% and 40%, respectively, at 1 year.

Conclusion.—In patients with newly diagnosed acute promyelocytic leukemia, ATRA followed by chemotherapy increases event-free survival. It is strongly suggested that ATRA be incorporated into front-line treatment for these patients.

▶ It seems clear that the combination of ATRA plus standard chemotherapy provides optimal treatment for patients with acute promyelocytic leukemia. Unanswered questions that remain have to do with dose and schedule of both.—P.H. Wiernik, M.D.

Four Years' Experience With the Treatment of All-Trans Retinoic Acid in Acute Promyelocytic Leukemia
Wu X, Wang X, Qien X, Liu H, Ying J, Yang Z, Yao H (Jin Ling Hosp, Nanjing,

China)
Am J Hematol 43:183–189, 1993

116-95-4–72

Background.—All-*trans* retinoic acid (ATRA) has been used since 1987 in the treatment of acute promyelocytic leukemia. Compared with untreated patients, patients treated with ATRA have had better results. However, some questions about ATRA treatment remain unresolved. One 4-year experience with ATRA treatment of patients with acute promyelocytic leukemia was reviewed.

Methods and Findings.—The cases of 43 patients treated between 1987 and 1992 were reviewed retrospectively. These patients were induced to differentiation using ATRA. In the early induction period, patients were at risk of severe hemorrhage, which was the primary cause of early death. Patients with abnormal coagulation received combined treatment with platelets and heparin or aminomethylbenzoic (PAMBA). Only 4 of 43 patients died of intracranial bleeding at 4–12 days, when WBC counts peaked. Combined ATRA and homoharringtonine and cytarabine chemotherapy decreased hyperleukocytosis during ATRA induction. None of the 7 patients receiving this treatment died at an early stage. The onset of remission at an early stage could be predicted through observations of the successive changes of karyotypes and morphology of the bone marrow and peripheral blood cells. In addition, ATRA could inhibit CFU-fibroblastoid growth. The overall leukemia-free survival after 4 years of follow-up was 80%. The relapse rate was 45%. Thirty-five patients are still alive and in remission, and 1 was alive in relapse. Five patients who had relapses on continued alternating ATRA and chemotherapy treatment were not induced by ATRA.

Conclusion.—In these patients with acute promyelocytic leukemia receiving induction therapy, the overall leukemia-free survival at 4 years was 80%. Many patients achieving remission with ATRA therapy relapsed within 1–3 years.

ACUTE LYMPHOCYTIC LEUKEMIA

Magnetic Fields and Cancer in Children Residing Near Swedish High-Voltage Power Lines

Feychting M, Ahlbom A (Karolinska Inst, Stockholm)
Am J Epidemiol 138:467–481, 1993

116-95-4–73

Background.—Previous studies have reported a correlation between increased cancer incidence and exposure to magnetic fields. There have been 2 major concerns with these studies: the validity of the exposure measurements and the potential for selection bias. The hypothesis that an increased incidence of childhood cancer is found in areas around high-voltage power lines was tested in a Swedish population.

Methods.—The Swedish population registry and cancer registry were compared to identify children who had cancer and who had lived within

300 m of any of the 220- and 400-kV power lines in Sweden between 1960 and 1985. Age-, sex-, and parish-matched controls were randomly selected for each patient with cancer. Magnetic field exposure was assessed by spot measurements in the home at the time of diagnosis and by both contemporary and historical calculations including line configuration, load, and distance from the house. Other data were collected from censuses, including socioeconomic status and an index of air pollution from road traffic.

Results.—There were 142 children identified and 558 controls. The largest category of cancer diagnosis was leukemia, especially acute lymphocytic leukemia, and then CNS tumors. Comparing leukemia diagnosis and calculated historical field exposure revealed a dose-dependent increased risk that was unaffected by any demographic factors but was confined to single-family homes. The data did not support a correlation between magnetic field exposure and development of CNS tumors.

Discussion.—The data support a correlation between exposure to magnetic fields and leukemia in children, even when introducing potential confounders, such as socioeconomic status and traffic-produced air pollution. The experimental methods are solid: use of the national registries minimized selection bias, and comparisons of the various methods of exposure assessment supported the validity of the calculated historical field exposure.

▶ This is the latest of a number of papers that suggest a relationship between childhood acute leukemia and the intensity of magnetic fields in the environment. Is a MRI a safe test for a child?—P.H. Wiernik, M.D.

Molecular Rearrangements on Chromosome 11q23 Predominate in Infant Acute Lymphoblastic Leukemia and Are Associated With Specific Biologic Variables and Poor Outcome
Chen C-S, Sorensen PHB, Domer PH, Reaman GH, Korsmeyer SJ, Heerema NA, Hammond GD, Kersey JH (Univ of Minnesota, Minneapolis; George Washington Univ, Washington, DC; Washington Univ, St Louis, Mo; et al)
Blood 81:2386–2393, 1993   116-95-4-74

Background.—In infants, acute lymphoblastic leukemia (ALL) generally has distinct biological characteristics and a poor prognosis. Cytogenetic research has indicated that many such leukemias have chromosome 11q23 translocations. Thirty infants with ALL were assessed for molecular defects of 11q23.

Methods and Findings.—Fourteen patients had cytogenetic 11q23 abnormalities. All of them had 11q23 rearrangements at the molecular level. Another 7 also had 11q23 molecular rearrangements, including 1 with normal cytogenetic findings. Molecular 11q23 abnormalities were significantly associated with adverse prognostic variables, such as age younger than 6 months, hyperleukocytosis, CD10⁻phenotype, and early treatment failure. Through molecular analysis, a group of infants with germline 11q23 with a very good treatment outcome was identified. The projected event-free survival for this group was 80% at a median follow-up of 46 months, compared with 15% in infants with 11q23 rearrangements.

Conclusion.—As many as 70% of infants with ALL may have 11q23 rearrangements. These rearrangements cannot always be detected by cytogenetic analysis. The presence of germline 11q23 DNA may be used to identify a subgroup of infants with ALL who have good outcomes using current treatment and who have a different underlying etiology.

▶ Karyotypic analysis is more difficult in ALL than in acute myeloid leukemia. In the former, chromosomes often appear short and fuzzy, which makes identification of subtle translocations difficult. Therefore, many more significant chromosome structural abnormalities have been identified in acute myeloid leukemia than in ALL. New molecular techniques allow for the identification of important chromosomal abnormalities in leukemia that would not be detected by standard cytogenetic methods, especially in ALL.—P.H. Wiernik, M.D.

Detection and Significance of *bcr-abl* mRNA Transcripts and Fusion Proteins in Philadelphia-Positive Adult Acute Lymphoblastic Leukemia

Tuszynski A, Dhut S, Young BD, Lister TA, Rohatiner AZ, Amess JAL, Chaplin T, Dorey E, Gibbons B (St Bartholomew's Hosp, London)
Leukemia 7:1504–1508, 1993   116-95-4–75

Purpose.—Patients with acute lymphoblastic leukemia (ALL) and the Philadelphia (Ph) translocation have a poor prognosis; it is important to identify them, as they can be offered myeloablative therapy with bone marrow transplantation as consolidation therapy in complete remission. The Ph chromosome carries a hybrid *bcr-abl* gene, which is transcribed into chimeric *bcr-abl* messenger RNA. Recent studies have suggested that the incidence of *bcr-abl* fusion may be higher than suspected on the basis of cytogenetic analysis. Polymerase chain reaction (PCR) analysis was used to assess the presence of the Ph translocation and *bcr-abl* messenger RNA in 84 consecutive adult patients with ALL.

Methods and Results.—Patients were tested prospectively by cytogenetic analysis and retrospectively by PCR. Overall, 20.3% of the patients were positive for *bcr/abl* or Ph chromosome, or both. Positivity for *bcr-abl* or Ph was most common in patients with ALL aged 31–50 years; it was less common in patients older than age 50 years. Of 10 *bcr-abl*-positive patients, 8 expressed the e1a2 messenger RNA transcript and 1 each expressed the b3a2 and b2a3 transcripts. When *bcr-abl* messenger

RNA transcripts were seen, the appropriate p190 or p210 bcr-abl protein was always expressed, as was the Ph chromosome.

Conclusion.—This study finds 100% concordance between cytogenetic study and PCR regarding the expression of the Ph chromosome or *bcr-abl* in adult patients with ALL. There are no significant clinical or karyotypic differences between patients with p190 or p210. The *abl* exon 2 may be absent in as many as 10% of *bcr-abl*–positive messenger RNA transcripts, which must be kept in mind when PCR is used for diagnostic purposes.

▶ This is a surprising result because Ph chromosome–negative *bcr-abl*–positive chronic myeloid leukemia is well described.—P.H. Wiernik, M.D.

Expression of the Multidrug Resistance-Associated P-Glycoprotein (P-170) in 59 Cases of De Novo Acute Lymphoblastic Leukemia: Prognostic Implications
Goasguen JE, Dossot J-M, Fardel O, Le Mee F, Le Gall E, Leblay R, LePrise PY, Chaperon J, Fauchet R (Université de Rennes, France; Laboratoire d'Hématologie et d'Immunologie, Rennes, France; Laboratoire de Cytogénétique, Rennes, France; et al)
Blood 81:2394–2398, 1993   116-95-4–76

Background.—Although there have been many studies of the multidrug resistance (MDR)1 gene expression in leukemic cells from acute lymphoblastic leukemias (ALLs) that attempted to demonstrate a correlation with treatment response or patient follow-up, most of them have involved a small number of patients and have combined patients at diagnosis with those at relapse. The presence of the MDR-associated membrane protein P-170 was investigated in 59 patients with ALL using an immunocytochemical alkaline phosphatase antialkaline phosphatase technique with 2 separate monoclonal antibodies, JSB1 and C219.

Patients.—The patients were 36 children and 23 adults with ALL. All were examined at the time of diagnosis. Immunophenotypes were obtained for all patients and karyotypes were analyzed for 37.

Findings.—Positive cells and cases were detected at comparable rates with JSB1 and C219. The staining intensity was greater with JSB1. The rate of the first complete remission differed between MDR-positive and MDR-negative adults. Of the 16 MDR-positive patients seen with a first complete remission, 81% had relapses, compared with 37% of MDR-negative patients. There was a greater relapse rate among MDR-positive patients than in MDR-negative patients when adults and children were analyzed separately. The survival rates were significantly higher in MDR-negative patients overall and in children and adults assessed separately. This trend was also seen in event-free survival curves. The percentage of second complete remission was only 15% in the MDR-positive group, compared with 38% for the MDR-negative group. Multivariate analysis indicated that these findings were independent of age, immuno-phenotypes, and karyotypes.

Conclusion.—The MDR-positive phenotype is clearly associated with a higher relapse rate, shorter duration of remission, and shorter median survival than the MDR-negative phenotype. These findings are indepen-dent of age, leukocyte count, immunophenotype (except for ALL with membrane immunoglobulin), and karyotype.

▶ Before drawing definitive conclusions from this study regarding the clini-cal significance of P-glycoprotein expression in ALL, its major potential pit-falls should be noted. The choice of antibodies recognizing intracellular epi-topes of P-glycoprotein, especially the selection of antibody C219, which has been proven to react with antigens other than P-glycoprotein, is a prob-lem. Also, an arbitrary cutoff point of 1% P-glycoprotein–positive cells in the absence of identification of blast cells by double-staining for P-glycoprotein and a blast cell–detecting antigen is a common potential problem in studies such as this one. The finding of such a low level of P-glycoprotein expression could be interpreted as indicative of potential for multidrug resistance if P-glycoprotein expression was determined by standardized techniques and pa-tients were uniformly treated.—P.H. Wiernik, M.D.

Outcome Prediction in Childhood Acute Lymphoblastic Leukaemia by Molecular Quantification of Residual Disease at the End of Induction

Brisco MJ, Condon J, Hughes E, Neoh S-H, Sykes PJ, Seshadri R, Toogood I, Waters K, Tauro G, Ekert H, Morley AA (Flinders Med Centre, Bedford Park, Australia; Women's and Children's Hosp, North Adelaide, Australia; Royal Children's Hosp, Parkville, Australia)
Lancet 343:196–200, 1994
116-95-4–77

Background.—In children with acute lymphoblastic leukemia (ALL), treatment for minimal residual disease (MRD) can be modified accord-ing to the prognostic factors seen at diagnosis. If methods of detecting and measuring MRD early in the course of ALL were available, treat-ment could be improved by identification of patients likely to relapse as well as those with a high probability of cure. A clone-specific polymerase chain reaction (PCR) was used to detect the rearranged immunoglobulin heavy-chain gene from the leukemic clone in patients with ALL.

Methods.—A total of 181 children with ALL were studied. The chil-dren, all with total leukocyte counts less than $100 \times 10^9/L$ at presenta-tion, were drawn from 2 randomized clinical trials. Bone marrow was aspirated for PCR both at diagnosis and after 35–42 days of induction therapy to determine whether quantifying MRD in first remission could predict long-term outcome. Limiting dilution analysis was used to quan-tify the leukemic cells.

Results.—Minimal residual disease was measured successfully in 88 of the children. Thirty-eight patients showed leukemic cells in their bone marrow at first remission, with counts ranging from 6.7×10^{-2} to 9.9×10^{-7} cells; 68% of these patients went on to relapse. The remaining 50 patients had no detectable MRD, and only 12% of them relapsed. Patients from the first trial relapsed at all levels of detected MRD. In patients from the second trial, in which more intensive treatment gave better results, there was a close relation between the level of MRD and the probability of relapse: 5 of 5 patients with greater than 10^{-3} MRD, vs. 2 of 26 with no detectable MRD.

Conclusion.—Molecular monitoring may be useful for early detection of leukemic cells after chemotherapy in children with ALL. This may allow prediction of outcome and individualized treatment, because the results of PCR give information on both the in vivo drug sensitivity of the leukemia and the number of cells that remain to be killed. With advances in molecular testing, it should eventually be possible to measure MRD in 80% to 90% of patients.

Long-Term Follow-Up of Residual Disease in Acute Lymphoblastic Leukemia Patients in Complete Remission Using Clonogeneic IgH Probes and the Polymerase Chain Reaction

Nizet Y, Van Daele S, Lewalle P, Vaerman JL, Philippe M, Vermylen C, Cornu G, Ferrant A, Michaux JL, Martiat P (Cliniques Universitaires Saint-Luc, Brussels, Belgium)
Blood 82:1618–1625, 1993 116-95-4–78

Background.—Polymerase chain reaction (PCR) and clonogenic probes derived from the TCR-γ-δ or the IgH-rearranged genes have been used to monitor minimal residual disease (MRD) in patients with acute lymphoblastic leukemia (ALL) in complete remission. A number of important questions about this technique remain, including the incidence of clinically relevant clonal for a given PCR strategy, the interval between an increase in MRD and relapse, and the relevant level of sensitivity. These questions were answered in a follow-up study of 25 patients with B-lineage ALL in complete remission and a PCR-detectable rearrangement of the immunoglobulin heavy-chain genes.

Methods.—Bone marrow samples were obtained by a simplified PCR strategy in which the PCR product was directly used as a clonogenic probe recognizing rearranged immunoglobulin heavy-chain sequences as a first approach. After the patients went into complete remission, bone marrow aspirates were obtained for serial study. In the 5 cases in which sensitivity was less than $1:10^4$, the PCR fragment was sequenced and a specific oligonucleotide was synthetized and used as a probe. When MRD became undetectable, TCRδ rearrangement or a specific translocation was used as a cross-control to avoid false negative results arising from clonal evolution.

Results. —The median follow-up was 30 months. All but 1 of 23 patients had detectable MRD within 3 months of complete remission. Of 21 patients, 19 still had detectable MRD at 6 months, regardless of long-term clinical outcome. For the 10 patients who were still in complete remission at the end of the follow-up, MRD decreased continuously until it became undetectable in 5 patients and remained detectable in 5. Two patients had an increase in MRD after cessation of treatment. All 8 patients with clinical relapse had persistent MRD, which increased 3–12 months before the relapse. One patient had clonal evolution of the VDJ heavy-chain region, with recurrence of MRD demonstrated by TCRδ rearrangement.

Conclusion. —The simplified PCR strategy is useful for the follow-up of MRD in most patients with ALL. Sequencing is sometimes necessary to achieve a relevant sensitivity. Any sample that becomes negative needs a cross-control to assess the possibility of clonal evolution. The long-term outcome may be predicted in patients receiving therapy by a sequential search for MRD. Further analysis is needed to determine whether patients who remain positive after cessation of treatment are at increased risk of relapse.

▶ It must be remembered that to date, the identification of MRD in acute leukemia has not led to an intervention that has been demonstrated to change clinical outcome.—P.H. Wiernik, M.D.

The Prognostic Significance of the Skeletal Manifestations of Acute Lymphoblastic Leukemia of Childhood

Heinrich SD, Gallagher D, Warrior R, Phelan K, George VT, MacEwen GD (Louisiana State Univ, New Orleans; Children's Hosp, New Orleans, La)
J Pediatr Orthop 14:105–111, 1994   116-95-4-79

Objective. —Leukemia is the most common malignancy of children. As many as 59% of children with acute leukemia have been reported to have bone and joint pain, and as many as 70% of those with acute lymphoblastic leukemia (ALL) have skeletal radiographic abnormalities at diagnosis. A retrospective analysis assessed the prognostic significance of musculoskeletal abnormalities in children with ALL.

Methods. —The review included the charts and radiographs of 83 children with ALL who had a skeletal survey at diagnosis. These surveys were reviewed for radiographic changes associated with acute leukemia, including osteopenia, metaphyseal bands, periosteal reactions, geographic lytic lesions, sclerosis, mixed sclerosis and lysis, and permeative destruction. Survival among children with a negative skeletal survey, those with 1–4 positive radiographic findings, and those with 5 or more positive findings were compared.

Findings.—Initially, 40% of the children had pain in the extremities and 31% had joint pain. Fifty-seven percent had radiographic skeletal abnormalities, and 75% of those had metaphyseal bands. About half had osteoporosis, periosteal reactions, diffuse permeative bone destruction, or some combination of these. The 5-year survival was 88% for children with radiographic bone involvement and 82% for those without. Among children with radiographic changes, the 5-year survival was 100% for those with 1–4 positive findings and 76% for those with 5 or more lesions. Symptoms lasted an average of 24 days before diagnosis in the patients with skeletal radiographic abnormalities compared with 22 days for those with 1–4 bone changes and 54 days for those with more than 5 bone changes. Children without radiographic skeletal abnormalities had a higher incidence of poor prognostic indicators.

Conclusion.—Patients with ALL without radiographic abnormalities on their initial skeletal survey appear to have an aggressive form of leukemia. Those with lesions have an indolent form of leukemia that is of short duration for patients with 1–4 skeletal lesions and of longer duration for those with 5 or more lesions. The children with skeletal lesions have a longer duration of symptoms before diagnosis, which decreases their survival to that of the aggressive form of leukemia. Physicians who care for children must be able to recognize the orthopedic and radiographic signs of acute leukemia.

Parental Psychopathology and Children's Adjustment to Leukemia
Brown RT, Kaslow NJ, Madan-Swain A, Doepke KJ, Sexson SB, Hill LJ (Emory Univ, Atlanta, Ga)
J Am Acad Child Adolesc Psychiatry 32:554–561, 1993   116-95-4-80

Background.—Although studies of children with moderate-risk cancers have shown that these children generally evidence healthy psychosocial features, some studies have indicated that a subset of these children and their parents do evidence psychiatric disorders. The relationship between parental psychopathologic disorders and the psychosocial functioning of children with acute lymphocytic leukemia (ALL) was examined.

Methods.—Standard tests and psychiatric interviews were used to determine levels of psychiatric dysfunction in 61 parent-child pairs. The parents were asked to evaluate themselves and their spouses in self-report measures of psychopathology and to evaluate internalizing and externalizing behavioral problems in the child. The children with ALL ranged in age from 2 to 17 years. Of the 61 children, 23 were old enough and competent enough to complete self-report instruments to measure levels of depressive and anxiety symptoms, internalizing and externalizing behavioral problems, and maladaptive attributional style (taking personal responsibility for causing negative events).

Results.—A significant number of the parents (34%) met criteria for at least 1 Axis I psychiatric disorder, and parents reported an Axis I disorder in 29% of the spouses. Those parents reported that their children showed more depressive and internalizing symptoms than did the parents who did not evidence a psychiatric disorder. The children of the parents who received a psychiatric disorder diagnosis self-reported higher levels of anxiety and a greater responsibility for negative events than did the other children.

Discussion.—Even within the group of children whose parents evidenced psychopathologic disorders, the measures of child psychopathology were within the normal range, although elevated. This may indicate that parental psychopathologic disorders may be a risk factor for development of psychopathologic disorders in the child, but that there is probably an interaction among a group of stressors that can predict or produce psychopathologic changes in the child. Further research should focus on the other psychiatric risk factors for chronically ill children, including disease parameters, level of adaptive behavior functioning, and psychosocial stressors. Further longitudinal studies of psychosocial functioning in children with ALL and their families could identify critical periods during which the child and family could require psychiatric intervention.

Improved Therapy for Children With Acute Lymphoblastic Leukemia and Unfavorable Presenting Features: A Follow-Up Report of the Childrens Cancer Group Study CCG-106

Gaynon PS, Steinherz PG, Bleyer WA, Ablin AR, Albo VC, Finklestein JZ, Grossman NJ, Novak LJ, Pyesmany AF, Reaman GH, Chappell RJ, Sather HN, Hammond GD (Univ of Wisconsin, Madison; Mem Sloan-Kettering Cancer Ctr, New York; MD Anderson Cancer Ctr, Houston; et al)
J Clin Oncol 11:2234–2242, 1993   116-95-4–81

Background.—Past Childrens Cancer Group (CCG) studies have demonstrated an event-free survival rate of 50% or less for children with acute lymphoblastic leukemia (ALL) and unfavorable initial features. A promising pilot experience with 2 intensive experimental regimens—Reg A, based on the Berlin-Frankfurt-Münster 1976 regimen, and Reg B, the New York regimen—prompted further study to examine the benefit and morbidity of these 2 regimens.

Methods.—Initially, 217 eligible children with ALL and unfavorable presenting features were included in the randomized study. These children, who entered the study from 1983 to 1984, were assigned to receive Reg A, Reg B, or Reg C, the control regimen. However, interim analyses revealed a significantly worse outcome for patients receiving Reg C; therefore, assignment to this group was halted. From 1984 to 1987, 328 more patients were randomized to receive either Reg A or Reg B.

Results.—Children receiving Reg A or Reg B had a 7-year event-free survival rate of more than 60% compared with 40% for children receiving Reg C. The difference in event-free survival rates remained greater than 20 percentage points at 7 years, and the difference in survival was 15 percentage points. The average hospitalization stay was 16 days longer with Reg A and 20 days longer with Reg B than with Reg C. Although the 2 intensive regimens offered similar event-free survival and survival rates, Reg B entailed more days of parenteral therapy and higher levels of exposure to anthracyclines and alkylating agents.

Conclusion.—Two intensive experimental chemotherapy regimens yielded a better outcome for children with ALL and unfavorable initial features than a control regimen. The 2 intensive regimens, which had similar outcomes, were more effective but more toxic; Reg A resulted in 78 additional hospital days per relapse prevented and Reg B in 101 days. The ongoing CCG trial for ALL with unfavorable initial features is based on Reg A.

▶ These results in unfavorable-prognosis childhood ALL are outstanding. The Berlin-Frankfurt-Münster study (1) of 1976 was a major contribution to ALL therapy.—P.H. Wiernik, M.D.

Reference

1. Henze G, et al: *Klin Padiatr* 193:145, 1983.

Severe Toxicity Limits Intensification of Induction Therapy for Acute Lymphoblastic Leukemia
Weiss M, Telford P, Kempin S, Kritz A, Sogoloff H, Gee T, Berman E, Scheinberg D, Little C, Gaynor J, Belanger C, Bertino J, Andreeff M, McKenzie S, Clarkson B (Mem Sloan-Kettering Cancer Ctr, New York)
Leukemia 7:832–837, 1993   116-95-4–82

Introduction.—With available chemotherapeutic regimens, 60% to 80% of patients with acute lymphoblastic leukemia (ALL) will achieve complete remission; however, only 20% to 30% of adult patients go on to be disease-free survivors. Some vincristine/prednisone-based induction regimens have been used along with intensified consolidation therapy and maintenance therapy; none has proven clearly better than the others. A regimen of further intensified induction therapy in adult patients with ALL was used in an effort to increase the number of patients with early complete remission and, consequently, long-term disease-free survival.

Methods and Results.—A dose-intense induction regimen was administered to 14 adult patients with newly diagnosed ALL and lymphoblastic lymphoma. Induction therapy consisted of vincristine, prednisone, intermediate-dose cytarabine, and idarubicin, all administered within the first week of treatment. In the first 8 patients, the intensive induction regimen resulted in considerable hepatic, gastrointestinal, infectious, and neurologic toxicity, with a treatment-related mortality of 29%. The latter 6 patients did not receive cytarabine during their induction regimen. Although gastrointestinal morbidity declined, infectious morbidity remained unacceptable, and this regimen was also terminated. Of 14 patients, 9 achieved complete remission, 3 died, and 2 had resistant disease. Of 6 relapses, 3 occurred in patients in whom persistent, severe toxicity prohibited the use of chemotherapy. Three patients are still alive at a minimum follow-up of 20 months.

Conclusion.—The intensive induction regimen explored in this study is too toxic for use in adult patients with ALL and lymphoblastic lymphoma. A high-dose cytarabine and anthracenedione induction regimen with G-CSF is currently being examined to determine its ability to promote myeloid recovery, thus continuing the exploration of whether increasing the proportion of patients who achieve early complete remission will lead to increases in the proportion of long-term survivors.

▶ It seems that unlike in childhood ALL, the next general improvement in the outcome of adult ALL must await the development of a new drug.—P.H. Wiernik, M.D.

Phase I Study of Topotecan, a New Topoisomerase I Inhibitor, in Patients With Refractory or Relapsed Acute Leukemia

Kantarjian HM, Beran M, Ellis A, Zwelling L, O'Brien S, Cazenave L, Koller C, Rios MB, Plunkett W, Keating MJ, Estey EH (Univ of Texas, Houston; Natl Cancer Inst, Bethesda, Md)
Blood 81:1146–1151, 1993   116-95-4–83

Objective.—Topotecan (hycamptamine) is a new topoisomerase I (topo I) inhibitor that may have selective antitumor activity. Animal studies have shown that it has a broad-spectrum activity, and phase I clinical studies identified myelosuppression as the dose-limiting toxicity. Responses to Topotecan have been observed in patients with lung and ovarian cancer. A phase I study of Topotecan in patients with leukemia was conducted to assess possible antitumor activity and to define the maximally tolerated dose (MTD) and the major toxicities of Topotecan.

Methods.—Included were 27 patients with refractory or relapsed acute leukemia, 17 with acute myelogenous or undifferentiated leukemia, 7 with acute lymphocytic leukemia, and 3 with chronic myelogenous leukemia in the blastic phase. Topotecan was administered by 5-day continuous infusion every 3–4 weeks in doses ranging from 3.5 to 18-mg/m² per course. The outcome assessment included a unique in vitro assay to measure Topotecan-stabilized topo I DNA in patient samples.

Results.—The dose-limiting toxicity was severe mucositis, occurring in 2 of 5 patients receiving a Topotecan dose of 11.8 mg/m^2 per course. Another patient in this group had prolonged myelosuppression. In contrast, severe mucositis developed in only 1 of 12 patients receiving the MTD of 10 mg/m^2 per course, although 5 had mild to moderate mucositis. Less common toxic effects included nausea, vomiting, diarrhea, and prolonged myelosuppression. The complete response rate was 11%; the partial response rate was 7%; and the hematologic improvement rate was 4%. For patients with acute myelogenous or undifferentiated leukemia, the overall complete plus partial response rate was 24%. The in vitro assay showed a variable ability of Topotecan to interact with topo I.

Conclusion.—For patients with refractory or relapsed acute leukemia, Topotecan has a MTD of 10 mg/m^2 per course when administered by continuous infusion for 5 days every 3–4 weeks. Higher doses are associated with severe mucositis. Further studies will identify the precise activity of this drug in different leukemia subgroups, compare its efficacy in combination with other antileukemic drugs, and correlate topo I–DNA complex formation with clinical response.

▶ Unfortunately, this may not be the new drug for acute lymphocytic leukemia, but the activity against acute myelogenous leukemia observed in a phase I study is impressive. Complete responses are rarely observed in phase I studies, and such major activity in a phase I study usually signals major activity for the agent under study.—P.H. Wiernik, M.D.

Outcome After Cessation of Therapy in Childhood Acute Lymphoblastic Leukaemia

Jankovic M, for the Associazione Italiana Ematologia ed Oncologia Pediatrica (AIEOP) (Università di Milano, Italy)
Eur J Cancer 29A:1839–1843, 1993　　　　　　　　116-95-4–84

Objective.—The long-term outcome of acute lymphoblastic leukemia (ALL) was examined in 2,192 children who had completed treatment, entered complete remission, and had a median 52 months of follow-up. The median age at the time of diagnosis was 4 years, 8 months.

Treatment.—Various multiple-drug regimens were used. Almost all patients received induction treatment with vincristine and prednisone and then maintenance treatment with 6-mercaptopurine plus methotrexate, reinforced by pulses of vincristine-prednisone therapy. Almost half of the patients received a third drug during induction or consolidation, or both, and in recent years, patients have received reinduction therapy. Most children received cranial irradiation. The median duration of treatment was 34 months. Twenty-seven patients had bone marrow transplantation.

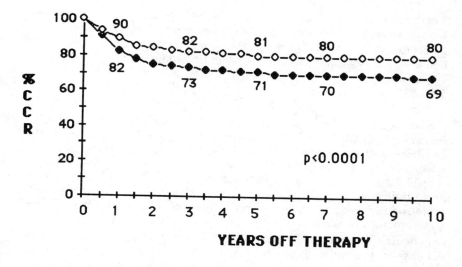

MALES N=1125 E=299
FEMALES N=1065 E=186

Fig 4–10.—Disease-free interval by gender after treatment suspension in childhood ALL. *Numbers above curve* represent the number of patients at risk for each period. (Courtesy of Jankovic M, for the Associazione Italiana Ematologia ed Oncologia Pediatrica (AIEOP): *Eur J Cancer* 29A:1839–1843, 1993.)

Results.—Seventy-six percent of patients remained alive in continuous complete remission, whereas 22% had at least 1 no-treatment relapse. Eleven patients had a solid malignancy while in complete remission, and 8 of them died. Most relapses involved the bone marrow and occurred in the first year without treatment. Boys were 1.5 times more likely than girls to relapse, and there was a significant gender-related difference in the duration of complete remission (Fig 4–10). Cranial irradiation did not influence the interval free of CNS relapse.

Conclusion.—About one fourth of the children with ALL who enter complete remission and discontinue treatment are at risk of relapsing, dying in continued remission, or having a solid malignancy.

▶ Women do better with adult acute myeloid leukemia also. In fact, the vast majority of our long-term disease-free survivors (more than 10 years) are women. This observation is entirely unexplained.—P.H. Wiernik, M.D.

Treatment of Late Bone Marrow Relapse in Children With Acute Lymphoblastic Leukemia: A Pediatric Oncology Group Study

Sadowitz PD, Smith SD, Shuster J, Wharam MD, Buchanan GR, Rivera GK (State Univ of New York, Syracuse; Univ of Chicago; Univ of Florida, Gainesville; et al)

Blood 81:602–609, 1993

116-95-4–85

Background.—Although survival for children with acute lymphoblastic leukemia (ALL) has gradually improved during the past 2 decades, the late bone marrow relapse rate after complete remission in children who have completed 2½–3 years of primary chemotherapy is still approximately 20%. In a randomized clinical trial, the efficacy of doxorubicin and prednisone (regimen 1) was compared with that of cytarabine and teniposide (regimen 2) administered as part of a multidrug retreatment chemotherapy program to patients with late bone marrow relapse.

Patients.—Between 1983 and 1989, 109 patients with a median age of 4.1 years at the initial diagnosis of ALL and a median age of 8.7 years at first bone marrow relapse were entered into the trial. Patients with previous bone marrow relapse or extramedullary relapse were excluded. The median duration of first remission was 53 months. Treatment consisted of reinduction therapy for 4 weeks, continuation therapy for 132 weeks that incorporated either regimen 1 or regimen 2, and a later intensification phase during which either regimen was administered again.

Results.—Of 105 assessable patients, 102 (97%) achieved a second complete remission and 100 patients received continuation therapy. Of 92 patients who completed continuation therapy, 46 subsequently had a bone marrow relapse. There was no significant difference in event-free survival between regimen 1 and regimen 2. The overall 4-year event-free survival was 37%. Analysis of the second remission duration showed that age younger than 10 years at diagnosis, duration of first remission from diagnosis of greater than 54 months, and a WBC count of less than 5,000/μL at relapse were independently associated with a more favorable outcome.

Conclusion.—The results of the trial as to which treatment regimen was superior were inconclusive. The finding that more than one third of children with late bone marrow relapse of ALL were successfully treated is encouraging.

The Role of Radiation Therapy in the Treatment of Acute Lymphoblastic Leukemia With Lymphomatous Presentation: A Report From the Childrens Cancer Group

Cherlow JM, Steinherz PG, Sather HN, Gaynon PS, Grossman NJ, Kersey JH, Johnstone HS, Breneman JC, Trigg ME, Hammond GD (Long Beach Mem Med Ctr, Calif; Mem Sloan-Kettering Cancer Ctr, New York; Univ of Southern

California, Los Angeles; et al)
Int J Radiat Oncol Biol Phys 27:1001–1009, 1993   116-95-4–86

Introduction.—In favorable-risk groups of children with acute lymphoblastic leukemia (ALL), cranial irradiation (CXRT) can be replaced by intrathecal methotrexate, avoiding the adverse effects of CXRT without decreasing survival. Patients with ALL with lymphomatous presentation who have bulk disease and a T-cell immunophenotype, high WBC count, or absence of anemia have a comparatively poor prognosis, with a high rate of CNS and other extramedullary recurrences. As part of Childrens Cancer Group study 123, the role of radiation therapy was studied in children with ALL with lymphomatous presentation.

Methods.—Included were 308 patients with ALL with lymphomatous presentation but without CNS disease. They were randomly divided into 3 treatment groups. Group A received Berlin-Frankfurt-Münster chemotherapy, which was designed for high-risk patients with ALL, along with CXRT, 1,800 centigray (cGy). Group B received LSA_2L_2 chemotherapy, which was designed for patients with non-Hodgkin's lymphoma, plus CXRT, 1,800 cGy, and 1,500 cGy of radiation to areas of extra-abdominal bulk disease. Group C received the same therapy as group B but without CXRT. All 3 groups received intrathecal methotrexate throughout therapy. The minimum follow-up was 52 months.

Results.—The 5-year actuarial CNS relapse rate was 7% in group B and 17% in group C. Event-free survival rates were 53% and 39%, respectively. Cranial irradiation was not helpful in patients with WBC counts of less than $50,000/mm^3$. The CNS relapse rate was the same in group A as in group B, but the event-free survival rate for group A was significantly higher at 68%. The event rate was lower for patients in groups B and C who completed chest irradiation compared with those who did not. The CNS relapse rates were the same for patients whose cranial fields did and did not encompass the entire meningeal surface.

Conclusion.—For patients with ALL with lymphomatous presentation treated with LSA_2L_2 chemotherapy—a less than optimal regimen—the addition of CXRT decreases CNS relapse rate and improves event-free survival. Cranial irradiation can be beneficial even when compliance with radiation volume guidelines is absent. The Childrens Cancer Group continues to use CXRT for this group of patients at high risk of CNS relapse.

Soluble Factor(s) Produced by Human Bone Marrow Stroma Increase Cytokine-Induced Proliferation and Maturation of Primitive Hematopoietic Progenitors While Preventing Their Terminal Differentiation
Verfaillie CM (Univ of Minnesota, Minneapolis)
Blood 82:2045–2053, 1993   116-95-4-87

Objective.—Previously, growing hematopoietic progenitor cells separated from the stromal layer in in vitro long-term bone marrow cultures (LTBMCs) resulted in greater conservation and differentiation of primitive human hematopoietic progenitors. Thus, soluble factors produced by the stroma may be mainly responsible for hematopoiesis. To define these soluble factors, early-acting cytokines were studied to determine whether they can also induce conservation and differentiation of primitive progenitors.

Methods.—Normal human lineage—/CD34+/HLA-DR− cells (DR−) were cultured either in the absence of a stromal layer (stroma-free) or in a culture system in which DR− cells were separated by a microporous membrane from the stromal layer (stroma-noncontact). Three times per week, both culture groups were supplemented with or without cytokines.

Results.—After 5 weeks in a stroma-free culture and supplementation with the early-acting cytokines IL-3, stem cell factor, leukemia-inhibitory factor, and G-CSF, DR− cells showed cell expansion similar to that of DR− cells in stroma-noncontact cultures supplemented by the same cytokines. Stroma-noncontact cultures supplemented with or without IL-3 showed much greater generation of committed progenitors and conservation of primitive LTBMC-initiating cells than stroma-free cultures supplemented with IL-3 alone or with all 4 early-acting cytokines.

Conclusion.—Soluble factors in human bone marrow stroma, alone or in synergy with certain cytokines, can conserve primitive LTBMC-initiating cells, induce early differentiation of some of the primitive progenitors, and prevent terminal differentiation of these cells. The soluble stromal factors of interest are probably not the 4 used in this study. Their identification could have important implications for in vitro stem cell expansion in cancer treatment and gene therapy.

Low Leukocyte Counts With Blast Cells in Cerebrospinal Fluid of Children With Newly Diagnosed Acute Lymphoblastic Leukemia

Mahmoud HH, Rivera GK, Hancock ML, Krance RA, Kun LE, Behm FG, Ribeiro RC, Sandlund JT, Crist WM, Pui C-H (St Jude Children's Research Hosp, Memphis, Tenn)
N Engl J Med 329:314–319, 1993   116-95-4–88

Objective.—Despite the availability of effective CNS therapy and aggressive attempts at salvage, more than half of the patients with acute lymphoblastic leukemia (ALL) and recurrent CNS leukemia die of their disease. Intensified CNS therapy is essential to improve the chances of cure. However, there is ongoing debate about the criteria for predicting the presence or risk of CNS leukemia and about the intensity and timing of treatment. The clinical significance of leukemic blast cells in the cere-

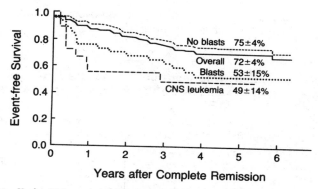

Fig 4–11.—Kaplan-Meier analysis of 5-year event-free survival according to findings in cerebrospinal fluid at presentation. One group of patients had no detectable blast cells, another group (*Blasts*) had fewer than 5 leukocytes per microliter and blast cells, and a third group had CNS leukemia. Survival was significantly better in the group with no blast cells than in the other 2 groups. *Plus-minus values* are means ± standard error. (Courtesy of Mahmoud HH, Rivera GK, Hancock ML, et al: *N Engl J Med* 329:314–319, 1993.)

brospinal fluid at the time of diagnosis of ALL was investigated in a randomized trial of intensive chemotherapy.

Methods.—Three hundred fifty-one children with ALL received intrathecal chemotherapy during the first year. Those with clinical and cytogenetic features predictive of relapse also received cranial irradiation and intrathecal chemotherapy 1 year after remission. Signs of CNS leukemia at diagnosis were 5 or more leukocytes per mL of cerebrospinal fluid with leukemic blast cells in cytocentrifuged preparations or cranial nerve palsy. Patients with these signs received additional intrathecal chemotherapy and cranial irradiation.

Results.—On retrospective analysis, 291 patients had no detectable blast cells in their cerebrospinal fluid, 42 had less than 5 leukocytes per μL and blast cells, and 18 met the criteria for CNS leukemia. The mean 5-year event-free survival was 72% (Fig 4–11). The 5-year probability of survival free of relapses confined to the CNS in patients with detectable blast cells and fewer than 5 leukocytes per μL of cerebrospinal fluid was lower than that in patients without blast cells, a mean of 87% vs. 96%, but it was not different from the probability in patients with CNS leukemia at diagnosis. All patients with detectable blast cells who had isolated relapses did so during the first year of treatment, before cranial irradiation was scheduled to begin. Multivariate analysis showed that the finding of blast cells in the cerebrospinal fluid with fewer than 5 leukocytes per μL was an independent risk factor for CNS relapse.

Conclusion.—Patients with leukemic blast cells in their cerebrospinal fluid are at increased risk for CNS relapse when cranial irradiation is delayed. These patients should receive intensified CNS therapy early in the course of treatment. A new classification system for risk of CNS relapse, based on the number of leukocytes in the cerebrospinal fluid and the presence of leukemic blast cells, is proposed.

Central Nervous System Treatment in Childhood Acute Lymphoblastic Leukemia: Long-Term Follow-Up of Patients Diagnosed Between 1973 and 1985
Gelber RD, Sallan SE, Cohen HJ, Donnelly M, Dalton V, Tobia F, Clavell LA, Tarbell NJ (Dana-Farber Cancer Inst, Boston; Univ of Rochester, NY; Univ of Puerto Rico, San Juan; et al)
Cancer 72:261–270, 1993   116-95-4–89

Patients.—Four treatment protocols were evaluated in 540 children treated for acute lymphoblastic leukemia (ALL) in 1973–1985. The group included 341 children considered to be at high risk. The 518 patients who achieved complete remission received specific treatment of the CNS.

Treatment.—Cranial radiation was begun at the time of complete remission. All patients were treated with lateral fields on a 4- or 6-MV linear accelerator. Most often, 2-Gy fractions were delivered 5 days a week. Four or 5 doses of methotrexate were administered intrathecally at the same time, and methotrexate was repeated every 18 weeks for the duration of treatment.

Outcome.—The overall 7-year event-free survival rate was 62%. It was 72% for standard-risk patients and 56% for those at high risk. Thirty-one patients, all but 5 of them in the high-risk group, had CNS relapse as an initial event, with or without concurrent bone marrow relapse. The cumulative incidence of CNS relapse was 6%, ranging from 2.5% for the standard-risk group to 8.2% in the high-risk group. Only 4 of the 31 patients with CNS relapse remained alive 25 months or longer after the event. The median survival after CNS relapse was 22 months.

Recommendations.—Intensive CNS treatment is warranted for high-risk patients with ALL because CNS relapse after cranial irradiation carries a poor prognosis. Currently, intrathecal methotrexate and cytosine arabinoside are administered to standard-risk patients, and 18 Gy of cranial radiation is added for high-risk patients. The value of hyperfractionated cranial irradiation is being studied.

Extended Triple Intrathecal Chemotherapy Trial for Prevention of CNS Relapse in Good-Risk and Poor-Risk Patients With B-Progenitor Acute Lymphoblastic Leukemia: A Pediatric Oncology Group Study
Pullen J, Boyett J, Shuster J, Crist W, Land V, Frankel L, Iyer R, Backstrom L, van Eys J, Harris M, Ravindranath Y, Sullivan M (Univ of Mississippi, Jackson;

Univ of Tennessee, Memphis; Univ of Florida, Gainesville; et al)
J Clin Oncol 11:839–849, 1993

116-95-4–90

Background.—Although preventive therapy directed toward the CNS is accepted as an essential part of therapy for childhood acute lymphoblastic leukemia (ALL), there is no consensus about which form it should take. Craniospinal irradiation plus intrathecal methotrexate is effective, but the radiation is toxic. The results are reported for the Pediatric Oncology Group acute leukemia in childhood 13 study, in which 2 treatment regimens using different forms of CNS chemoprophylaxis were tested in children with ALL.

Methods.—The analysis included 1,152 children older than age 1 year with non-T, non-B ALL and no apparent CNS disease at diagnosis. One group was randomized to receive standard therapy, consisting of 6 injections of intrathecal methotrexate, hydrocortisone, and cytarabine during intensification therapy. These patients also received additional doses at 8-week intervals during maintenance therapy, for a total of 17 additional doses. The other group received standard and methotrexate pulses (SAM). These patients also received the same dose of triple intrathecal chemotherapy during intensification. During maintenance therapy, they received pulses of intermediate-dose parenteral methotrexate, 1 g/m². The first 4 pulses were accompanied by a low-dose intrathecal methotrexate boost. The 2 groups, which were stratified for risk group and immunophenotype, received the same systemic therapy.

Results.—The estimated 5-year rate of continuous complete remission was about 61% in each group. The 5-year probability of an isolated CNS relapse for good-risk children was 3% in the standard-therapy group vs. 10% in the SAM group. The probability for poor-risk children was 8% in the standard-therapy group and 13% in the SAM group. The overall probability of CNS relapse was 5% in the standard-therapy group vs. 11% in the SAM group. About one third of the isolated CNS relapses in poor-risk patients occurred before the initiation of preventive therapy at week 9. The advantage of standard therapy was significant for good-risk children but not for poor-risk children. Neither CNS preventive regimen offered any significant advantage in general outcome.

Conclusion.—In children being treated for ALL, triple intrathecal chemotherapy throughout intensification and maintenance offers better prevention of CNS leukemia than intermediate-dose methotrexate pulses. The results of standard treatment appear to be comparable to those of other reported forms of CNS preventive therapy. For patients with B-progenitor ALL, extended triple intrathecal chemotherapy is a reasonable alternative to CNS irradiation plus upfront intrathecal methotrexate.

Treatment of CNS Relapse in Children With Acute Lymphoblastic Leukemia: A Pediatric Oncology Group Study

Winick NJ, Smith SD, Shuster J, Lauer S, Wharam MD, Land V, Buchanan G, Rivera G (Univ of Texas, Dallas; Univ of Chicago; Univ of Florida, Gainesville; et al)

J Clin Oncol 11:271–278, 1993   116-95-4–91

Introduction.—Most studies of outcome in children with acute lymphoblastic leukemia after isolated CNS relapse have had relatively few patients. A total of 120 patients enrolled on protocol 8304 of the Pediatric Oncology Group who had an isolated CNS relapse despite previous CNS prophylaxis were described.

Methods.—None of the children had CNS disease at diagnosis; all had received prophylactic CNS therapy during their initial treatment. The protocol after CNS relapse consisted of systemic reinduction, cranial radiation (24 Gy), triple intrathecal therapy, and continuation chemotherapy with 6-week cycles of mercaptopurine-methotrexate and vincristine-cyclophosphamide, with randomization to intervening pulses of prednisone-doxorubicin or teniposide-cytarabine for a total of 88 weeks.

Results.—All patients achieved a second complete remission with the treatment protocol. There were 61 protocol failures, including bone marrow relapse in 35 children, a second isolated CNS relapse in 13, and a testicular relapse in 10. One child died in remission. At 4 years, the overall event-free survival was 46%. Leukoencephalopathy, which occurred in 20 patients, was the most important toxic effect of therapy. There was a trend toward superior event-free survival in favor of teniposide-cytarabine over prednisone-doxorubicin pulses. No significant correlation was found between symptoms at the time of relapse and subsequent event-free survival. An evaluation of radiation therapy found a major deviation in dose, field, or modality in 28 patients, but such deviations did not appear to affect the overall outcome or the incidence of a second CNS relapse.

Conclusion.—Long-term disease-free survival is possible after CNS relapse in children with acute lymphoblastic leukemia. The modest degree of myelosuppression and limited nonhematopoietic toxicities observed in these patients suggest that the chemotherapy program can be intensified. Future protocols must intensify systemic therapy to prevent bone marrow relapse.

▶ The first paper (Abstract 116-95-4–88) of these 4 (Abstracts 116-95-4–88 to 116-95-4–91) is a very important one that demonstrates the importance of examination of cytocentrifuged cerebrospinal fluid at diagnosis in childhood ALL. It is clear that occult cerebrospinal fluid blasts can be demonstrated by cytocentrifuge in adult acute myelocytic leukemia also, but it is not clear that they have the same significance in acute myelocytic leukemia as in ALL. Perhaps that is because cytarabine is always a component of induction therapy in the former in a dose and schedule that achieve therapeutic levels in the cerebrospinal fluid. The report by Pullen et al. (Abstract 116-95-4–90) demonstrates the inferiority of intermediate-dose parenteral methotrexate to triple intrathecal therapy in children with ALL, but others have demonstrated that CNS prophylaxis with parenteral intermediate-dose methotrexate alone is sufficient for adults with ALL (1).—P.H. Wiernik, M.D.

Reference

1. Wiernik PH, et al: *Leukemia* 7:1236, 1993.

5 Bone Marrow Transplantation

Acute Leukemia and Myelodysplasia

Prospective Comparative Study of Bone Marrow Transplantation and Postremission Chemotherapy for Childhood Acute Myelogenous Leukemia

Amadori S, for the Associazione Italiana Ematologia ed Oncologia Pediatrica Cooperative Group (Univ La Sapienza, Rome)
J Clin Oncol 11:1046–1054, 1993

116-95-5-1

Objective.—The results of allogeneic bone marrow transplantation (BMT), autologous BMT, and sequential postremission chemotherapy were compared in 161 children younger than 15 years of age who were in first remission of acute myelogenous leukemia (AML).

Study Plan.—The patients, all with newly diagnosed AML, initially received 2 courses of daunorubicin and standard-dose cytarabine therapy. Consolidation treatment consisted of a course of daunorubicin, cytarabine, and thioguanine (DAT regimen). Patients who remitted completely were then randomized to either autologous BMT or sequential postremission chemotherapy, except for those with an HLA-matched sibling, who were assigned to allogeneic BMT. Sequential chemotherapy con-

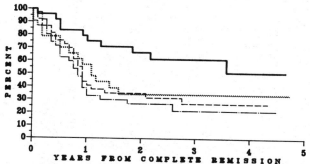

Fig 5–1.—Probability of disease-free survival by intended postremission therapy: BMT (*solid line, n* = 24); autologous BMT (*solid line with dots, n* = 35); sequential postremission chemotherapy (*dashed line, n* = 37); and nonrandomized (*slashed line, n* = 31). (Courtesy of Amadori S, for the Associazione Italiana Ematologia ed Oncologia Pediatrica Cooperative Group: *J Clin Oncol* 11:1046–1054, 1993.)

sisted of 3 further courses of DAT, followed by 3 pairs of drugs administered sequentially for a total of 6 cycles.

Results.—The complete remission rate was 79%. The estimated overall survival at 5 years was 42%, and the estimated event-free survival rate at 5 years was 25%. The median follow-up was 28 months. Complete responders had a disease-free survival rate of 31% at 5 years; the cumulative risk of relapse was 64%. Among patients who remitted completely, those undergoing allogeneic BMT had a 5-year disease-free survival of 51%, which was significantly higher than the rate for patients who underwent autologous BMT (21%) or sequential postremission chemotherapy (27%) and for the 31 nonrandomized patients (Fig 5–1). In all groups, marrow relapse was the most common cause of failure after complete remission. No deaths were ascribed to drug toxicity.

Conclusion.—Allogeneic marrow transplantation is clearly the best means of preventing relapse and extending disease-free survival in children in first remission of AML.

▶ This is a very small study, but the conclusions drawn have major implications. Therefore, a study of similar design with greater statistical power seems imperative.—P.H. Wiernik, M.D.

Intensively Timed Induction Therapy Followed by Autologous or Allogeneic Bone Marrow Transplantation for Children With Acute Myeloid Leukemia or Myelodysplastic Syndrome: A Childrens Cancer Group Pilot Study
Woods WG, Kobrinsky N, Buckley J, Neudorf S, Sanders J, Miller L, Barnard D, Benjamin D, DeSwarte J, Kalousek D, Shina D, Hammond GD, Lange BJ (Univ of Minnesota, Minneapolis; Childrens Cancer Group, Arcadia, Calif)
J Clin Oncol 11:1448–1457, 1993   116-95-5–2

Background.—Although significant advances have been made in the treatment of acute myeloid leukemia (AML), only about one third of patients will be long-term survivors. The best treatment for children with myelodysplastic syndrome (MDS) is unknown. This pilot study—Childrens Cancer Group protocol 2861—examined the feasibility of aggressively timed induction therapy and then autologous or allogeneic bone marrow transplantation (BMT) as the only postremission therapy for children with AML or MDS.

Methods.—Included were 142 patients younger than 21 years of age with newly diagnosed AML or MDS. All received a timing-intensive course of 5-drug induction chemotherapy consisting of dexamethasone, cytarabine, thioguanine, etoposide, and daunorubicin. This regimen was administered for 4 days, and then 6 days later for a second cycle, regardless of the patient's hematologic status. Patients who went into remission were eligible for bone marrow ablative therapy with busulfan and cyclophosphamide, then 4-hydroperoxycyclophosphamide–purged autologous or allogeneic BMT rescue.

Results.—Seventy-six percent of patients achieved remission. Of the rest, 13% died of complications of their leukemia or chemotherapy, and 11% did not achieve remission. Bone marrow transplantation was performed in 75 patients: 58 autologous, 16 allogeneic rescue, and 1 from an unrelated donor. The 3-year actuarial disease-free survival rate was 51% for patients receiving autologous rescue with 4-hydroperoxycyclophosphamide–purged grafts vs. 55% for those receiving allogeneic grafts. The overall 3-year actuarial survival rate was 45%, and the event-free survival rate was 37%. The elevated WBC count and CNS leukemia at the time of AML diagnosis were identified as adverse prognostic factors.

Conclusion.—For children and adolescents with newly diagnosed AML or MDS, aggressively timed induction therapy and then marrow ablation and autologous or allogeneic BMT rescue appear to be a feasible and effective form of treatment. This postremission approach appears to have acceptable toxicity and high efficacy. Evidence of CNS disease at the diagnosis of AML may be a marker of more or resistant disease.

A Prospective Randomized Comparison of Total Body Irradiation-Etoposide Versus Busulfan-Cyclophosphamide as Preparatory Regimens for Bone Marrow Transplantation in Patients With Leukemia Who Were Not in First Remission: A Southwest Oncology Group Study

Blume KG, Kopecky KJ, Henslee-Downey JP, Forman SJ, Stiff PJ, LeMaistre CF, Appelbaum FR (Stanford Univ, Calif; Southwest Oncology Group Statistical Ctr, Seattle; Univ of Kentucky, Lexington; et al)
Blood 81:2187–2193, 1993   116-95-5–3

Objective.—In late 1986, the Southwest Oncology Group began a phase III trial evaluating 2 new preparatory regimens designed to condition patients with leukemia to receive allogeneic bone marrow from a histocompatible sibling.

Patients.—The 122 patients with leukemia enrolled in the trial were stratified by age and classified as "good-risk" patients (in second complete remission of acute leukemia or in the accelerated phase of chronic myelogenous leukemia) or "poor-risk" patients (more advanced leukemia).

Management.—Half of the patients were randomized to receive the FTBI/VP-16 regimen, consisting of 1,320 centigray of total body irradiation and a single dose of 60 mg of etoposide per kg. The remaining patients received the BU/CY regimen, consisting of 16 mg of busulfan per kg administered orally in 16 doses in 4 days, and 120 mg of cyclophosphamide per kg in 2 equal doses administered intravenously on successive days. Subsequently, 114 patients received bone marrow from histo-compatible siblings. Cyclosporine and prednisone were used for immunosuppression.

Results.—All but 1 of the marrow transplant recipients lived at least 1 month and exhibited marrow engraftment. Thirty-five patients were known to be alive a median of 31 months after entry. Thirty-one of 114 transplanted patients are in continued complete remission. Thirty-eight patients died without evidence of relapse. The degree of risk significantly influenced survival and relapse, but age did not. The type of preparative regimen used did not significantly influence the risk of acute or chronic graft-vs.-host disease developing.

Conclusion.—The FTBI/VP-16 and BU/CY regimens are comparably effective and safe when used to condition patients with leukemia for al-logeneic bone marrow transplantation.

Autologous Bone Marrow Transplantation After a Long First Remission for Children With Recurrent Acute Lymphoblastic Leukemia
Billett AL, Kornmehl E, Tarbell NJ, Weinstein HJ, Gelber RD, Ritz J, Sallan SE (Dana-Farber Cancer Inst, Boston; Children's Hosp, Boston; Harvard Med School, Boston; et al)
Blood 81:1651–1657, 1993   116-95-5-4

Introduction.—The prognosis for children with newly diagnosed acute lymphoblastic leukemia (ALL) remains poor. Allogeneic bone marrow transplantation (BMT) from matched sibling donors improves survival after relapse, but matched sibling donors are often not available. The safety and efficacy of purged autologous BMT were assessed in children with ALL who were in second or subsequent remission after a first re-mission of at least 24 months.

Patients.—Autologous BMT was done in 51 children with ALL aged 3–18 years. Patients with a first remission of less than 24 months were excluded. Bone marrow was harvested and treated with 3 cycles of monoclonal antibodies and complement specific for leukemia-associated antigens. All patients underwent ablative chemotherapy and then total body irradiation before autologous BMT. The median time from bone marrow harvest to reinfusion was 13 days.

Results.—Five patients died of treatment-related complications, 18 relapsed, 1 patient died of a second malignancy, and 27 remained in continuous complete remission for a median of 39 months. The overall survival was 63% at 3 years, 55% at 4 years, and 47% at 7 years. The 3-year event-free survival was 53%, and the 3-year leukemia-free survival was 58%. Multivariate analysis showed that the duration of the longest remission before autologous BMT was the most significant predictor of both event-free and leukemia-free survival; remission duration immedi-ately before autologous BMT was the next most significant predictor of event-free survival; and cell dose of marrow reinfused was the next most significant predictor of leukemia-free survival.

Conclusion.—Autologous BMT is an effective alternative therapy for most children in second or subsequent remission after relapse of ALL for whom an appropriate donor for allogeneic BMT is unavailable.

▶ Further evidence that the bone marrow microenvironment may be important in leukemogenesis is suggested by the fact that leukemia may rarely develop in donor cells after BMT and by the finding of evidence of viral infection of the marrow microenvironment in some patients (1).—P.H. Wiernik, M.D.

Reference

1. Payne CM, et al: *Exp Hematol* 15:143, 1987.

Burkitt-Type Acute Lymphoblastic Leukemia in Donor Cells After Allogeneic Bone Marrow Transplantation for Acute Nonlymphoblastic Leukemia

Cransac M, Boiron J-M, Merel P, Cony-Makhoul P, Marit G, Bernard P, Ferrer J, Reiffers J (Hôpital Haut-Lévêque, Pessac, France; Université de Bordeaux II, France; Centre Regional Transfusion Sanguine, Bordeaux, France)

Transplantation 56:120–123, 1993

116-95-5-5

Background.—Secondary leukemias rarely develop after bone marrow transplantation (BMT) for acute nonlymphoblastic leukemia. Among the 13 reported cases of secondary leukemia in donor cells, most were acute lymphoblastic leukemia (ALL). A patient with secondary Burkitt's type ALL that developed in donor cells after allogeneic BMT for acute nonlymphoblastic leukemia was reported.

Case Report.—Woman, 37, underwent BMT during complete remission of acute nonlymphoblastic leukemia. Despite standard prophylaxis, graft-vs.-host disease that was refractory to steroid and cyclosporine-thalidomide therapies developed. Hyperleukocytosis reappeared 3 years after BMT. Sternal bone marrow aspirate was consistent with type 3 ALL, with 90% peroxidase-negative leukoblasts. Polyclonal surface immunoglobulins were apparent on 70% of malignant cells. The immunophenotype was HLA-DR in 82%, CD19 in 80%, CD20 in 70%, CD24 in 89%, and CD9 in 88%. The CD10, T, and myeloid markers as well as CD21 and CD25 surface markers were negative. In situ hybridization using a biotinized probe did not reveal the Epstein-Barr virus genome, although Epstein-Barr virus serology was weakly positive. The discontinuance of immunosuppressive therapy did not influence disease progression; weekly vincristine and corticosteroid therapies were ineffective. The patient died of infectious and hemorrhagic complications 3 weeks after a single course of methotrexate. Typing of DNA at locus D10S28 revealed a specific band that disappeared at 3 and

36 months after BMT, suggesting that all leukemic cells, including the Burkitt-type blast cells, originated in the donor.

Conclusion.—Less than 5% of leukemias secondary to allogeneic BMT for acute or chronic leukemia originate in the donor. Although the etiology is unknown and may involve multiple mechanisms, great precautions must be taken to identify tumor cell origin. Molecular analysis may be more reliable than cytogenetic studies, which are often equivocal.

Busulfan-Based Regimens and Allogeneic Bone Marrow Transplantation in Patients With Myelodysplastic Syndromes
Ratanatharathorn V, Karanes C, Uberti J, Lum LG, de Planque MM, Schultz KR, Cronin S, Dan ME, Mohamed A, Hussein M, Sensenbrenner LL (Wayne State Univ, Detroit)
Blood 81:2194–2199, 1993   116-95-5-6

Background.—The myelodysplastic syndromes (MDSs) are a category of clonal hematologic disorders in which dysplastic changes are followed by progressive hematopoietic failure. Some patients ultimately have treatment-resistant acute myeloid leukemia develop. Marrow transplantation remains the only possible means of curing MDSs.

Methods and Patients.—A preparative regimen including busulfan was administered before allogeneic bone marrow transplantation (BMT) in 27 consecutive patients with MDS. The 17 male and 10 female patients had a median age of 33 years. Sixteen patients had primary MDS, whereas 11 either had preceding hematologic disorders or had MDS develop after receiving cytotoxic drugs or radiation therapy, or both. Six patients with leukemic transplantation received antileukemic treatment before BMT. Complex chromosomal abnormalities were identified in 13 patients, and simple abnormalities in 5.

Treatment.—The most frequent preparative regimen, used in 24 patients, consisted of 4 mg of busulfan per kg, administered orally each day for 4 days; 4 intravenous doses of cytosine arabinoside, 2 g/m^2, administered at 12-hour intervals; and intravenous cyclophosphamide, 60 mg/kg for 2 days. Eighteen patients received bone marrow from a genotypically matched sibling.

Results.—Engraftment occurred promptly in all but 1 of the patients. Of the 27 patients, 17 remain alive without evidence of disease. The disease-free survival was significantly better in patients receiving bone marrow from genotypically matched donors (Fig 5-2). Twelve patients had acute graft-vs.-host disease, and 4 of them subsequently had chronic disease.

Conclusion.—Preparative regimens that include busulfan are effective in patients with MDS who undergo BMT. It is possible to achieve lasting

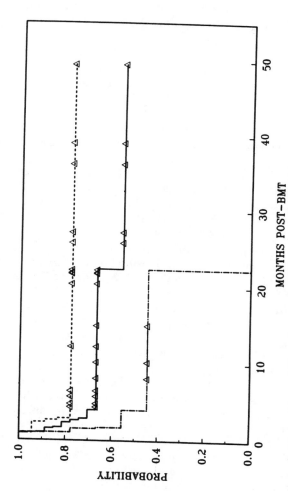

Fig 5–2.—Kaplan-Meier product-limit estimates of disease-free survival: *solid line,* entire group (27 patients); *dashed line,* 18 patients with genotypically matched donors; *dots and dashes,* 9 patients with nongenotypic matched donors. (Courtesy of Ratanatharathorn V, Karanes C, Uberti J, et al: *Blood* 81:2194–2199, 1993.)

disease-free survival even in patients who have had leukemic transplantation and in those with complex chromosomal abnormalities.

▶ This paper, and a previous one from Seattle (1), suggest that BMT is the most effective therapy for young patients with myelodysplasia. Unfortunately, only a minority of patients with myelodysplasia are candidates for the procedure, primarily because of age.—P.H. Wiernik, M.D.

Reference

1. Appelbaum FR, et al: *Ann Intern Med* 112:590, 1990.

Chronic Myelogenous Leukemia

Bone Marrow Transplantation for Chronic Myeloid Leukemia: Long-Term Results
Gratwohl A, for the Chronic Leukemia Working Party of the European Group for Bone Marrow Transplantation (Kantonsspital Basel, Switzerland)
Bone Marrow Transplant 12:509–516, 1993   116-95-5-7

Background.—Chronic myeloid leukemia (CML) currently is the most frequent single indication for bone marrow transplantation (BMT). The results of BMT were reviewed in the 1,480 patients undergoing BMT for CML in 1979–1990 who were entered in the European Group for Bone Marrow Transplantation registry.

Patients.—A total of 1,082 transplants were done in the initial chronic phase of CML; 88 in the higher chronic phase; 251 in the accelerated phase; and 59 in blast crisis. Marrow donors were HLA-identical siblings in 1,373 instances and syngeneic twins in another 28.

Results.—The best outcome was noted when patients were transplanted at an early stage of disease. To date, no patient transplanted during blast crisis has lived for more than 5 years. Almost half (47%) of 947 patients who received their first marrow transplant in the first chronic phase from an HLA-identical sibling donor were alive at 8 years. The relapse rate at 5 years was 33% in this group, and the transplant-related mortality was 42%. Depletion of T cells was a major factor in both leukemia-free survival and the relapse incidence. Patients younger than 20 years of age at the time of BMT had a relatively good leukemia-free survival rate. On multivariate analysis, the combination of a female donor and a male recipient predicted a poorer leukemia-free survival rate.

Conclusion.—A substantial number of patients with CML can now achieve a complete, lasting remission without maintenance treatment. The overall median survival of patients in this series is 6 years after BMT, and almost half of the group remained alive at 8 years. The best results are obtained when an HLA-identical donor is available and when BMT is done as soon after diagnosis as is possible. Currently, patients in blast crisis are not routine candidates for BMT.

▶ Although these results are excellent, the absence of a plateau on the survival curve is troublesome and suggests that transplantation does not cure this disease. The usefulness of transplantation in this setting is limited by the fact that the median age for patients wtih CML is well above the current age limitations for the procedure. Are current transplant results better than those obtained with α-interferon in young patients? There has never been a prospective, controlled trial asking that question.—P.H. Wiernik, M.D.

Frequent Detection of BCR-ABL Specific mRNA in Patients With Chronic Myeloid Leukemia (CML) Following Allogeneic and Syngeneic Bone Marrow Transplantation (BMT)

Gaiger A, Lion T, Kalhs P, Mitterbauer G, Henn T, Haas O, Födinger M, Kier P, Forstinger C, Quehenberger P, Hinterberger W, Jäger U, Linkesch W, Mannhalter C, Lechner K (Univ of Vienna; St Anna-Kinderspital, Vienna)
Leukemia 7:1766–1772, 1993

116-95-5–8

Background.—In patients with chronic myeloid leukemia (CML) who have undergone bone marrow transplantation (BMT), polymerase chain reaction (PCR) is highly sensitive in detecting minimal residual disease. However, the clinical significance of this test is questionable as not all PCR-positive patients will go into hematologic relapse. Polymerase chain reaction was used to study many samples during an extended period in 30 BMT recipients with CML.

Methods.—A total of 440 peripheral samples of blood or bone marrow, or both, were studied by a 2-step PCR to detect *bcr-abl*–specific messenger RNA. A mean of 15 samples was obtained per patient during a median observation time of 29 months. Twenty-eight patients received non–T-cell–depleted allogeneic marrow, whereas 2 received syngeneic marrow.

Findings.—Half of the patients had *bcr-abl*–specific messenger RNA after BMT. A positive sample was found in only 2 of 11 patients who were in remission for at least 40 months. Five patients, all in complete hematologic remission, had PCR positivity on only 1 occasion. Of 10 patients with PCR positivity in 2 or more consecutive samples, 5 subsequently had hematologic relapse. A *bcr-abl* positivity was seen in 11 of 15 patients without graft-vs.-host disease vs. 4 of 15 patients with graft-vs.-host disease.

Conclusion.—For patients with CML who undergo BMT, transient hematologic relapse does not follow *bcr-abl* positivity in most cases. In contrast, patients wtih a positive PCR in 2 or more consecutive samples are at high risk for relapse. The finding that most patients without graft-vs.-host disease are *bcr-abl* positive supports the possible antileukemic action of the donor cells.

▶ We need these kind of data in Philadelphia chromosome–positive acute lymphoblastic leukemia.—P.H. Wiernik, M.D.

Unrelated-Donor Bone Marrow Transplantation for Philadelphia Chromosome-Positive Chronic Myelogenous Leukemia in Children
Gamis AS, Haake R, McGlave P, Ramsay NKC (Univ of Minnesota, Minneapolis)
J Clin Oncol 11:834–838, 1993   116-95-5-9

Background.—When bone marrow from matched-sibling donors is administered to patients with Philadelphia chromosome–positive (Ph[1]) chronic myelogenous leukemia (CML), the chance of disease-free survival is 55% to 64%. Trials of unrelated-donor bone marrow transplantation (BMT) performed chiefly in adults with CML were reviewed and compared.

Patients and Treatment.—The results of marrow transplantation with unrelated-donor bone marrow in a group of 11 children were compared with those of MSD transplantation in a group of 11 other children with Ph[1] CML. Ten of the unrelated-donor marrow recipients had advanced CML. Three of them received fully matched bone marrow. Transplantation was performed a median of 2.6 years after diagnosis. Of the 11 patients receiving matched-donor bone marrow, 5 had advanced CML. The median interval from diagnosis to BMT was .7 year. All the children received cyclophosphamide and fractionated total-body radiation before the infusion of non–T-cell–depleted bone marrow.

Results.—Engraftment times were comparable in the 2 groups. Two of the grafts from unrelated marrow donors failed. Patients in this group had more severe acute graft-vs.-host disease and more persistent chronic disease. The estimated disease-free survival rates at 3 years were 45% in the unrelated-donor group and 78% in the patients receiving matched-donor marrow. All patients except 1 in the unrelated-donor group had Karnofsky scores indicating a good ability to function in daily life.

Conclusion.—Transplantation of bone marrow from unrelated donors has produced unexpectedly favorable results in children with Ph[1] CML.

▶ The mortality rate for unrelated-donor transplants approaches 50% in adults.—P.H. Wiernik, M.D.

Induction of Graft-Versus-Host Disease as Immunotherapy for Relapsed Chronic Myeloid Leukemia
Porter DL, Roth MS, McGarigle C, Ferrara JLM, Antin JH (Harvard Med

School, Boston; Univ of Michigan, Ann Arbor)
N Engl J Med 330:100–106, 1994

116-95-5-10

Background.—Allogeneic bone marrow transplantation can cure chronic myeloid leukemia (CML) by both the conditioning regimen and the antileukemic effects of the lymphocytes in grafted marrow. The ability of interferon-α2b and infusions of mononuclear cells from the marrow donor to induce a graft-vs.-leukemia response was investigated in patients with CML in relapse after bone marrow transplantation.

Methods.—Interferon-α2b and infusions of mononuclear cells were given to 11 patients with relapsed CML after allogeneic bone marrow transplantation. Toxic effects, hematologic and cytogenetic reactions, and elimination of cells with the *bcr-abl* messenger RNA transcript characteristic of leukemic cells were noted.

Findings.—Six of 8 patients with stable CML after relapse had complete remissions; no cells with *bcr-abl* messenger RNA transcripts were found. Three patients with accelerated CML after relapse did not have a remission. In 8 patients, myelosuppression was prominent. Six patients had grade I and 3 patients had grade III acute graft-vs.-host disease. Five patients had limited chronic graft-vs.-host disease.

Conclusion.—Induction of a graft-vs.-leukemia response with interferon-α2b and infusions of donor mononuclear cells is an effective antileukemic treatment in patients with CML in relapse after bone marrow transplantation. This treatment may offer an alternative to a second bone marrow transplantation.

Salvage Immunotherapy Using Donor Leukocyte Infusions as Treatment for Relapsed Chronic Myelogenous Leukemia After Allogeneic Bone Marrow Transplantation: Efficacy and Toxicity of a Defined T-Cell Dose

Drobyski WR, Keever CA, Roth MS, Koethe S, Hanson G, McFadden P, Gottschall JL, Ash RC, van Tuinen P, Horowitz MM, Flomenberg N (Med College of Wisconsin, Milwaukee; Blood Ctr of Southeastern Wisconsin, Milwaukee; Univ of Michigan, Ann Arbor)
Blood 82:2310–2318, 1993

116-95-5-11

Background.—Allogeneic bone marrow transplantation (BMT) has been the only successful treatment modality for patients with Philadelphia chromosome (Ph)–positive chronic myelogenous leukemia (CML). There is, however, a significant incidence of relapse. Studies have reported achieving remissions in patients with relapsed CML with the administration of donor leukocyte infusions, although these studies have also documented severe toxicity. Both the antileukemic effect and the toxicity are thought to be caused by T cells. The efficacy and toxicity of T-cell infusion in patients with relapsed CML were assessed.

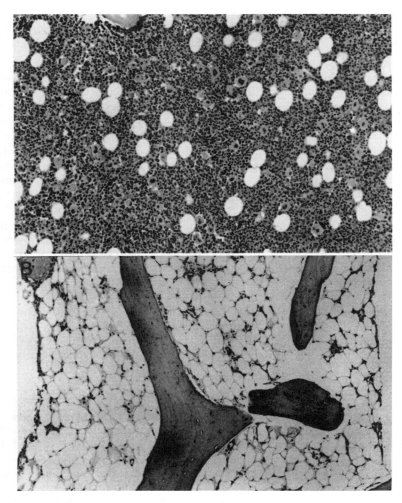

Fig 5–3.—A, bone marrow biopsy (UPN 364) obtained 4 weeks after leukocyte infusions showing a hypercellular marrow with granulocytic hyperplasia consistent with persisting morphologic relapse. **B,** biopsy obtained 7 months after infusion shows a markedly hypocellular marrow with eradication of leukemia. (Courtesy of Drobyski WR, Keever CA, Roth MS, et al: *Blood* 82:2310–2318, 1993.)

Methods.—Eight patients with CML who had a relapse after receiving allogeneic BMT grafts from HLA-matched siblings were enrolled. No patients had active graft-vs.-host disease or had a history of moderate to severe graft-vs.-host disease. Immunosuppressive and cytotoxic agents were discontinued in all patients. Each patient received a predetermined dose of T cells derived from leukocyte collections from the original BMT donors; the T cells were infused every other day for 1–2 weeks.

Results.—Of the 8 patients, 6 were in the accelerated phase and 2 were in blast crisis. Both of the patients in blast crisis died; the remaining 6 have been in hematologic and cytogenetic remission for periods exceeding their initial remission period. The onset of remission varied greatly. Seven of 8 patients had graft-vs.-host disease. One patient had fatal-grade intravenous graft-vs.-host disease, 1 had grade III graft-vs.-host disease and required prolonged treatment, and the remaining 5 had grade I graft-vs.-host disease and continued with low-dose prednisone treatment. Four of the patients with accelerated-phase disease had marrow aplasia (Fig 5–3) at a median of 130 days after infusion.

Discussion.—Infusion of T cells had a potent antileukemic effect in patients treated in the accelerated phase of disease. Although an antileukemic response was observed soon after infusion, remission occurred gradually. This suggests that leukocyte infusions must be used at an early stage in CML relapse to be effective. Because most of the included patients had only mild graft-vs.-host disease in contrast to more severe toxicity in patients in studies using T-cell infusion at the time of BMT, the infusion delay may minimize the severity of graft-vs.-host disease. Donor myeloid deficiency may be implicated in the development of marrow aplasia. Further research should determine the minimal number of T cells required to achieve remission.

▶ Why not skip the transplant and treat initially with interferon and donor mononuclear cell infusions?—P.H. Wiernik, M.D.

Hodgkin's and Non-Hodgkin's Lymphoma

Autologous Bone Marrow Transplantation for Pediatric Hodgkin's Disease: A Case-Matched Comparison With Adult Patients by the European Bone Marrow Transplant Group Lymphoma Registry
Williams CD, Goldstone AH, Pearce R, Green S, Armitage JO, Carella A, Meloni G (Univ College Hosp, London; Princess Margaret Hosp, Swindon, England; Univ of Nebraska, Omaha; et al)
J Clin Oncol 11:2243–2249, 1993   116-95-5-12

Background.—In both children and adults who fail to respond to chemotherapy or combined treatment for Hodgkin's disease, the response to salvage therapy is poor. However, high-dose therapy, with or without total body irradiation and then rescue autologous bone marrow transplantation (ABMT) may yield better responses to salvage therapy. No studies have specifically compared the outcome of this therapy in adults vs. children.

Methods.—A case-control study was conducted on the outcome of ABMT in pediatric and adult patients with Hodgkin's disease. The pediatric group consisted of 81 patients, median age 14 years at diagnosis, who underwent ABMT. They were matched to a group of 81 adult patients, median age 26 years at diagnosis, who also had ABMT. The

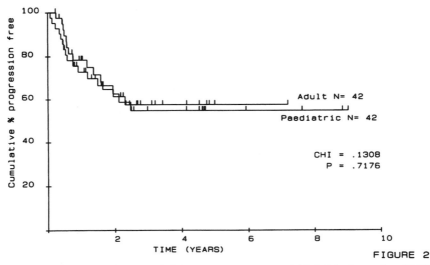

Fig 5–4.—Progression-free survival of chemosensitive patients with Hodgkin's disease after ABMT: comparison between pediatric and matched adult patients. $\chi = .1308$; $P = .7176$. (Courtesy of Williams CD, Goldstone AH, Pearce R, et al: *J Clin Oncol* 11:2243–2249, 1993.)

groups were matched after identification by multivariate analysis of the main prognostic factors for progression-free survival.

Results.—The progression-free survival rate was comparable for the 2 groups—39% for the pediatric group and 48% for the adult group. The overall relapse and progression rate was 52% for the pediatric group and 40% for the adult group; the difference was not significant (Fig 5-4). There were no significant differences in site of relapse or in incidence or causes of procedure-related morbidity or mortality. The pediatric group did have a slightly quicker neutrophil recovery. The interval between diagnosis and transplant was unrelated to outcome at ABMT in the pediatric group.

Conclusion.—Similar results were found for ABMT in pediatric and adult patients with Hodgkin's disease. Suitability for transplantation should be judged using the same criteria for children and adults. Further study is needed to identify the long-term side effects and complications of high-dose chemotherapy and irradiation.

Allogeneic, Syngeneic, and Autologous Marrow Transplantation for Hodgkin's Disease: The 21-Year Seattle Experience

Anderson JE, Litzow MR, Appelbaum FR, Schoch G, Fisher LD, Buckner CD, Petersen FB, Crawford SW, Press OW, Sanders JE, Bensinger WI, Martin PJ, Storb R, Sullivan KM, Hansen JA, Thomas ED (Fred Hutchinson Cancer Re-

search Ctr, Seattle; Univ of Washington, Seattle)
J Clin Oncol 11:2342–2350, 1993

116-95-5-13

Background.—About half of patients with stage III or IV Hodgkin's disease either fail to achieve complete remission or relapse after their first complete remission. Some studies have used high-dose chemoradiation therapy and then bone marrow transplantation for patients with relapsed or refractory Hodgkin's disease, but the choice between allogeneic and autologous marrow transplantation has not been fully investigated.

Methods.—A 21-year experience with myeloablative therapy and then marrow transplantation was analyzed for 127 patients with relapsed or refractory Hodgkin's disease. Preparative treatment consisted of high-dose chemotherapy for all patients, with total body irradiation in 61 patients and not in the other 66. Patients with less advanced Hodgkin's disease and no history of chest radiation therapy generally received cyclophosphamide and 12 Gy of total body irradiation. Those with more advanced disease were enrolled in studies evaluating different radiation dose schedules or different combination chemotherapy regimens before total body irradiation. Twenty-three patients were treated for primary refractory disease, 34 were treated in early first relapse or second complete remission, and 70 were treated for refractory first relapse or disease after their second complete remission. Autologous marrow transplantation was administered to 68 patients, allogeneic marrow to 53, and syngeneic marrow to 6.

Results.—The overall 5-year actuarial probability of survival was 21%. At the same time, the actuarial event-free survival rate was 18%, the relapse rate was 65%, and the nonrelapse mortality rate was 49%. For patients receiving allogeneic bone marrow, the 5-year actuarial survival was 20% and the actuarial event-free survival was 22%. All 12 survivors in this group received marrow from an HLA-identical sibling. In the autologous marrow group, the 5-year actuarial survival rate was 13%, and the actuarial event-free survival rate was 14%. One syngeneic marrow recipient was alive and free of disease. Survival, event-free survival, and nonrelapse mortality rates were not significantly different for patients receiving HLA-identical vs. autologous marrow, although the relapse rate was higher in the autologous marrow group. The allogeneic marrow group was more likely to have adverse clinical characteristics before transplantation. Multivariate analysis showed that higher performance status and absence of bulky disease predicted improved event-free survival and lower relapse rates. The event-free survival and nonrelapse mortality rates were also better in patients with fewer previous treatment regimens.

Conclusion.—Transplantation in Hodgkin's disease is more likely to be successful if performed early after relapse, when disease burden is lower, tumor sensitivity to chemotherapy is greater, and performance status is likely to be better. The relapse rate is lower with HLA-identical marrow; therefore, it may be preferred to autologous marrow.

One Hundred Autotransplants for Relapsed or Refractory Hodgkin's Disease and Lymphoma: Value of Pretransplant Disease Status for Predicting Outcome

Rapoport AP, Rowe JM, Kouides PA, Duerst RA, Abboud CN, Liesveld JL, Packman CH, Eberly S, Sherman M, Tanner MA, Constine LS, DiPersio JF
(Univ of Rochester, NY)
J Clin Oncol 11:2351–2361, 1993   116-95-5–14

Objective.—Experience with 100 consecutive autologous bone marrow transplantation procedures in 96 patients with refractory or relapsed Hodgkin's disease and non-Hodgkin's lymphoma was reviewed in an attempt to find pretransplantation factors that helped predict the outcome. Transplants were conducted in 47 patients with Hodgkin's disease and 53 with non-Hodgkin's lymphoma.

Treatment.—For the most part, patients were prepared with high-dose carmustine, etoposide, cytarabine, and cyclophosphamide (BEAC regimen). Rescue with unpurged autologous stem cells was then done. Twenty-six patients who had evidence of disease at the time of transplantation received post-transplantation radiation therapy of 20–40 Gy to the involved field.

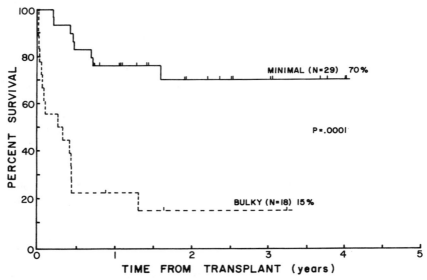

Fig 5–5.—Actuarial event-free survival according to whether patients had minimal or bulky disease (P = .0001). (Courtesy of Rapoport AP, Rowe JM, Kouides PA, et al: *J Clin Oncol* 11:2351–2361, 1993.)

Observations.—Patients with Hodgkin's disease had a median follow-up of 2 years and a 3-year actuarial event-free survival rate of 49%. Those with non-Hodgkin's lymphoma had a median follow-up of 19 months and an event-free survival rate of 40%. The absence of any area of disease measuring 2 cm or more at admission correlated with an improved event-free survival. For patients with Hodgkin's disease, bulky disease decreased the projected event-free survival rate from 70% to 15% (Fig 5–5). For patients with non-Hodgkin's lymphoma, the event-free survival rate decreased from 48% to 25% if bulky disease was seen at admission. Post-transplantation radiation therapy correlated with improved event-free survival for patients with non-Hodgkin's lymphoma. Preparative treatment was well tolerated by patients who had minimal disease when admitted, but it produced significant toxicity in patients with bulky disease.

Conclusion.—The initial extent of Hodgkin's disease or non-Hodgkin's lymphoma is a useful predictor of event-free survival rate in patients who undergo autotransplantation. The BEAC preparative regimen used is effective and safe, particularly in patients without bulky disease. Post-transplantation irradiation of the involved field may improve the outcome in selected patients with non-Hodgkin's lymphoma.

▶ There is no question that patients with relapsed Hodgkin's disease who would otherwise be lost have been saved with bone marrow transplantation (BMT). In my experience, patients with Hodgkin's disease are more likely to be truly salvaged with BMT than are patients with other lymphomas.—P.H. Wiernik, M.D.

Escalating Dose of Mitoxantrone With High-Dose Cyclophosphamide, Carmustine, and Etoposide in Patients With Refractory Lymphoma Undergoing Autologous Bone Marrow Transplantation
Attal M, Canal P, Schlaifer D, Chatelut E, Dezeuze A, Huguet F, Payen C, Pris J, Laurent G (Purpan Hosp and Claudius Regaud Ctr, Toulouse, France)
J Clin Oncol 12:141–148, 1994   116-95-5–15

Purpose.—Various high-dose chemotherapy regimens have been used to prepare patients with malignant lymphoma for autologous bone marrow transplantation (ABMT). A dose-finding study was conducted for mitoxantrone administered in combination with high-dose cyclophosphamide, carmustine, and etoposide to patients with refractory lymphoma undergoing ABMT.

Methods.—Twenty patients aged 23–58 years were treated during a 5-day period with escalating doses of mitoxantrone and high-dose carmustine. Six patients had refractory Hodgkin's disease and 14 had non-Hodgkin's lymphoma. All patients had been unresponsive to conventional chemotherapy before undergoing ABMT, and 7 patients also had received mediastinal irradiation. Plasma mitoxantrone concentrations were measured using high-performance liquid chromatography.

Results.—The mean duration of neutropenia was 24.4 days, and the mean duration of thrombocytopenia was 19.7 days. Twelve patients (60%) achieved a complete remission and 6 (30%) a partial remission, for an overall response rate of 90%. The maximum tolerated mitoxantrone dose was 75 mg/m². Toxic deaths or major organ toxicities did not occur, but 2 of 5 patients treated with mitoxantrone doses of 90 mg/m² had severe organ failure. The probability of survival 2 years after ABMT was 34%.

Conclusion.—Combination therapy with mitoxantrone, up to 75 mg/m², and etoposide, when used to prepare patients with refractory lymphoma for ABMT, has an acceptable toxicity and a promising complete remission rate.

▶ Mitoxantrone has been underused in lymphoma. This is only 1 representative study that suggests mitoxantrone deserves study in initial treatments for lymphoma. Keating and associates at M.D. Anderson Hospital have studied a combination of mitoxantrone plus fludarabine in low-grade lymphoma that seems especially promising.—P.H. Wiernik, M.D.

High-Dose Chemotherapy and Autologous Hematopoietic Stem-Cell Transplantation for Aggressive Non-Hodgkin's Lymphoma

Vose JM, Anderson JR, Kessinger A, Bierman PJ, Coccia P, Reed EC, Gordon B, Armitage JO (Univ of Nebraska, Omaha)
J Clin Oncol 11:1846–1851, 1993   116-95-5–16

Background.—Previous studies have shown high-dose chemotherapy combined with stem cell transplantation to be a successful treatment modality for patients with recurrent non-Hodgkin's lymphoma. The impact of this treatment combination on clinical and tumor progression was assessed in patients with intermediate-grade recurrent non-Hodgkin's lymphoma.

Methods.—During an 8-year period at a single center, 158 patients with intermediate-grade, relapsed, or primary refractory non-Hodgkin's lymphoma received high-dose chemotherapy and either autologous bone marrow transplantation (ABMT) or peripheral stem-cell transplantation (PSCT). A prognostic model was developed and the cohort was divided into a good-prognosis group and a poor-prognosis group based on tumor size and the presence of 1 (good prognosis) or more (poor prognosis) of the following adverse conditions: 3 or more previous chemotherapy regimens, an above normal lactate dehydrogenase level, or chemoresistance. The effects of each transplantation type on failure-free survival were assessed with each group. Immunophenotype was analyzed in 138 of the patients.

Results.—Patients with a B-cell immunophenotype had a lower failure-free survival rate than did those with a T-cell immunophenotype. Of the 158 patients, 51 had achieved failure-free survival at 21 months (compared with a 29% actuarial failure-free survival rate). The effects of the transplantation types were differential. There was no difference between ABMT and PSCT effects in the poor-prognosis group, whereas in the good-prognosis group, the 3-year failure-free survival rate was more than twice as high for those who received PSCT as for those who received ABMT (70% vs. 32%).

Discussion.—The success of this treatment regimen on the good-prognosis group sugggests that patients should not be denied transplantation based on only 1 adverse indication. The data also suggest that chemoresistance, although important, may be related to other prognostic factors. The comparatively high success rate with PSCT compared with ABMT in the good-prognosis group is important and may indicate that the timing of treatment correlates with maximal peripheral stem cell effectiveness.

▶ The PSCT may well replace ABMT as the preferred cell-support therapy for lymphoma patients undergoing high-dose chemotherapy.—P.H. Wiernik, M.D.

Outcome and Complications

Experiences of the First 493 Unrelated Marrow Donors in the National Marrow Donor Program
Stroncek DF, Holland PV, Bartch G, Bixby T, Simmons RG, Antin JH, Anderson KC, Ash RC, Bolwell BJ, Hansen JA, Heal JM, Henslee-Downey PJ, Jaffé ER, Klein HG, Lau PM, Perkins HA, Popovsky MA, Price TH, Rowley SD, Stehling LC, Weiden PL, Wissel ME, McCullough J (Univ of Minnesota, Minneapolis; Sacramento Med Found Blood Ctr, Calif; Univ of Pittsburgh, Pa; et al)
Blood 81:1940–1946, 1993   116-95-5-17

Background.—Previous reports suggest that bone marrow donation rarely results in life-threatening complications or death, but information on minor complications and on the long-term consequences of marrow donation is insufficient. More than 410,000 individuals participated in the National Marrow Donor Program (NMDP) until late 1991; more than 850 volunteers had donated marrow.

Study Population.—Donor complications and marrow recovery times were examined in the first 493 individuals donating bone marrow through the NMDP. The donors, seen at 42 centers, had a median age of 38 years. The median volume of bone marrow collected was 1,050 mL. Nearly 90% of the donors received autologous red cells, but only 3 donors (.6%) received allogeneic blood.

Complications.—Six percent of donors had acute complications related to marrow collection, but only 1 had a serious complication—apnea occurring during anesthesia. Tiredness, pain at the collection site, and low-back pain were frequently reported when donors were questioned 2 days after discharge. The mean time to complete recovery was 16 days, but in 10% of donors, more than a month passed before all symptoms resolved. The duration of the collection procedure correlated with subsequent pain and fatigue. The amount of marrow collected appeared to be less important than either the collection time or the duration of anesthesia. Multivariate analysis showed that only the marrow collection time correlated significantly with the time to recovery.

Discussion.—Donating bone marrow is generally well tolerated and produces few complications. The recovery period may be minimized by decreasing the time needed to collect marrow and, probably, the volume collected as well.

▶ It is reassuring to know that marrow donation is safe, but what are the results with these donations? How many potential donors were worked up to provide the 850 donations, and what is the outcome of the resultant transplants?—P.H. Wiernik, M.D.

Extended Follow-Up in 212 Long-Term Allogeneic Bone Marrow Transplant Survivors: Issues of Quality of Life
Schmidt GM, Niland JC, Forman SJ, Fonbuena PP, Dagis AC, Grant MM, Ferrell BR, Barr TA, Stallbaum BA, Chao NJ, Blume KG (City of Hope Med Ctr, Duarte, Calif; Stanford Univ Hosp, Calif)
Transplantation 55:551–557, 1993   116-95-5–18

Objective.—Quality of life was evaluated in 212 patients who underwent allogeneic bone marrow transplantation (BMT) and at least 1 year of follow-up. There were 162 adults and 50 pediatric patients included. Most were interviewed over the phone using an instrument that covered health status and treatment-related symptoms, level of activity and functioning, and qualitative aspects of daily life.

Observations.—More than two thirds of adults who previously had been employed or were in school full time had returned to full-time activity at the time of assessment. Ninety percent of the children had returned to school or were working full time. All of the children and 89% of the adults had Karnofsky performance ratings of 90 or 100. A number of symptoms, including those of chronic graft-vs.-host disease, were more prevalent in adults. Cataracts frequently developed in children who received total body irradiation in conjunction with BMT. When the overall quality of life was rated on a scale of 1 to 10, adults had a median score of 9, and children, 9.5 (10 being the highest rating). Poor self-ratings by adults were associated with both sexual dissatisfaction and the need for regular medication.

Conclusion.—Most adult and pediatric survivors of BMT have good quality of life.

▶ A generally encouraging survey.—P.H. Wiernik, M.D.

Acute Graft-Versus-Host Disease Prophylaxis With Methotrexate and Cyclosporine After Busulfan and Cyclophosphamide in Patients With Hematologic Malignancies
von Bueltzingsloewen A, Belanger R, Perreault C, Bonny Y, Roy D-C, Lalonde Y, Boileau J, Kassis J, Lavallee R, Lacombe M, Gyger M (Université de Montréal)
Blood 81:849–855, 1993   116-95-5–19

Background.—Combined treatment with methotrexate and cyclosporine produced significantly less morbidity and mortality after allogeneic bone marrow transplantation (BMT), but the additive toxic effects of ablative preparative measures may preclude optimal immunoprophylaxis.

Objective.—The feasibility of methotrexate-cyclosporine prophylaxis was examined in 101 consecutive patients with hematologic malignancy who received HLA-matched bone marrow transplants and busulfan and cyclophosphamide.

Treatment.—Busulfan, 4 mg/kg/day, and cyclophosphamide, 50 mg/kg/day, were administered for 4 days. Post-transplant immunosuppression consisted of methotrexate in a dose of 15 mg/m² on day 1 and 10 mg/m² on days 3, 6, and 11 combined with intravenous cyclosporine in a dose of 1.5 mg/kg every 12 hours. Nearly three fourths of the patients received a full course of methotrexate and achieved a therapeutic cyclosporine concentration of 250–600 ng/mL.

Results.—The frequency of grade II–IV acute graft-vs.-host disease was 9.2% overall and 5.5% in patients receiving optimal prophylaxis. Of 89 patients who lived for at least 100 days after BMT, 48% subsequently had chronic graft-vs.-host disease. The estimated rate of relapse was 29% overall and 15% in low-risk patients after a median follow-up of about 2 years. Relapse was associated with both high-risk features and the absence of chronic graft-vs.-host disease. Disease-free survival was significantly greater in patients receiving optimal prophylaxis, reflecting fewer early deaths from acute graft-vs.-host disease and infection.

Conclusion.—A combination of methotrexate and cyclosporine is quite effective in preventing acute graft-vs.-host disease in patients with hematologic malignancy who are to undergo BMT. Treatment-related deaths are less frequent as a result, and disease-free survival is significantly improved.

Veno-Occlusive Disease of the Liver and Multiorgan Failure After Bone Marrow Transplantation: A Cohort Study of 355 Patients

McDonald GB, Hinds MS, Fisher LD, Schoch HG, Wolford JL, Banaji M, Hardin BJ, Shulman HM, Clift RA (Fred Hutchinson Cancer Research Ctr, Seattle; Univ of Washington, Seattle)

Ann Intern Med 118:255–267, 1993   116-95-5–20

Introduction.—Surviving bone marrow transplantation involves recovery from cytoreductive treatment, successful grafting, avoidance of infections and graft-vs.-host disease, and cure of the primary disorder. One complication of this type of surgery is veno-occlusive disease (VOD) of the liver, which appears to be related to a patient's having hepatitis at the time of transplant. The incidence, clinical course, and risk factors of VOD in patients undergoing bone marrow transplantation were studied.

Methods.—All 355 surviving patients undergoing bone marrow transplantation in 1 year were examined for VOD, which included an assessment of hyperbilirubinemia, hepatomegaly or right upper quadrant liver-related pain, and sudden weight gain within 20 days of transplant surgery.

Results.—Of the 355 patients, 190 had VOD, for an incidence rate of 54%. Fifty-four invididuals had severe VOD, 92 had moderate VOD, and 44 had mild VOD. Eighty-six patients had "no liver disease." The elevated serum transaminase concentrations correlated highly with the severity of VOD. Severe VOD appeared related to specific cytoreductive therapy methods such as total body irradiation, busulfan plus cyclophosphamide treatment, cyclophosphamide, 1,3-bis[2-chloroethyl]-1-nitrosourea, and etoposide combination treatment. Administering either vancomycin or amphotericin simultaneously with cytoreductive treatments increased platelet transfusion requirements, organ failure, dying before day 100, and significant sudden weight gain associated with severe VOD, whereas GM-CSF appeared to protect against this disease.

Conclusion.—Veno-occlusive disease developed in more than half of the bone marrow transplant recipients and sometimes led to renal and cardiopulmonary failure. An increase in the pretransplant transaminase level, the occurrence of persistent fever, and the use of high-dose cytoreductive therapy can help to predict the development of severe veno-occlusive disease in these patients.

▶ Severe VOD occurred in 15% of the transplant series and was fatal in all but 1 patient. This is a major complication of bone marrow transplantation. This paper suggests methods by which the incidence of VOD may be reduced such as selection of patients with normal hepatic function and no previous abdominal irradiation. It also suggests that mismatched or unrelated-donor transplants should be considered very carefully and that such transplants should not be considered routine.—P.H. Wiernik, M.D.

Naturally Occurring Anticoagulants and Bone Marrow Transplantation: Plasma Protein C Predicts the Development of Venocclusive Disease of the Liver

Faioni EM, Krachmalnicoff A, Bearman SI, Federici AB, Decarli A, Gianni AM, McDonald GB, Mannucci PM (Univ of Milan, Italy; Fred Hutchinson Cancer Research Ctr, Seattle; Milan Cancer Inst, Italy)
Blood 81:3458–3462, 1993   116-95-5-21

Background.—Veno-occlusive disease (VOD) of the liver is the major dose-limiting complication of bone marrow transplantation (BMT) for malignant diseases. Recent reports have indicated that hemostatic mechanisms are involved in the development of VOD. The status of protein C, antithrombin III, and protein S in patients undergoing BMT for hematologic malignancies was investigated, and an early predictive marker for the development of VOD was sought.

Methods.—Fifty patients participated. All were undergoing BMT for hematologic malignancies. Measurements of naturally occurring anticoagulants, protein C, protein S, and antithrombin III were made from blood samples drawn at 4 times: before starting cyclophosphamide, after cyclophosphamide, after total body irradiation, and after BMT. The patients were categorized as having either VOD of the liver or no liver disease after cytoreductive therapy.

Results.—Of the 50 patients originally enrolled, 29 experienced VOD. Measurement of blood samples revealed that protein C decreased from before cytoreductive therapy to post-transplant, but levels of protein S and antithrombin III did not change. Patients undergoing BMT who had VOD develop had lower baseline protein C levels than patients in whom VOD did not develop. Specificity of baseline protein C for predicting VOD was 87%; sensitivity was 69%. No correlation was found between baseline protein C levels less than 88% and severity of VOD. Comparison of protein C with other risk factors for VOD revealed that 5 of 7 patients with no known risk factors who contracted VOD were identified by low baseline protein C levels. Although 7 of 16 patients without VOD had at least 1 risk factor, protein C levels in these patients were normal.

Conclusion.—Protein C was the only hemostatic variable found to predict the development of VOD of the liver in patients undergoing BMT. Low levels of protein C may play a part in the pathogenesis of VOD. Further trials are now required to investigate the prophylaxis or treatment of VOD with protein C concentrates in high-risk patients.

▶ The comment here is that VOD of the liver remains a major obstacle in BMT. The authors present some information that suggests that a reduction in protein C may be responsible for the hypercoagulable state. Somewhat problematic is the fact that protein S is not reduced in this study. Both protein C and protein S are synthesized in the liver. Why is only 1 of these proteins reduced after the cytoreductive chemotherapy?—W.R. Bell, M.D.

The Spectrum of Non-*Candida* Fungal Infections Following Bone Marrow Transplantation

Morrison VA, Haake RJ, Weisdorf DJ (Univ of Minnesota, Minneapolis)
Medicine 72:78–89, 1993   116-95-5–22

Background.—Severely immunocompromised cancer patients are especially vulnerable to fungal infection, which is a major cause of morbidity and mortality. The incidence, progress, and outcome of non-*Candida* fungal infections were examined in patients who received bone marrow transplantation (BMT).

Methods.—In a single-center, 15-year study, 1,186 patients who underwent BMT were evaluated for non-*Candida* fungal infection. Infections were treated and the outcome was assessed.

Results.—Significant infection developed in 11% of patients, with 6% of the infected patients being affected by multiple fungal isolates. Seventeen fungal isolates were identified, and the infections produced 4 clinical expressions: minor skin or soft tissue infections, single-organ or single-site infections, disseminated fungemia, and isolated fungemia. The most common isolates were *Aspergillus* and then *Fusarium* and *Alternaria* (table). Mortality was highest among patients infected with *Aspergillus, Chrysosporium, Fusarium, Mucor,* or *Scopulariopsis.* These isolates were also significantly associated with invasive (affecting organs, especially pulmonary involvement) or disseminated disease. *Acremonium, Alternaria, Penicillium,* and *Saccharomyces* were among the generally nonlethal isolates and were associated with either isolated fungemia or localized skin or soft tissue infection.

Clinical Subtype of Infection and Fungal Isolates

| | | Clinical Subtype of Infection | | | |
| | | | Number (%) | | |
Fungal Isolate	Total n=138	Minor Skin & Soft Tissue n=7	Single Organ or Single Site n=61	Disseminated n=58	Isolated Fungemia n=12
Acremonium	3 (2)	—	—	—	3 (25)
Alternaria	6 (4)	—	6 (10)	—	—
Aspergillus	97 (70)	5 (71)	49 (80)	43 (74)	—
Chrysosporium	1 (1)	—	—	1 (2)	—
Curvularia	1 (1)	—	1 (2)	—	—
Fusarium	10 (7)	—	2 (2)	7 (12)	1 (8)
Hansenula	1 (1)	—	—	—	1 (8)
Histoplasma	3 (2)	—	—	3 (5)	—
Malassezia	1 (1)	—	—	—	1 (8)
Mucor	3 (2)	—	1 (2)	2 (3)	—
Penicillium	2 (1)	—	—	—	2 (17)
Phialophora	1 (1)	—	1 (2)	—	—
Phoma	1 (1)	1 (14)	—	—	—
Rhodotorula	1 (1)	—	—	—	1 (8)
Saccharomyces	2 (1)	—	1 (2)	—	1 (8)
Scopulariopsis	2 (1)	1 (14)	—	1 (2)	—
Trichosporon	3 (2)	—	—	1 (2)	2 (17)

(Courtesy of Morrison VA, Haake RJ, Weisdorf DJ: *Medicine* 72:78–89, 1993.)

Discussion.—Effective treatment of non-*Candida* fungal infections is challenging, and clinical outcome is poor. Prolonged treatment with amphotericin B is best. However, CSFs, especially macrophage CSFs, may improve the outcome in patients with invasive fungal infections. Because diagnosis usually is not made until these infections are well established, improved prophylactic techniques must be developed.

▶ A well-written, exhaustive review of this problem at 1 major transplant center.—P.H. Wiernik, M.D.

Viridans Streptococcal Shock in Bone Marrow Transplantation Patients

Steiner M, Villablanca J, Kersey J, Ramsay N, Haake R, Ferrieri P, Weisdorf D (Univ of Minnesota, Minneapolis)
Am J Hematol 42:354–358, 1993   116-95-5-23

Background.—The marked immune suppression that accompanies bone marrow transplantation (BMT) leaves the recipients very susceptible to infection. The viridans streptococci that inhabit the oropharynx and bowel have low infective potential in ordinary circumstances, but a rapidly progressive and frequently fatal shock syndrome has been seen in association with viridans streptococcal sepsis in some recipients of BMT.

Objective.—The prevalence of viridans streptococcal infection and of shock was examined in 832 patients undergoing BMT at 1 center between 1976 and 1988.

Findings.—Blood or CSF cultures were positive for viridans streptococci in 123 of the 832 recipients of BMT. Ten of the patients with sepsis (8%) had clinical shock within a month of transplantation. A single streptococcal strain was responsible in 9 patients; 1 also had *Staphylococcus, epidermidis* bacteremia. All patients who had shock were children (median age, 8.6 years). All were neutropenic at the time bacteremia developed, and most remained so for days to weeks after the initial positive culture. The most frequent viridans streptococcal species, isolated from 7 patients, was *Streptococcus mitis*. None of the isolates had unusual antibiotic sensitivity profiles.

Course and Outcome.—All but 2 of the 10 patients required inotropic support and vasodilators, and all of them required ventilatory support. Seven patients had marked neurologic disorder, including 5 with encephalopathy, 2 with symptoms of elevated intracranial pressure, and 1 with hemorrhagic infarction. Six patients died of shock or of secondary complications a median of 15 days after the onset of symptoms. The 4 surviving patients recovered completely clinically and microbiologically. The institution of antibiotic therapy before symptoms of shock developed, even with a regimen including vancomycin, did not improve survival. All

4 autopsies revealed severe lung damage with hyaline membrane formation and diffuse alveolar injury.

Conclusion.—Certain strains of viridans streptococci may trigger a state of fulminant shock in immunocompromised recipients of BMT.

▶ An important newly discovered cause of failure after BMT, especially in young patients.—P.H. Wiernik, M.D.

High-Dose Cyclophosphamide-Induced Myocardial Damage During BMT: Assessment by Positron Emission Tomography

Gardner SF, Lazarus HM, Bednarczyk EM, Creger RJ, Miraldi FD, Leisure G, Green JA (Case Western Reserve Univ, Cleveland, Ohio)
Bone Marrow Transplant 12:139–144, 1993   116-95-5–24

Background.—High-dose cyclophosphamide is a key part of chemotherapeutic preparative regimens for patients undergoing bone marrow transplantation (BMT), even though it has significant myocardial toxicity. Predicting this cardiotoxicity has been a clinical problem, with conventional techniques (e.g., ECG or echocardiography) demonstrating insufficient sensitivity. This prospective study compared serial ECG and positron emission tomography (PET) in the prediction of cyclophosphamide cardiotoxicity.

Methods.—The study sample included 12 patients scheduled for autologous BMT, all of whom underwent serial ECGs and PET scans before and after high-dose cyclophosphamide administration. Possible alterations in ^{13}N-ammonia perfusion and ^{18}F-2-deoxyglucose metabolism were sought in an attempt to define a cellular expression of cardiotoxicity. Eight healthy volunteers were also studied to identify any possible pre-BMT difference that predisposed to the development of cyclophosphamide cardiotoxicity.

Results.—In the patients, there were no significant global or regional changes in either myocardial N-13 ammonia or 18-fluorodeoxyglucose from baseline to follow-up. There were no significant differences between either of the patient studies and the control studies. One of the patients did have ^{13}N-ammonia perfusion in the inferior region at the same time as ECG T-wave inversions in the inferior leads, possibly because of alterations in myocardial blood flow or membrane permeability. Reductions in summed voltage on the ECG occurred in the absence of clinical cardiotoxicity.

Conclusion.—Positron emission tomography scans appear unable to predict cardiotoxicity in BMT patients receiving high-dose cyclophosphamide. Further prospective studies are needed in the subgroup of patients who have ECG changes. Several patients could not tolerate PET scanning because of hip pain from lying on the scanner table.

Cataract Formation After Bone Marrow Transplantation

Tichelli A, Gratwohl A, Egger T, Roth J, Prünte A, Nissen C, Speck B (Univ Hosps, Basel, Switzerland)
Ann Intern Med 119:1175–1180, 1993   116-95-5–25

Introduction.—Cataract formation is among the most common of late complications of total body irradiation in patients undergoing bone marrow transplantation. Single-dose total body irradiation of 10 Gy or more consistently produces cataracts, whereas fractionating the radiation dose results in cataract formation in fewer than 20% of patients after 4 years of follow-up.

Study Population.—One hundred ninety-seven patients undergoing allogeneic or autologous bone marrow transplants at least 6 months earlier were examined to identify factors associated with cataract formation. Indications for marrow transplantation included malignant hematologic disorders and severe aplastic anemia. The 105 males and 92 females had a median age of 25 years. Seventy-four patients received single-dose total body irradiation, 90 received fractionated total body irradiation, and 33 received only chemotherapy in preparation for marrow transplantation.

Observations.—Cataracts developed in 36% of patients a median of 38 months after bone marrow transplantation. Twenty-three percent of the patients required surgery for their cataracts. The frequency of cataract was 69% in patients prepared with single-dose total body irradiation but only 20% in those receiving fractionated radiation. Only 1 of the 33 patients receiving chemotherapy alone had cataract develop after marrow transplantation. On multivariate regression analysis, prednisone treatment for longer than 3 months doubled the risk of cataract developing, but chronic graft-vs.-host disease was not a significant factor.

Conclusion.—The rarity of isolated ocular relapse of leukemia suggests that shielding the lens be considered when patients receive total body irradiation in preparation for bone marrow transplantation.

▶ An important quality-of-life issue.—P.H. Wiernik, M.D.

Prophylactic Use of Ganciclovir for Allogeneic Bone Marrow Transplant Recipients

von Bueltzingsloewen A, Bordigoni P, Witz F, Bene MC, Schmitt C, Lacour B, Sommelet D (Hôpital d'Enfants, Nancy, France; Faculté de Medicine, Nancy, France)
Bone Marrow Transplant 12:197–202, 1993   116-95-5–26

Background.—Cytomegalovirus (CMV) infection is a major cause of morbidity and mortality in 30% to 50% of patients undergoing bone marrow transplantation (BMT). The use of ganciclovir to decrease CMV infection in high-risk patients was investigated.

Patients and Methods.—Study participants included 40 BMT recipients with hematologic malignancies or inherited diseases. Twenty-nine were CMV seropositive and 11 were seronegative with a seropositive donor. Ganciclovir was administered prophylactically before or after transplantation, or both, to all CMV-seropositive patients and seronegative patients with seropositive donors. All patients were transfused with screened blood products, and 33 also received CMV hyperimmune globulin. An historical group of 39 patients who had received significantly more unscreened blood products and fewer HLA-mismatched marrow transplants served as controls.

Results.—The toxicity of ganciclovir was hematologic, and in 7 patients neutropenia was responsible for cessation of the drug. Transfusion requirements were higher in the ganciclovir group than in controls. The cumulative incidence of CMV infection in the first 120 days post-transplant was 2.5% in the treated group and 59% in the nontreated control patients. There were no cases of CMV pneumonitis in the treated group, but 4 occurred in the untreated group. Twenty-three patients in the untreated group had CMV infection after a median of 45 days post-transplant, but no cases of CMV infection were found in the treated group after cessation of ganciclovir. Eighteen patients in the ganciclovir group died within the first year post-transplant. The causes of death were related to regimen-induced toxicity and chronic graft-vs.-host disease; none were related to CMV. In contrast, there were 6 deaths within the first year after transplant in the control group, 3 of which were CMV related.

Conclusion.—The prophylactic administration of ganciclovir prevents CMV pneumonitis and considerably decreases the incidence of CMV infection in high-risk BMT recipients. However, despite the reduction in CMV infection, the overall survival was not improved in the patients taking ganciclovir. This may be the result of a significantly higher proportion of patients being transplanted with advanced disease and of using HLA-nongenoidentical transplants. Further studies are needed to define more precisely the role of ganciclovir in the prevention of CMV infection after BMT.

▶ The toxicity of the agent should preclude its routine prophylactic use.—P.H. Wiernik, M.D.

Metabolic Evidence of Cobalamin Deficiency in Bone Marrow Cells Harvested for Transplantation From Donors Given Nitrous Oxide
Carmel R, Rabinowitz AP, Mazumder A (Univ of Southern California, Los Angeles; Kenneth J Norris Jr Comprehensive Cancer Ctr, Los Angeles)
Eur J Haematol 50:228–233, 1993   116-95-5–27

Background.—Nitrous oxide exposure beyond 4–6 hours inactivates cobalamin. However, shorter exposure appears to produce no hematologic effects and the metabolic deficiency is quickly reversed. The metabolic viability of bone marrow cells harvested from donors anesthetized with nitrous oxide was examined.

Methods.—Bone marrow cells were harvested from 9 donors. Five were anesthetized using nitrous oxide; 4 received other anesthetic agents and served as controls. The deoxyuridine suppression test, which indicates cobalamin deficiency, was performed on the cells the day of harvesting and again on subsequent days. The cells were further tested with the addition of vitamins (hydroxocobalamine, methyl tetrahydrofolate [MTHF], and folinic acid).

Results.—In 4 of the 5 specimens, the cells exhibited profound deoxyuridine suppression. The addition of vitamins yielded mixed results. The addition of MTHF brought no improvement in any specimen. As is characteristic of cobalamin deficiency, the in vitro addition of cobalamin brought only slight or no improvement. Although there was no evidence of folate deficiency, folinic acid did produce significant improvement in 2 samples. Deoxyuridine suppression testing on subsequent days revealed that the deficiency persisted on the second day and was reversed in 1 sample on the third day. After 3 weeks of cryopreservation, the cells were completely normal.

Conclusion.—Nitrous oxide impairs cobalamin metabolism even with brief exposure. The defect is reversed after 2 days of cryopreservation. Marrow that is stored for autologous transplantation will probably be normal when it is used. However, cells that are infused immediately in allogeneic transplants may be impaired. These data support the screening of vitamin levels for all surgical patients when nitrous oxide is to be used; this will prevent the exacerbation of an already established cobalamin deficiency.

▶ These results suggest that nitrous oxide anesthesia should never be used for bone marrow harvesting. Nitrous oxide is a potential antileukemic agent. It selectively reduces the proliferation of rat leukemia cells (1), increases the proportion of early S-phase cells in normal human bone marrow (2), and has demonstrated antileukemic activity in patients (3). The effect of nitrous oxide on the cell cycle might make it worthy of study with a cell-cycle–specific antileukemic agent such as cytarabine.—P.H. Wiernik, M.D.

References

1. Ermenz AAM, et al: *Cancer Lett* 45:123, 1989.
2. Cullen MH, et al: *Br J Haematol* 42:527, 1979.
3. Eastwood PW, et al: *N Engl J Med* 268:297, 1963.

Factors Influencing Third Party Payer Costs for Allogeneic BMT

Griffiths RI, Bass EB, Powe NR, Anderson GF, Goodman S, Wingard JR
(Johns Hopkins Med Institutions, Baltimore, Md; Johns Hopkins Univ,
Baltimore, Md; Emory Univ, Atlanta, Ga)
Bone Marrow Transplant 12:43–48, 1993   116-95-5–28

Objective.—Although several studies have looked at the costs of bone marrow transplantation (BMT), there are few data on how patient characteristics relate to costs, changes in BMT costs, or costs associated with major complications. Third-party payers are increasingly hesitant to cover new ancillary therapies for BMT recipients unless they prove beneficial at reasonable cost. The association between payer costs for allogeneic BMT and patient characteristics and clinical complications was examined.

Methods.—The retrospective analysis included 402 patients undergoing allogeneic BMT between 1980 and 1987 at a university-based BMT center. The investigators looked at total inpatient costs, both hospital and physician, and number of hospitalized days in the first 6 months after BMT. The analysis focused on how payer costs for BMT have changed with time, as well as how such costs relate to patient characteristics and the occurrence of complications.

Results.—All costs were expressed in 1990 dollars. Inpatient payer costs for the first 180 days after BMT averaged $208,410. Adjusted for inflation, these costs increased from $227,806 in 1980 to $308,545 in 1983, then decreased to $156,163 by 1987. Multivariate analysis suggested that costs were strongly associated with cytomegalovirus infection, with an increase of $53,517; acute graft-vs.-host disease, an increase of $46,500; and malignant disease, decrease of $36,633. These associations remained even after adjustment for length of survival and year of BMT. Patient age, sex, and race had no effect on inpatient payer costs.

Conclusion.—Inpatient payer costs for patients undergoing allogeneic BMT have decreased significantly over the years. However, complications (e.g., cytomegalovirus infection and acute graft-vs.-host disease) are associated with very high costs to third-party payers. Attempts to reduce the costs of BMT should focus on reducing these complications.

6 Transfusion Medicine

Introduction

Having just completed my annual excursion through the literature of transfusion medicine, I can happily report to you that the discipline continues to grow, its influence has become wider, and its contributions are increasingly multidisciplinary. If you wander through the selected articles, you will note my continuing bias toward selecting articles of potential clinical relevance. Of interest, however, is the fact that much of the transfusion literature represents collaboration between full-time transfusion medicine practitioners and clinical or basic science partners who have come together to address an acknowledged problem affecting patient care. This healthy trend will continue to bring fertile ideas to new and old problems in the evolving arena of transfusion medicine concerns.

The section on Blood Component Collection and Preparation has a number of intriguing offerings. A paper on apheresis technology in red cell collection has broad implications for the systems by which we procure blood components. A second paper on a new freezing technology is equally exciting and may make cryopreservation more user-friendly. A selection on leukodepletion at the bedside is one of many in the chapter discussing the available methods and rationale of white cell removal. Finally, an article on the use of cytokines to prime granulocyte donors may return white cell transfusions to the forefront of therapy for infected, granulocytopenic patients.

In the Red Cell Immunology section, 2 interesting aspects of our enhanced knowledge of the Rh blood group are featured. One article demonstrates the progress made by cell biologists in understanding the enigmas of the protein. A second selection demonstrates the utility of polymerase chain reaction in determining prenatal Rh to facilitate management of patients at risk for hemolytic disease of the newborn.

The Platelet Immunology and Transfusion section is well stocked this year. Our understanding of platelet activation is being applied to the issues of alloimmune thrombocytopenia. A series of contributions is offered that describe the use of leukocyte filters in the reduction of transfusion reactions to platelets, the potential role of cytokines produced by white cells in enigmatic platelet transfusion reactions, and the continuing problems faced in trying to prevent septic platelet transfusion reactions. Patients with refractory thrombocytopenia may benefit from the wisdom of an article on platelet crossmatching. Treatment of the refractory patient with protein A column therapy is advocated by another article; whether this approach works and what the true incidence of adverse effects is may be answered in coming years.

The Autologous Transfusion section is also large, with articles promoting and advocating restraint with this transfusion strategy. Two articles on the use of perioperative EPO to enhance autologous collection suggest a limited rather than a broad role to prevent surgical transfusions. The continuing growth of autologous transfusions is aptly demonstrated by a study advocating its use in radical prostatectomy, another study suggesting that cell salvage is safe in patients with hepatocellular carcinoma, and 2 orthopedic studies suggesting that preoperative donation is cost-effective in joint replacement but postoperative salvage is probably not worth the effort. The year would not be complete without additional confusion about the role of transfusion in immunomodulation. One article suggests that autologous donation has adverse immunomodulatory effects, whereas another claims that autologous blood prevents infectious complications after colorectal cancer surgery. The widely promoted use of autologous platelet-rich plasma could not withstand the careful scrutiny of study at the Mayo Clinic, where its efficacy in cardiac surgery could not be verified.

The Adult Transfusion Practice section has an unusual potpourri of medical citations. Erythropoietin seems to have some benefit in the perioperative period, and aprotinin facilitated reduced blood loss in hip replacement surgery. A number of protocols are featured to propose rational transfusion approaches to postoperative patients. One study suggests that we may undertransfuse patients who might benefit, whereas another documents the costs of overtransfusion for patients with little likelihood of positive outcomes. Porcine factor VIII is promoted for patients with acquired hemophilia, and leukodepletion is offered as a cost-effective adjuvant to leukemia therapy. Two opposing views of component use are offered: a study from Europe suggests that platelets and cryoprecipitate are not required for liver transplantation, whereas a study from Oregon suggests that the use of component therapy increases donor exposures in massively transfused trauma victims.

The Pediatric Transfusion Therapy section offers a positive study on the use of EPO to prevent late anemia in recipients of intrauterine transfusions for hemolytic disease of the newborn. A useful protocol for the treatment of severe anemia in children and a careful evaluation of the efficacy of prophylactic platelet transfusions in premature infants should be of value to the pediatric hematologists. Finally, a study of inhibitor development in young hemophiliacs treated only with cryoprecipitate may provide a useful baseline for comparison with other populations treated with recombinant factor VIII in whom inhibitor development is a continuing concern.

In the Transplantation and Immunomodulation section, a long-awaited prospective study of tumor recurrence in patients transfused during colorectal surgery for cancer is featured. It is doubtful that this single study will quiet the enthusiasts or satisfy the skeptics, so additional reports should be anticipated. Several carefully performed animal studies may shed some light on this difficult area that is of continuing concern to clinicians and researchers.

The Adverse Effects of Transfusion section continues to be a large component of this annual review. One encouraging study suggests that undertransfusion is more risky than receiving blood for severe anemia. A review of transfusion-associated AIDS by the Centers for Disease Control demonstrates the current low risk. An approach to viral inactivation for platelets demonstrates HIV eradication by photochemical methods. A number of articles describe current dilemmas in our efforts to decrease the risk of post-transfusion HTLV-II, hepatitis C, and cytomegalovirus infection in transfusion recipients. An interesting case report answers a question often proposed by hematologists about whether leukodepletion techniques can eliminate the risk of transfusion-associated graft-vs.-host disease. The answer is no, so irradiation of cellular components remains critical for patients at risk for this lethal transfusion complication.

Paul M. Ness, M.D.

Blood Component Collection and Preparation

Red Cell Collection by Apheresis Technology

Meyer D, Bolgiano DC, Sayers M, Price T, Benson D, Slichter SJ (Puget Sound Blood Ctr, Seattle; Univ of Washington, Seattle)

Transfusion 33:819–824, 1993   116-95-6–1

Background.—Apheresis may increase the volume of blood components collected per donor visit, thereby limiting patient exposure to multiple donors. Adherence to safety considerations may enhance collection of RBCs with apheresis. The feasibility and acceptability of using apheresis to collect 450 mL of RBCs from whole blood donors were evaluated.

Methods.—Twenty whole-blood donors gave a unit of whole blood bimonthly; 20 apheresis donors gave 450 mL of RBCs every fourth month. Adverse reactions or symptoms were recorded by donors in a daily diary and by a phlebotomist during each donor visit.

Results.—No adverse effects occurred during whole blood donations. Mild-to-moderate numbness or tingling of the face or extremities was noted in 83% of apheresis procedures; these symptoms resolved spontaneously or responded to calcium ingestion or plasma return rate reduction. Faintness, nausea, chills, diaphoresis, chest tightness, and hypotension occurred in 20% of the symptomatic apheresis procedures. These symptoms resolved within 10 minutes of saline administration or plasma-return rate reduction. The primary symptom noted by all donors was tiredness after donation. Male donors recovered more quickly than female donors; among apheresis donors, males recovered by day 3 and females recovered by day 4. Seventy percent of apheresis donors considered the procedure acceptable and 15% considered it unacceptable. The remainder were undecided.

Conclusion.—Apheresis technology enables the collection of 2 units of RBCs at a single session. Although apheresis is associated with more symptoms and greater inconvenience than whole blood donation, appropriate modifications to reduce side effects and resolution of scheduling problems should increase the usefulness of apheresis for RBC collection.

▶ The possibility of collecting red cells by apheresis technology is exciting for a number of reasons. From a donor with adequate blood volume and hematocrit, it will be possible to collect 2 units of red cells at the same time. These red cells should be standardized in terms of quantity in a unit and will be "better" red cells because the lesion of collection will not destroy the original aliquot of red cells subjected to excess anticoagulant with current phlebotomy methods. The blood center can benefit by collecting red cells from group O and B donors, particularly Rh-negative donors, and by collecting plasma or platelets from AB donors. The blood recipient would also receive the advantages of reduced donor exposure and a more standardized red cell product. For autologous donors, it may be possible to reduce the number of visits to the blood center. The availability of this technology may revolutionize blood collection procedures.—P.M. Ness, M.D.

Refrigerated Storage of Lyophilized and Rehydrated, Lyophilized Human Red Cells

Sowemimo-Coker SO, Goodrich RP, Zerez CR, Tanaka KR (Cryopharm Corp, Pasadena, Calif; Univ of California, Los Angeles)
Transfusion 33:322–329, 1993   116-95-6-2

Introduction.—Currently, human RBCs are refrigerated in citrate-phosphate preservative solution, allowing a shelf life of 35–42 days. Storage at $-65°C$ or below extends the shelf life for as long as 10 years but requires a low-temperature freezer and extensive washing of the thawed cells to remove glycerol. Storage in the lyophilized state may be a useful alternative.

Objective and Methods.—The effects of lyophilization of RBCs on their metabolic and rheologic properties were examined by collecting human RBCs in citrate-phosphate-dextrose-adenosine (CPDA)-1 and then freeze-drying them in lyoprotective solution. The lyophilized cells were stored at $-20°C$ for 7 days before being rehydrated and washed in dextrose-saline. The cells then were resuspended in final wash solutions of ADSOL, CPDA-1, or a special solution containing glucose, citrate, phosphate, adenine, and mannitol. Resuspended cells were stored at 4°C for another week.

Results.—The reconstituted lyophilized RBCs maintained levels of adenosine triphosphate (ATP), 2,3-diphosphoglycerate (2,3-DPG) and lactate that were at least equal to those in control nonlyophilized cells stored for a similar period in CPDA-1. Osmotic deformability profiles were also similar. Levels of ATP and 2,3-DPG were better maintained in reconstituted lyophilized RBCs stored at 4°C after rehydration than in control RBCs stored in the same solutions for comparable periods.

Conclusion.—Human RBCs may be successfully lyophilized for storage in standard blood bank preservatives. Their rheologic properties and levels of ATP and 2,3-DPG are well maintained even without rejuvenation at 4°C after rehydration.

▶ Although most transfusion needs for red cells can be met acceptably with liquid storage for the currently allowable 42 days, the storage of rare units and occasional cases of autologous transfusion require longer periods of storage capability achievable with frozen blood. Current methodologies of red cell freezing are costly and cumbersome. If a technology were available to provide long-term red cell storage relatively inexpensively with a technique that would quickly make stored red cells available for transfusion, the indications for long-term storage would probably broaden. These techniques using lyophilized and rehydrated red cells may meet these requirements. If this procedure pans out, one could envision stockpiling red cells at times of peak donor availability in the spring and fall for use in periods of chronic donor shortages such as the summer.—P.M. Ness, M.D.

Quality Control of Red Cell Filtration at the Patient's Bedside
Sirchia G, Rebulla P, Parravicini A, Marangoni F, Cortelezzi A, Stefania A (Ospedale Maggiore, Milan, Italy)
Transfusion 34:26–30, 1994

116-95-6-3

Objective.—Concern has been raised about the quality of bedside filtration, in particular that filtration protocol violations could result in unpredictable WBC removal. Filtration with the latest generation of flatbed polyester filters was evaluated in the laboratory and clinical settings.

Methods.—In the laboratory, 25 RBC units were suspended for 1–2 days and 10 units for 14 to 21 days in additive solution. The units were then filtered through each filter, after which an automated complete blood count and a manual WBC count were made in 2 samples per unit. One sample was collected from a segment clamped at 5 and 25 cm below the filter along the line connecting the prefiltration and postfiltration bag, and the other was collected from the postfiltration bag. In the hematology outpatient clinic, nurses administered 25 RBC units stored for 1–2 days through each type of filter to patients. After transfusion, a blood sample was collected from the transfusion set for a WBC count, without filter priming or saline rinsing.

Results.—After laboratory filtration, WBC counts in the segment samples were comparable to those from the filtration bags. White blood cell counts were also similar in the segments collected at bedside, except for 14- to 21-day-old RBCs filtered in the laboratory through 1 of the filters; these filters produced slightly higher WBC counts in the segments than in the postfiltration bags. The WBC count in the postfiltration bag was never higher than that in the segment. Nurses were easily trained in the use of bedside filtration, which resulted in no adverse effects.

Conclusion.—Bedside RBC filtration might be as good as that performed in the laboratory. It is, at least in settings in which blood transfusion is a familiar practice and in which nurses have adequate training. Quality control of RBC bedside filtration is both feasible and simple.

▶ The many controversies surrounding the clinical indications for leukodepleted blood are being resolved by studies in the literature and ongoing investigations. However, another area of controversy is the best method of providing leukodepleted blood components for those patients likely to benefit. The principal options are prestorage leukodepletion in a blood bank or bedside filtration by nurses or other clinical unit personnel. Many blood bankers would share my bias that prestorage leukodepletion is better because it can be performed under standardized conditions amenable to quality control procedures. This investigation from Italy implies that similar results can be obtained with bedside filters if appropriate training programs are instituted and maintained.—P.M. Ness, M.D.

The Effects of Daily Recombinant Human Granulocyte Colony-Stimulating Factor Administration on Normal Granulocyte Donors Undergoing Leukapheresis
Bensinger WI, Price TH, Dale DC, Appelbaum FR, Clift R, Lilleby K, Williams B, Storb R, Thomas ED, Buckner CD (Fred Hutchinson Cancer Research Ctr, Seattle; Univ of Washington, Seattle; Puget Sound Blood Ctr, Seattle)
Blood 81:1883–1888, 1993   116-95-6–4

Background.—Difficulties in collecting adequate granulocyte quantities from normal donors and the short half-life of transfused granulocytes have precluded granulocyte transfusion to patients who are infected and neutropenic. Recombinant human G-CSF (rhG-CSF) increases the granulocyte count and may facilitate collection of large quantities from normal donors. The effects of daily administration of rhG-CSF to normal donors were evaluated.

Methods.—Five syngeneic and 2 HLA-identical bone marrow donors and 1 haploidentical son who had not donated marrow received a mean daily dose of rhG-CSF, 5 μg/kg/day, for as long as 14 days. Granulocytes were collected a mean of 7.6 times. Complete blood cell counts, including a 200-cell WBC differential, were performed daily before and after collection and before rhG-CSF administration.

Results.—Peripheral WBC counts increased rapidly after rhG-CSF administration; bands, promyelocytes, metamyelocytes, and myelocytes became apparent in peripheral circulation by day 4. Administration of rhG-CSF significantly increased the quantity of granulocytes collected compared with untreated donors, producing overall a sixfold increase in granulocytes collected. The mean granulocyte quantity was 3 times greater compared with unstimulated donors until day 3, and 13 times greater on day 9. Recipients of granulocytes collected after rhG-CSF had fivefold to tenfold increases in mean peripheral-blood granulocyte counts 18–24 hours after transfusion, with an overall 19-fold increase in the mean granulocyte level compared with historical controls. Neither donors administered rhG-CSF nor recipients of their granulocytes had adverse effects from rhG-CSF.

Conclusion.—These results suggest that rhG-CSF may be safely administered to normal individuals, that rhG-CSF significantly increases granulocyte collection, and that it provides significant levels of circulating granulocytes in recipients who are neutropenic. Additional studies are needed to evaluate rhG-CSF in normal granulocyte donors.

▶ The enthusiasm of many hematologists for the use of granulocyte transfusions has waned over the past 10 years with the development of improved antibiotics and the realization of the inadequacy of the dose of granulocytes generally collected from healthy hemapheresis donors. This paper suggests that rhG-CSF may change that perception. These dramatic results show a major increase in yield in treated donors and no adverse effects in the donors or the granulocyte recipients. As this treatment becomes more available, we may witness greater demand for granulocyte transfusions and greater efficacy for difficult-to-treat cases of bacterial or fungal sepsis in patients with bone marrow failure.—P.M. Ness, M.D.

Red Cell Immunology

Structure and Expression of the RH Locus in the Rh-Deficiency Syndrome

Chérif-Zahar B, Raynal V, Le Van Kim C, D'Ambrosio A-M, Bailly P, Cartron J-P, Colin Y (Institut Natl de Transfusion Sanguine, Paris)
Blood 82:656–662, 1993

116-95-6–5

Background.—The Rh-deficiency syndrome is a rare hemolytic anemia caused by RBC deficiency of Rh proteins. It is associated with morphologic and functional erythrocyte abnormalities, including significant reductions of additional RBC membrane proteins. A Rh deficiency results from either homozygosity for a silent allele at the RH locus (Rh_{null} amorph type) or for a recessive inhibitor at an unlinked locus (Rh_{null} regulator or Rh_{mod}). The Rh genes (*CcEe* and *D*) were recently cloned, allowing Southern blot analysis of mutant DNA structure in affected individuals.

Subjects.—Blood samples were collected from 3 Rh$_{null}$ regulator, 1 Rh$_{null}$ amorph, and 1 Rh$_{mod}$ patients and compared with samples with common Rh phenotypes by immunologic and DNA analysis.

Results.—Membrane preparations from the Rh-deficiency samples were subjected to sodium dodecyl sulfate polyacrylamide gel electrophoresis (SDS-PAGE) and then reacted with anti-Rh antibodies. The immunostaining results indicated that Rh-deficient cells from all mutant types have neither the Cc/Ee nor the D proteins. Immunostaining revealed that Rh-deficient cells also lack LW and membrane glycoproteins. As expected, Southern blot DNA analysis demonstrated that Rh$_{mod}$ and Rh$_{null}$ regulator individuals do not have large alterations in the Rh genes. More surprisingly, the same was true in a Rh$_{null}$ individual. Although the level of Rh messenger RNA was very low, polymerase chain reaction amplification of Rh messenger RNAs did not detect a mutation in the coding region of this gene. This suggests that in this individual, the Rh gene mutation may affect transcriptional activity.

Conclusion.—Various mutations that decrease expression of the Rh genes alter the expression of a variety of erythrocyte surface components. This suggests that the Rh proteins may be a necessary component of an erythrocyte membrane complex that includes several peptides.

▶ It is unlikely that many of us will encounter the Rh-deficiency syndrome (chronic hemolytic anemia with stomatocytosis), but this was such a nice piece of science by Dr. Cartron's group, which has led the way in this field, that I was compelled to include it. As it turns out, Rh$_{null}$ and Rh$_{mod}$ individuals, although unable to express Rh antigens, have no alterations in their Rh genes. Moreover, the defective expression of these genes is associated with the defective expression of a number of other red cell membrane blood group antigens, suggesting that the Rh proteins are necessary either for the transport or stable membrane expression of these other blood group antigens.—J.L. Spivak, M.D.

Immunochemical Characterization of Rhesus Proteins With Antibodies Raised Against Synthetic Peptides
Hermand P, Mouro I, Huet M, Bloy C, Suyama K, Goldstein J, Cartron JP, Bailly P (Institut Natl de Transfusion, Sanguine, Paris; Lindsley F Kimball Research Inst, New York)
Blood 82:669–676, 1993   116-95-6–6

Background.—The importance of Rh blood group antigens has long been recognized. However, the biochemical and molecular biology of these vital proteins has only recently been elucidated. Rh-positive individuals express the major RhD antigen and carry both D and *CcEe* genes at the RH locus, whereas Rh-negative individuals encode the single *CcEe* gene and do not produce D antigen. The antigenic specificity of the *CcEe* gene transcript was examined using polyclonal antibodies directed

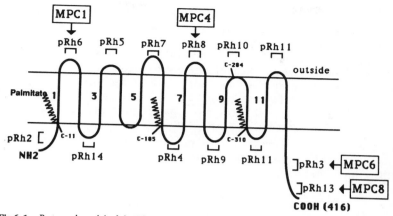

Fig 6–1.—Proposed model of the Rh mature protein encoded by the RhIXb cDNA clone. Schematic drawing showing the topology of the Rh protein within the cell membrane, with both NH2 and COOH termini located intracellularly. Regions corresponding to synthetic peptides used in this study are mentioned, as well as the polyclonal antibodies (*boxes*) specific for the indicated peptides. The surface-exposed cysteine 284 involved in the immunoreactivity of Rh proteins and cysteines 11, 185, and 310 containing a potential palmitate fatty acid chain are indicated. (Courtesy of Hermand P, Mouro I, Huet M, et al: *Blood* 82:669–676, 1993.)

against synthetic peptides. These were chosen on the basis of hydropathy plots and antigenicity index calculations from the predicted coding sequence.

Methods.—The following peptides were chemically synthesized: peptides pRh6 encoding amino acids 33–45, pRh4 spanning residues 185–202 with a Leu substituted Asn residue at position 197, $pRh4_1$ with 2 additional substitutions, a Glu substituted Lys at 192 and a Thr substituted Asn at residue 200, pRh3 encoding for residues 390–404, pRh13 transcribing amino acids 408–416, pRh8 coding for residues 224–233, $pRh8_1$ with a Pro substituted Ala at position 225, and $pRh8_2$ with an Ala to Pro and a Glu to Gln substitution at positions 225 and 232 (Fig 6–1). Polypeptides were probed with human monoclonal antibodies and rabbit polyclonal antibodies harvested during a course of 8 injections of peptide conjugates.

Results.—Specificity for authentic Rh polypeptides was noted for all antibodies. All reacted on Western blot with Rh proteins immunoprecipitated with human monoclonal anti-RhD, -c, and -E. The antibody MPC1, but no other, agglutinated all human erythrocytes save for Rh_{null} and Rh_{mod} cells, which entirely lack or are seriously deficient in Rh proteins, respectively. Immunoblots with membrane proteins from common and rare variants demonstrated that MPC1 and MPC8 reacted in Western blot with 32-Kd Rh polypeptides from all common RBCs containing full, unmodified Rh proteins, implying a ubiquitous distribution of peptide regions 33–45 and 408–416 in several and perhaps all Rh proteins, regardless of blood group specificity. The antibody MPC4 reacted with membrane preparations from cells carrying the E antigen only, whereas MPC6 recognized the Rh proteins from E and Ee preparations. The MPC6 and MPC8 antibodies bound only to the cytoplasmic side of the erythrocyte membrane after immunoadsorption assays using inside-out or right-side-out sealed vesicles from DccEE RBCs as competing antigens. Attempts to transiently or stably express the Rh complementary DNA in eukaryotic cells were unsuccessful, indicating that expression of the Rh antigen at the cell membrane may require proper transport or folding of the Rh proteins, or both.

Conclusion.—In contrast to some previous findings, the topologic evidence supports an intracellular location for the 27 C-terminal residues of the Rh polypeptides.

▶ This paper is one of many attempts to dissect the nature of the Rh protein on the red cell membrane. One of the targets of these studies is to understand why this protein is so immunogenic for Rh-negative recipients. The proposed configuration (Fig 6–1) of the Rh protein should be of interest.—P.M. Ness, M.D.

Prenatal Determination of Fetal RhD Type by DNA Amplification
Bennett PR, Le Van Kim C, Colin Y, Warwick RM, Chérif-Zahar B, Fisk NM, Cartron J-P (Queen Charlotte's and Chelsea Hosp, London; Institut Natl de Transfusion Sanguine, Paris)
N Engl J Med 329:607–610, 1993   116-95-6–7

Introduction.—Administration of anti-RhD antibodies has greatly decreased the incidence of Rh alloimmunization. Even when sensitization has occurred, recent advances in in utero diagnosis and treatment offer improved outcome in affected fetuses. An early and safe method of determining Rh status is desirable in those cases in which alloimmunization is a risk factor and the father is thought to be heterozygous. The currently used methods, fetal-blood sampling and serial aminocentesis, carry the risks of invasive procedures. Whether the fetal RhD genotype could be reliably determined in amniotic fluid cells and chorionic villus cells using DNA amplification was investigated.

Methods.—The RhD type was determined in 15 fetuses using the polymerase chain reaction (PCR) in amniotic cells and serologic methods in fetal blood collected simultaneously. Blood sampling and amniocentesis were clinically indicated in all patients, either by structural markers of aneuploidy or for suspected alloimmunization in RhD-negative mothers. In another 15 fetuses, the RhD type determined from chorionic villus–biopsy samples was compared with that identified by typing of DNA from the fetus itself.

Results.—Analysis of the 2 groups of fetuses was done simultaneously at different laboratories. Investigators at the 2 sites were unaware both of the results from the other site and of the serologic results. The 2 laboratories were in complete agreement on the results of DNA typing. Of 10 fetuses with RhD-negative mothers, 4 were identified as RhD-negative and 6 as RhD-positive. Of 5 fetuses with RhD-positive mothers, 4 were identified as RhD-positive and 1 as RhD-negative. Results of RhD typing of DNA from chorionic-villus samples and from fetal tissue were also in complete agreement. Eleven fetuses were RhD-positive and 4 were RhD-negative. Four RhD-positive fetuses had RhD-negative mothers; 3 RhD-negative fetuses had RhD-positive mothers.

Conclusion.—It is possible to determine fetal RhD type in amniotic cells early in pregnancy and without invading the fetomaternal circulation. None of the samples from RhD-negative fetuses was contaminated by maternal RhD-positive DNA. However, clinicians and laboratory technicians should be aware of the extreme sensitivity of PCR and the dangers of sample contamination. Because the quantity of amniotic fluid required is small, amniocentesis late in the first or early in the second trimester is advocated for fetal Rh typing.

▶ Blood samples can be obtained from infants at risk for hemolytic disease of the newborn, but the invasive procedures required can stimulate alloimmunization or increase the titer of an antibody through an anamnestic response. This paper describes a method that can determine the fetal RhD type of cells from amniotic fluid or chorionic villus biopsy that does not require sampling from the fetal-maternal circulation. As with any PCR method, caution must be used to avoid contamination with maternal cells.—P.M. Ness, M.D.

Platelet Immunology and Transfusion

Characterization of Platelet Activation Induced by HLA Antibodies Associated With Alloimmune Thrombocytopenia

Christie DJ, Leja DN, Carlson DL, Swinehart CD (Univ of Minnesota, Minneapolis)
J Lab Clin Med 121:437–443, 1993   116-95-6–8

Background.—Antibodies to HLAs may lead patients with leukemia bone marrow transplantation recipients, and others requiring intensive platelet support to be refractory to transfused platelets. Alloantibodies from multiply transfused patients can lead to energy-dependent platelet aggregation in vitro and the release of dense granule contacts.

Objective and Methods.—The platelet-activating properties of HLA antibodies were examined in 8 patients who were severely thrombocytopenic and were receiving multiple platelet transfusions. A patient with post-transfusion purpura and 2 women whose newborn infants had alloimmune thrombocytopenia were also included. Antibodies were characterized by their cytotoxic effects on lymphocytes and by a monoclonal antibody antigen-capture enzyme-linked immunoassay.

Results.—Plasma from each patient induced dose-dependent platelet aggregation and the release of adenosine triphosphate (ATP) with antigen-positive platelet-rich plasma. Plasma samples from 3 patients induced normal aggregation and ATP release with platelet-rich plasma from donors who had taken platelet inhibitors such as aspirin. These platelets failed to release ATP when stimulated with adenosine diphosphate. Using a murine monoclonal antibody specific for P-selectin and radiolabeled IgG, samples from each patient induced P-selectin expression at about half the level seen with thrombin.

Conclusion.—Human leukocyte antigen antibodies mediate the expression of P-selectin on the platelet surface and, like thrombin, can activate platelets previously exposed to platelet-inhibiting agents such as aspirin.

▶ Whereas HLA antibodies have been implicated in cases of transfusion failure for many years, the exact mechanism by which these antibodies produce the platelet-refractory state has not been clearly identified. These studies demonstrate that anti-HLA antibodies or platelet-specific antibodies activate the platelet as efficiently as thrombin and mediate the expression of activation markers on the platelet surface. In addition, an intact Fc portion of the immunoglobulin molecule appears to be required for this process. If alloimmunization prevention strategies fail, studies of this type may result in other therapies to treat the refractory state.—P.M. Ness, M.D.

Prevalence of Platelet Transfusion Reactions Before and After Implementation of Leukocyte-Depleted Platelet Concentrates by Filtration
Goodnough LT, Riddell J IV, Lazarus H, Chafel TL, Prince G, Hendrix D, Yomtovian R (Case Western Reserve Univ, Cleveland, Ohio)
Vox Sang 65:103–107, 1993   116-95-6–9

Introduction.—Leukocyte-associated reactions are a common cause of morbidity after transfusion of blood components. An intervention that could decrease such complications would decrease both the morbidity and expense associated with transfusion. Routine use of a Pall PL 50 filter to leukocyte-deplete random donor platelet concentrates was instituted. Platelet transfusion reactions were examined to determine the effectiveness of this regimen.

Study Design.—Platelet transfusion reactions were examined for the 6-month period before (interval 1) and for a 6-month period of leukodepletion filtration (interval 2).

Results.—During interval 1, 1.7% of random, pooled platelet transfusions resulted in blood bank transfusion reaction workups. During interval 2, 5.3% of platelet transfusions resulted in workups. This difference was highly significant. There were no differences between the 2 intervals in the rate of platelet transfusion discontinuation, rate of premedication, percentage of direct antiglobulin test-positive reactions, percentage with icteric/hemolyzed serum, or reactions caused by RBC incompatability.

Conclusion.—The use of an expensive platelet filtration device did not decrease either morbidity from random, pooled platelet transfusions or the prevalence of blood bank transfusion workups.

▶ Advocates of newer leukodepletion filters suggest that reduction of transfusion reactions may be an important benefit of this expensive technology. These investigators showed that platelet transfusion reactions from randomdonor concentrates were not reduced in a time interval following implementation of routine filtration practice. The observation that the reported reaction rate actually increased substantially with the filters was not addressed, but a likely explanation is a change in reporting requirements and practice in the hospital. Although I do not advocate routine supplemental platelet filtration, a controlled study without historical controls would have removed this confounding factor.—P.M. Ness, M.D.

Cytokine Generation in Stored Platelet Concentrates
Stack G, Snyder EL (Yale Univ, New Haven, Conn; Veterans Affairs Med Ctr, West Haven, Conn)
Transfusion 34:20–25, 1994   116-95-6–10

Introduction.—Cytokines have a variety of immunologic, inflammatory, and hematopoietic effects. There is increasing evidence that cytokines may have a central role in mediating transfusion reactions. If so, the cytokines could be synthesized by recipient WBCs in response to transfusion or by donor WBCs either after transfusion or during storage before transfusion. The third possibility was examined.

Methods.—Enzyme immunoassays were used to test the plasma portion of stored platelet concentrates for the presence of various cytokines: IL-1β, IL-6, and IL-8, and tumor necrosis factor-α (TNF-α). One hundred twenty samples were tested from the inventory of a regional blood center, 30 samples each from 2-, 3-, 4-, and 5-day-old units. Seventeen individual platelet concentrates were sampled sequentially during 7 days of storage.

Results.—Fifty-nine percent of samples contained detectable IL-8, including 30% of 2-day-old and 83% of 5-day-old units. The median IL-8 concentration in these samples ranged from undetectable in the 2-dayold units to 1,100 pg/mL in 5-day-old units. The mean IL-8 concentrations at these ages were 116 and 11,600 pg/mL, respectively. Units stored for the longest times and those with the highest WBC counts tended to have the highest IL-8 levels—as much as 200,000 pg/mL. At sequential sampling, IL-8 levels increased progressively with time. Units with high IL-8 concentrations showed parallel but smaller increases in IL-1β. Ten percent of 5-day-old platelet concentrate units showed TNF-

α, but never in concentrations of more than 55 pg/mL. Two 5-day-old units with high WBC counts had detectable levels of IL-6; IL-6 was not detected in 21 additional units with WBC counts of 9,200/μL or storage times of 2 days or less. White blood cell reduction with third-generation filters on the first day of storage prevented production of IL-8 and IL-1β.

Conclusion.—Some stored units of platelet concentrate appear to contain IL-8 levels sufficient to cause physiologic changes. Further studies are needed to determine whether infusing these cytokines in platelet concentrate recipients has potential adverse effects; if so, prestorage reduction of WBCs could be beneficial.

▶ Transfusion reactions to platelets are common events in hematologic practice. When one attempts to categorize these reactions as to the cause, the leading culprit is usually alloantibody to white cells causing febrile reactions and transfusion failures, allergic reactions to plasma constituents, or septic reactions due to bacterial contaminants. A number of reactions occur where a clear-cut etiology cannot be established, suggesting other unexplained mechanisms. This paper is one of a series of studies suggesting that previously unexplained platelet transfusion reactions may be attributable to cytokines generated in platelet concentrates from contaminating white cells; these cytokines could accumulate during storage, perhaps explaining why older platelet concentrates are more commonly associated with clinical events. Although proof that white cells cause cytokines to accumulate in stored platelets has not been established, confirmation of this phenomenon and direct evidence of a role in transfusion reactions could justify leukodepletion of platelet concentrates in the future.—P.M. Ness, M.D.

A Prospective Microbiologic Surveillance Program to Detect and Prevent the Transfusion of Bacterially Contaminated Platelets
Yomtovian R, Lazarus HM, Goodnough LT, Hirschler NV, Morrissey AM, Jacobs MR (Case Western Reserve Univ, Cleveland, Ohio; Univ Hosps, Cleveland, Ohio; American Red Cross Blood Services, Cleveland, Ohio)
Transfusion 33:902–909, 1993   116-95-6–11

Background.—Bacterial contamination of blood components is a significant cause of transfusion-associated morbidity and mortality. A prospective surveillance program was instituted to assess the incidence of platelet bacterial contamination. How platelet storage duration influences the frequency and magnitude of bacterial contamination was also examined, and the usefulness of a pretransfusion Gram stain in avoiding bacterially contaminated platelets was evaluated.

Methods.—Surveillance period I involved taking 1–2-mL samples of all random-donor platelet pools and single-donor apheresis platelet units, which were then submitted for Gram's staining and microbiological culture. During this period, the results of tests were not available before transfusion. This policy was changed during surveillance period II, whereby platelet concentrates could not be released unless Gram's stain results on all pools and single-donor apheresis units were proved negative. The procedure was further modified later to require prospective Gram's staining before release from the blood bank only of random-donor pools and single-donor apheresis units stored for 4 and 5 days.

Results.—During 12 months, 3,141 random-donor platelet pools and 2,476 single-donor apheresis units were cultured. All single-donor apheresis units were sterile, but 6 random-donor pools were bacterially contaminated. One unit of 5 in the pool was the source in each case. Contaminants included 4 cases of *Staphylococcus epidermidis*, 1 case of *Bacillus cereus*, and 1 case of *Staphylococcus aureus* at counts of .5 $\times$ 10^2 to 10^{11} CFUs per mL in platelet pools, and 10^3 to 10^{13} CFUs per mL in source units. Units transfused at 4 days or less showed a lower rate of contamination than those kept for 5 days. Similarly, the magnitude of contamination was less in those stored for 4 days or less. Pretransfusion Gram's staining on 4- and 5-day-old platelet pools was 100% sensitive, and 99.93% specific in detecting contamination.

Conclusion.—The extent and magnitude of platelet bacterial contamination were shown, and the efficacy of the pretransfusion Gram staining of platelet units stored for 4 or 5 days was shown in the prevention of the transfusion of contaminated units. The risk of platelet contamination is associated with the duration of component storage. Such risk can be decreased by selecting shorter platelet outdates or screening older platelets with a pretransfusion Gram stain.

▶ Septic platelet transfusion reactions are a serious problem and account for a significant number of transfusion-related deaths. Their prevention is made difficult by the lack of reliable assays to measure contaminating bacteria in low amounts and the relative rarity of positive tests. These investigators used the Gram stain to screen random-donor platelets stored for 4–5 days and suggest that they prevented most serious reactions at their hospital. I have a number of problems with this approach. First, it is doubtful that most microbiology labs would achieve similar sensitivity and specificity with the Gram stain for this situation in view of the vast number of expected negatives. Second, clinically significant transfusion reactions can occur with platelets stored for shorter periods of time. Until a better method than the Gram stain comes along, the most practical solution is the use of single-donor platelets that limit the number of donor exposures and the chances that a bacteremic donor or a skin contaminant may result in sufficient bacterial growth to cause a deadly consequence.—P.M. Ness, M.D.

Platelet Crossmatches of Single-Donor Platelet Concentrates Using a Latex Agglutination Assay

Ogden DM, Asfour A, Koller C, Lichtiger B (Univ of Texas, Houston)
Transfusion 33:644–650, 1993   116-95-6-12

Background.—Alloimmunization to antigens presented on transfused cells in patients undergoing bone marrow transplantation has become problematic. Seventy percent of patients with leukemia and almost 100% of patients with aplastic anemia experience this problem. Some patients have initially responded to HLA-matched, single-donor platelets, whereas in other patients, HLA matching may not have been a reliable predictor of the outcomes of such transfusions. Additional studies have been done to determine which platelet tests would provide a successful transplant outcome. None of these studies could demonstrate a suitable test. An attempt was made to develop a rapid and sensitive latex agglutination assay that would provide a list of compatible donors for alloimmunized recipients.

Patients and Methods.—A crossmatch assay was performed on 79 transfusions administered to 50 patients. These results were retrospectively correlated with the transfusion outcome to establish the assay's limits of compatibility. Part I of the prospective study involved 50 patients who received 143 transfusions. Part II involved 105 transfusions administered to 43 of those patients. These were patients for whom there was no documentation related to nonimmune factors implicated in poor transfusion response. These include fever of more than 38°C, active bleeding, concurrent infection, or disseminated intravascular coagulation.

Results.—In part I, a positive crossmatch was associated with an unsuccessful transfusion outcome in 96% of patients. A negative crossmatch predicted a satisfactory platelet increment in 84% of patients. The assay characteristics yielded the following scores: sensitivity, 62%; specificity, 99%; and overall predictability, 87%. In part II, a positive crossmatch was 96% effective in predicting an unsuccessful transfusion. After 89% of the transfusions, a negative crossmatch was associated with an adequate platelet increment. For part II, the assay characteristics scores were sensitivity, 72%; specificity, 99%; and overall predictability, 91%.

Conclusion.—The latex agglutination assay is a simple, cost-effective test that requires little laboratory equipment and yields quick crossmatching information.

▶ This paper describes a relatively simple assay for use in platelet crossmatching and the results of its use at a single institution. The assay can use stored platelets coated to latex beads with no loss of immunoreactivity for several months. This type of assay has potential advantages over costly HLA matching programs and deserves further study.—P.M. Ness, M.D.

Treatment of Refractoriness to Platelet Transfusion by Protein A Column Therapy

Christie DJ, Howe RB, Lennon SS, Sauro SC (Univ of Minnesota, Minneapolis)

Transfusion 33:234–242, 1993

116-95-6-13

Background.—Leukemia therapy, bone marrow transplantation, and other disorders that require multiple transfusions of platelets to prevent bleeding can be seriously complicated by refractoriness to platelet transfusion. The effectiveness of protein A column therapy for improving platelet counts and refractoriness to platelet transfusion in patients with a history of unresponsiveness to platelet transfusion treatment was studied.

Patients and Methods.—Ten patients with thrombocytopenia and platelets at less than 10 to 24 × 10^9/L were evaluated. Of these, 9 had been previously treated with steroids, intravenous immune globulin, and other forms of immunosuppressive therapy with no noted improvement in transfusion response. All patients had received multiple platelet transfusions, with none demonstrating 1-hour corrected count increments (CCIs) of 7,500 or more. Antibodies that reacted with platelets and were directed against HLA class I antigens, ABO antigens, and platelet-specific alloantigens were noted in 8 patients. Treatment included taking 500–2,000 mL of plasma from each patient. Plasma was passed over a protein A silica gel column and then returned to the patient. One to 14 treatments were performed. A positive response to therapy was defined as at least a doubling of the pretreatment platelet count or 2 successive 10- to 120-minute post-transfusion CCIs of 7,500 or more.

Results.—Six patients responded with daily platelet counts that averaged 48 × 10^9/L after plasma treatments, in contrast to pretreatment counts of 16 × 10^9/L. In 4 of these patients, post-transfusion CCI values averaged 2,480 pretreatment and 10,010 post-treatment. Among the 4 unresponsive patients, the average platelet counts were 10 and 13 × 10^9, respectively. In these same patients, post-transfusion CCIs were 700 pretreatment and 1,520 post-treatment.

Conclusion.—Protein A column treatments may be a useful means of increasing platelet counts and responsiveness to platelet transfusions in select patients refractory to platelet transfusion because of platelet reactive antibodies.

▶ The treatment of patients who become refractory to platelet transfusions is difficult, with many patients failing to respond to platelets selected by HLA factors or platelet crossmatching. An effective method to handle this problem would be very important for these patients because intravenous immunoglobulin, splenectomy, immunosuppressive agents, and plasmapheresis have had limited success. The protein A column has been promoted as an effective therapy for this condition; unfortunately, this study suggests some benefit but lacks a sufficient number of patients or a concurrent control group to establish efficacy. Many patients lose their antibody and platelet refractoriness without therapy, limiting uncontrolled observations to the status of interesting anecdotes. The column has potential toxicity that also must be considered.—P.M. Ness, M.D.

Autologous Transfusion

A Phase III Trial of Recombinant Human Erythropoietin Therapy in Nonanemic Orthopedic Patients Subjected to Aggressive Removal of Blood for Autologous Use: Dose, Response, Toxicity, and Efficacy
Goodnough LT, Price TH, Friedman KD, Johnston M, Ciavarella D, Khan N, Sacher R, Vogler WR, Wissel M, Abels RI (Washington Univ, St Louis, Mo; Univ of Washington, Seattle; United Blood Services, Albuquerque, NM; et al)
Transfusion 34:66–71, 1994   116-95-6–14

Objective.—Recombinant human EPO has been found to facilitate autologous blood donation and reduce the need for allogeneic blood transfusion among autologous blood donors who are anemic at the time of their first donation. The efficacy of EPO in avoiding allogeneic blood in nonanemic donors remains to be defined. This randomized, controlled, multicenter, dose-escalation trial investigated the role of EPO therapy in autologous blood donors with an initial hematocrit of more than 39%.

Methods.—The study sample included 116 autologous blood donors scheduled for an elective orthopedic operation. All had an initial hematocrit between 39% and 51%. The patients received either EPO (150, 300, or 600 U/kg, intravenously) or placebo at 6 phlebotomy visits during the 3-week period. Outcome measures included number of units donated, marrow RBC production, and number of units of allogeneic blood transfused.

Results.—Fourteen percent of patients did not complete the study because of either adverse events or personal reasons. There were 2 serious adverse events, 1 each in the EPO and placebo group. There were 91 evaluable patients. All of the EPO groups donated significantly more units of blood than the placebo group. Additional RBC production was 440 mL for the placebo group compared with 621 mL in the group receiving 150 units/kg, 644 mL in the group receiving 300 units/kg, and 856 mL in the group receiving 600 units/kg. However, 9% of all EPO and all placebo recipients still received allogeneic blood.

Conclusion.—In nonanemic autologous blood donors, EPO can increase preoperative red cell production. However, there is no apparent clinical benefit in terms of reducing the use of allogeneic blood transfusion. Real reduction of allogeneic blood exposure might be better achieved by physician education in transfusion practices rather than autologous blood-ordering practices.

▶ This paper is a significant addition to the literature on the use of EPO as an adjunct to patients undergoing elective orthopedic surgery who also elect to be autologous donors. It is essentially a negative study in that no clinical benefit could be shown for patients who were not anemic. Although perioperative red cell production was enhanced, allogeneic transfusion requirements did not differ in treated patients compared with controls. The authors conclude that better physician education is more likely to decrease bank blood transfusions in these patients than the expensive administration of EPO.—P.M. Ness, M.D.

The Efficacy of Subcutaneous Recombinant Human Erythropoietin in the Correction of Phlebotomy-Induced Anemia in Autologous Blood Donors

Biesma DH, Kraaijenhagen RJ, Marx JJM, van de Wiel A (Eemland Hosp, De Lichtenberg, Amersfoort, The Netherlands; Univ Hosp, Utrecht, The Netherlands)
Transfusion 33:825–829, 1993   116-95-6–15

Background.—Preoperative collection of autologous blood is limited by restrictions on the storage of red cells and by the patient's erythropoi-

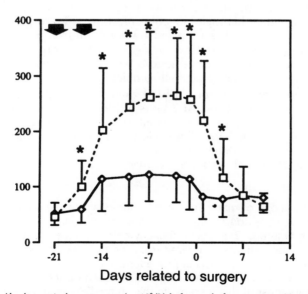

Days related to surgery

Fig 6–2.—Absolute reticulocyte counts ($\times 10^9/L$) before and after surgery in 20 autologous blood donors receiving rhEPO (EPO group, *squares*) and in 20 autologous blood donors not treated with rhEPO (control group, *diamonds*). Measurements were performed twice a week for 3 weeks, at admission, and on days 1, 4, 7, and 10 after surgery. Patients underwent phlebotomy on days −21 and −17 (*arrows*). *$P < .05$. (Courtesy of Biesma DH, Kraaijenhagen RJ, Marx JJM, et al: *Transfusion* 33:825–829, 1993.)

esis. Because the contribution of even 2 units of autologous blood may induce anemia in donors, support from recombinant human EPO (rhEPO) therapy has been investigated. The application of rhEPO has made it possible to collect more than 4 units of blood for autologous use, thereby decreasing the need for additional allogeneic transfusions. The efficacy of rhEPO in the recovery of preoperative hemoglobin concentrations was examined in 40 patients undergoing total hip replacement surgery.

Methods.—Forty autologous blood donors donated 2 units of blood before scheduled primary hip replacement surgery. Twenty donors received 500 units of rhEPO per kg administered subcutaneously twice per week in the 3 weeks before surgery. The 20 patients in the control group were not treated. The recovery of preoperative hemoglobin concentrations within the 3-week period was monitored.

Results.—In the group treated with EPO, the initial hemoglobin concentration was completely recovered before surgery. In the control group, hemoglobin concentration decreased after blood donation. The preoperative reticulocyte count increased sixfold in the EPO group compared with a twofold-to-threefold increase in the control group (Fig 6–2). Iron levels assessed by serum ferritin decreased less in the treated group than in the control group. The EPO-treated group had a postoperative serum EPO concentration significantly lower than the control group, but it did not differ from the pretreatment value and it was attended by a higher hemoglobin concentration after surgery. Some patients treated with rhEPO reported transient flu-like symptoms. There were no adverse events and no changes in blood pressure or platelet counts in either group. One autologous blood donor treated with rhEPO and 7 untreated patients needed allogeneic blood.

Conclusion.—Subcutaneous rhEPO therapy was safe and efficacious in compensating for the loss of 2 units of blood within a 3-week period. Although the patient sample was small, these results suggest that rhEPO may decrease the need for allogeneic blood. However, the expense of rhEPO treatment mandates strict criteria for its use; other blood conservation techniques such as intraoperative cell salvage should be investigated.

▶ This study is one of many attempts to demonstrate the efficacy of EPO in the perioperative period in patients who elect to donate autologous blood. As shown in Figure 6–2, a brisk reticulocytosis developed in the EPO-treated group, and these patients recovered from the red cell loss noted in the non-treated group before the surgical procedure. There was a small difference in the amount of bank blood transfused as well. The unresolved problem remains the high cost of this therapy. In this study, EPO cost $2,000. Because the cost of delivering a unit of red cells in the United States is approximately $150 and the risk of infectious complications is currently remote, the cost-benefit ratio of EPO use is difficult to support, at least in this setting.—P.M. Ness, M.D.

Efficacy of Preoperative Donation of Blood for Autologous Use in Radical Prostatectomy

Toy PTCY, Menozzi D, Strauss RG, Stehling LC, Kruskall M, Ahn DK (Univ of California, San Francisco; Univ of Iowa, Iowa City; State Univ of New York, Syracuse; et al)
Transfusion 33:721–724, 1993   116-95-6–16

Background.—The use of autologous blood donated preoperatively by patients undergoing elective surgery effectively reduces transfusion-related infectious and immunologic risks. In many centers, standard practice is to collect 2 units of blood before surgery. The amount of blood lost, the number of transfusions needed, and the efficacy of preoperative autologous blood donation were determined in patients undergoing radical prostatectomy.

Methods and Findings.—The records of 163 patients treated at 4 university and 3 community hospitals between 1987 and 1991 were reviewed. The mean red cell volume loss was calculated to be 1,003 mL, corresponding to 44% of the total red cell volume. Preoperative autologous blood donation reduced the rate of allogeneic blood transfusion from 66% to 20%. Thirty-two percent of patients donating 1–2 units received allogeneic blood, compared with 14% of those donating 3 units. The preoperative donation of 4 units decreased the allogeneic transfusion rate to 11%. However, as the number of units donated increased, the units not transfused also increased.

Conclusion.—Autologous blood donation effectively minimizes the transfusion of allogeneic blood to patients undergoing radical prostatectomy. However, many patients do not donate enough units before surgery. Three units should be donated before radical prostatectomy.

▶ This multicenter trial demonstrates that patients undergoing radical retropubic prostatectomy procedures use less bank blood when they donate autologous blood preoperatively. As one would expect, if more autologous units are available, less bank blood will be required by the patient, but the likelihood of wastage of autologous blood also increases. This study generally confirms our findings at Johns Hopkins, where the radical retropubic prostatectomy approach was developed and autologous blood for these patients was pioneered.—P.M. Ness, M.D.

Efficacy of Autotransfusion in Hepatectomy for Hepatocellular Carcinoma

Fujimoto J, Okamoto E, Yamanaka N, Oriyama T, Furukawa K, Kawamura E, Tanaka T, Tomoda F (Hyogo College of Medicine, Nishinomiya, Japan)
Arch Surg 128:1065–1069, 1993   116-95-6–17

Background.—Autologous blood transfusion decreases the need for banked blood in many surgical procedures and eliminates infectious risk. Although concerns of metastasis have contraindicated intraoperative blood salvage in patients with cancer, the procedure has been safely used in this patient group. The safety and clinical usefulness of autoinfusion in hepatectomy for hepatocellular carcinoma were evaluated.

Methods.—Among 104 patients undergoing hepatectomy for hepato-cellular carcinoma, 54 received autologous blood transfusion and 50 received homologous blood. Physical examination, chest radiography, hematology, and ultrasonography were performed quarterly until patient death or December of 1991.

Results.—Of the mean 831 mL of autotransfused blood used, 392 mL were obtained by preoperative donation and 439 mL were obtained by intraoperative salvage. Fifteen patients who received autologous blood transfusion required no homologous blood components during the operation, and 11 avoided homologous blood products during the entire hospitalization. Despite comparable intraoperative blood losses, auto-transfusion patients required significantly less homologous blood (814 mL) compared with homologous transfusion patients (3,466 mL). The groups had similar mean postoperative hemoglobin levels, platelet counts, prothrombin times, and partial thromboplastin times. A cytology study performed using 5 samples from 20 autotransfusion patients revealed all class 1 specimens. Seventeen autotransfusion patients remained disease-free 32 months after follow-up. Intrahepatic or extrahepatic recurrence rates and 3-year cumulative survival rates were comparable for the 2 groups. Extrahepatic metastasis did not occur in the absence of intrahepatic metastasis in autotransfusion patients.

Conclusion.—Autotransfusion is safe, effective, and practical when used in liver surgery for hepatocellular carcinoma. Additional study is required to determine the long-term safety and potential benefits.

▶ Intraoperative blood salvage procedures are generally considered to be contraindicated in cases of tumor resection surgery where the hematogenous spread of cancer cells from the operative field remains a concern. There are no data to suggest that this concern is justified. This study in patients undergoing hepatic resection for hepatocellular carcinoma failed to demonstrate enhanced tumor recurrence after salvage procedures. Other similar studies have been published in other cancer surgery series. Although the authors conclude that blood salvage is safe in this procedure, some statistical analysis of the number of patients required to prove the lack of risk would help to convince me of the wisdom of their conclusions.—P.M. Ness, M.D.

The Cost-Effectiveness of Preoperative Autologous Blood Donation for Total Hip and Knee Replacement

Birkmeyer JD, Goodnough LT, AuBuchon JP, Noordsij PG, Littenberg B (Dart-

mouth-Hitchcock Med Ctr, Lebanon, NH; Washington Univ, St Louis, Mo)
Transfusion 33:544–551, 1993   116-95-6–18

Background.—The frequency of preoperative autologous blood donation is increasing dramatically. However, the cost-effectiveness of this procedure has not been fully explored. A decision analysis was done to determine the cost-effectiveness of autologous blood donation for hip and knee replacement.

Methods.—Data on red cell use in 629 patients having surgery at 2 tertiary care centers were used. Cost-effectiveness was expressed as cost per quality-adjusted year of life saved.

Findings.—At centers 1 and 2, autologous blood donation for bilateral and revision joint replacement cost $40,000 and $241,000, respectively, per quality-adjusted year of life saved. For primary unilateral hip replacement, autologous blood donation cost $373,000 and $740,000 per quality-adjusted year of life saved at centers 1 and 2, respectively. The procedure was least cost-effective for primary unilateral knee replacement. Variations among procedures in the cost-effectiveness of autologous blood donation were explained by the differences between autologous blood collections and transfusion requirements. The poorer cost-effectiveness documented at center 2 was a result of higher transfusion rates in autologous blood donors than in nondonors.

Conclusion.—Autologous blood donation is not as cost-effective as other accepted medical procedures. Avoiding excessive collection and transfusion of autologous blood may greatly improve its cost-effectiveness.

▶ Although preoperative autologous blood collection programs have proliferated in the wake of the AIDS epidemic and their benefits have been routinely accepted by clinicians and mandated by some governmental agencies, they have not been scrutinized for cost-effectiveness. This study suggests that these programs are costly and are not as beneficial as other accepted medical practices. This conclusion is derived in part from current low rates of infectious transmission and significant numbers of autologous blood collections for patients who do not need these units. If one considers that many patients who receive autologous blood could probably have tolerated postoperative anemia without consequence, these conclusions about the cost-effectiveness for these specific orthopedic procedures and other common surgeries would be even stronger.—P.M. Ness, M.D.

Survival and Half-Life of Red Cells Salvaged After Hip and Knee Replacement Surgery

Umlas J, Jacobson MS, Kevy SV (Harvard Med School, Boston; Children's Hosp of Boston)

Transfusion 33:591–593, 1993   116-95-6–19

Background.—Studies of RBC survival after intraoperative salvage have not included hip and knee arthroplasty. Postoperative salvage and transfusion of unwashed hip and knee drainage may reduce the need for allogeneic blood. Only small volumes of RBCs are lost after hip and knee replacement; therefore, it would be important to know RBC viability. The survival and half-life of salvaged and peripheral RBCs were compared in 6 patients undergoing hip or knee replacement.

Methods.—Joint drainage was collected in an unanticoagulated bag for 3 hours after hip or knee arthroplasty; RBCs were labeled with radioactive ^{51}Cr and Ascorbate. A sample of peripheral venous blood was drawn and labeled with nonradioactive ^{52}Cr. Both labeled specimens were transfused and venous samples were drawn at 10, 15, and 20 minutes within the subsequent 18–24 hours and after 2, 3, 5, 7, and 14 days.

Results.—The average survival and half-life of both sets of RBCs were slightly less than normal. Nevertheless, RBC survival and half-life were comparable in salvaged and venous blood.

Conclusion.—The amount of RBCs salvaged during the first 6 hours after hip and knee arthroplasty is generally small, representing only a small part of the total perioperative RBC loss. Therefore, it may not be medically effective to collect RBCs after these procedures even though their survival and durability are normal. The potentially life-threatening, profound hypotension and upper-airway edema associated with the use of unwashed, postoperatively salvaged blood provide additional arguments against routine use of this material.

▶ The question of whether red cells salvaged from wound sites after knee and hip replacement surgery should be transfused has engendered divergent opinions. The practice has been marketed aggressively to orthopedic surgeons who believe it is efficacious and can provide anecdotal evidence of its utility. Blood bankers suggest that the amounts of blood available for salvage are generally small and that the potential for contamination with infectious agents or wound debris is large. Another concern that has been raised is whether these salvaged cells will survive post-transfusion. This paper shows that the cells will survive the rigors of the collection process and circulate normally, but the other concerns about minimal dosage and untoward effects remain important issues.—P.M. Ness, M.D.

Safety and Efficacy of Preoperative Donation of Blood for Autologous Use by Patients With End-Stage Heart or Lung Disease Who Are

Awaiting Organ Transplantation

Goldfinger D, Capon S, Czer L, Leibfreid J, Trento A, Ross D, Waters P, Klapper E, Pepkowitz S (Cedars-Sinai Med Ctr, Los Angeles)
Transfusion 33:336–340, 1993 116-95-6-20

Introduction.—The donation of autologous blood preoperatively can significantly limit the exposure of surgical patients to random-donor blood components. Transplant recipients who receive potent immunosuppressive agents may particularly benefit from autologous blood donation because of the lowered risk of contracting infectious disease.

Study Population.—The efficacy and safety of autologous blood donation were studied in patients with end-stage cardiac or pulmonary disease who were awaiting an organ transplant. Forty-eight consecutive heart transplant candidates and 24 patients awaiting lung transplantation were included.

Results.—Of the 72 patients, 64% were able to donate blood for autologous use. Four of them provided only half-units. There were no apparent demographic or clinical differences between patients who donated and those who failed to donate for nonmedical reasons. The heart transplant recipients who donated blood received a median of 6 units, and the lung transplant recipients who donated blood received a median of 4 units (table). Only about half of the autologous blood donors required more blood components than they donated. Adverse effects of autologous blood donation were rare.

Implications.—These preliminary findings suggest that many prospective organ transplant recipients, even those who are seriously ill, are able to donate blood that they may later require perioperatively.

▶ This paper describes another facet of an aggressive and comprehensive autologous blood collection program where patients awaiting cardiac or pulmonary transplants have been offered autologous transfusions. Because many of the patients required other components than red cells, homologous exposures could not be eliminated totally, although the average number of donor exposures was reduced. Adverse reactions were uncommon even in this high-risk population. Whether this process meets the test of appropriate risk-to-benefit ratio is unclear. One offshoot to this approach deserves comment: because some of these patients are undergoing therapeutic phlebotomy resulting from secondary polycythemia while awaiting their transplant, freezing of the units would certainly make sense rather than simply discarding their autologous cells.—P.M. Ness, M.D.

Perioperative Blood Transfusions Per Patient

	Heart transplant recipients		Lung transplant recipients	
	Donors (n = 24)	Nondonors (control) (n = 8)	Donors (n = 11)	Nondonors (control) (n = 6)
Packed red cells	2 (0–24)	2.5 (0–8)	2 (0–30)	1.5 (0–7)
Fresh-frozen plasma	3 (0–42)	3 (0–12)	0 (0–11)	0 (0–2)
Platelet concentrate	0 (0–43)	1 (0–12)	0 (0–7)	0 (0–1)
Cryoprecipitate	0 (0–20)	0 (0–10)	0 (0–10)	0
Total units	6 (0–129)	7 (0–42)	4 (0–58)	2 (0–8)
Total allogeneic component exposures	1 (0–117)†	7 (0–42)†	0 (0–53)‡	2 (0–8)‡
Patients exposed to allogeneic blood components§	13 (54)‖	7 (88)‖	5 (45)¶	6 (100)¶

Note: Values given as median (range).
† P = .0141.
‡ P = .1871.
§ Values given as number of patients (%).
‖ P = .0968.
¶ P = .0418.
(Courtesy of Goldfinger D, Capon S, Czer L, et al: *Transfusion* 33:336–340, 1993.)

Blood Donation Leads to a Decrease in Natural Killer Cell Activity: A Study in Normal Blood Donors and Cancer Patients

Marquet RL, Hoynck van Papendrecht MA, Busch OR, Jeekel J (Erasmus Univ, Rotterdam, The Netherlands)
Transfusion 33:368–373, 1993   116-95-6-21

Introduction.—Organ transplant recipients are known to benefit from transfusion-induced immunosuppression, but recent retrospective studies suggest that blood transfusions may have adverse effects on patients with cancer. Autologous blood is an increasingly popular alternative to allogeneic blood. The use of autologous blood to avoid immunosuppression assumes that the procedure is immunologically neutral.

Objective and Methods.—This assumption was examined by monitoring 33 normal blood donors after taking 1 unit of blood and 16 patients with colorectal cancer who donated 2 units at an interval of 3–4 days. The patients were in 1 arm of a randomized trial comparing the effects of allogeneic and autologous blood on the prognosis of cancer.

Findings.—On flow cytometric analysis, neither group had significant changes in the proportions of B cells, T cells, or natural killer (NK) cells. Total lymphocyte counts were significantly reduced in normal donors 12 days after donation. Phytohemagglutinin stimulation indicated no significant change in T-cell function in either group. However, the normal donors had significantly depressed NK cell function, as shown by a human erythroleukemic cell assay, on days 2 and 5 after donation but normal activity on day 12. In patients with cancer, NK cell activity on day 12 after the first donation was 54% of baseline. The 2 groups had comparable baseline NK cell activity. The number of NK cells correlated significantly with NK cell activity before but not after donation.

Conclusion.—Blood donation, particularly donating 2 units, seems to decrease NK cell activity. Confirmation of this finding could have important implications for patients with cancer who are scheduled for surgery.

▶ This paper adds another element of confusion to the evolving story of immunomodulation by blood transfusion. Many retrospective and a few prospective studies have produced results suggesting that transfusions of allogeneic blood components result in immunomodulation that may lead to higher rates of cancer recurrence or postoperative infection in susceptible recipients. Because many similar studies have not confirmed these adverse effects, investigations are now turning to controlled, prospective trials of transfusion recipients. Because patients who need blood cannot go without transfusions just to serve as controls, a logical control group would appear to be autologous blood recipients. This study, however, implies that autologous blood donation has its own set of immunologic consequences with resulting decreases in NK cell activity. If these results are confirmed, it may ultimately be impossible to separate out the immunomodulatory effects of transfusion from the effects of other invasive procedures, perhaps as trivial as phlebotomy for the samples required to run the assays, or even from the effects of noninvasive procedures.—P.M. Ness, M.D.

Beneficial Effect of Autologous Blood Transfusion on Infectious Complications After Colorectal Cancer Surgery
Heiss MM, Mempel W, Jauch K-W, Delanoff C, Mayer G, Mempel M, Eissner H-J, Schildberg F-W (Ludwig Maximilians Univ, Munich)
Lancet 342:1328–1333, 1993   116-95-6–22

Background.—Homologous blood transfusion increases the risk of postoperative infectious complications. The clinical consequences of this apparent immunosuppressive effect of homologous blood were evaluated.

Methods.—One hundred twenty patients with apparently curable colorectal cancer who were able to donate blood before surgery for autologous transfusion were enrolled in the controlled trial. Fifty-eight patients were assigned to receive homologous blood if transfusion was needed during surgery, and 62 were assigned to receive their own blood followed, if needed, by homologous blood.

Findings.—Postoperative infection rates differed significantly between the homologous and autologous blood groups, despite between-group similarity in factors known to affect the postoperative infection risk. Noninfectious complications occurred at similar rates between groups. The patients in the autologous blood group, probably because preoperative donation resulted in lower hemoglobin concentrations, were more likely to need transfusion than patients in the homologous blood group. Thirty-five percent of the patients needed homologous as well as autologous blood. In a multivariate analysis adjusting for the many infection-related variables, the only significant risk factors were tumor location, preoperative American Society of Anesthesiologists physical status index, and study group assignment.

Conclusion.—Blood transfusions have an independent, clinically relevant effect on the incidence of infections after surgery in patients with curable colorectal cancer. The rate of infectious complications was strongly associated with homologous blood transfusion, increasing with the number of units transfused.

► This study is another clinical investigation suggesting that homologous blood is associated with increases in the frequency of postoperative infection. The strong points of the paper are the use of an autologous vs. homologous design and a healthy discussion of some of the limitations of this kind of clinical study. Because many of the patients in the autologous group also received homologous blood and some patients in the homologous group were not transfused with any blood components, the final conclusions may be somewhat clouded.—P.M. Ness, M.D.

Autologous Platelet-Rich Plasma Does Not Reduce Transfusion of Homologous Blood Products in Patients Undergoing Repeat Valvular Surgery

Ereth MH, Oliver WC Jr, Beynen FMK, Mullany CJ, Orszulak TA, Santrach PJ, Ilstrup DM, Weaver AL, Williamson KR (Mayo Clinic, Rochester, Minn)
Anesthesiology 79:540–547, 1993   116-95-6–23

Background.—Patients who undergo cardiopulmonary bypass often require transfusion of homologous blood products and are subsequently exposed to the risk of transfusions. The administration of autologous platelet-rich plasma is thought to reduce homologous transfusion and minimize risks. The effect of autologous platelet-rich plasma on perioperative coagulation profiles, bleeding, and transfusion requirements was investigated in patients undergoing valvular surgery.

Methods.—Fifty-six patients undergoing repeat valvular surgery were enrolled. They were randomized to 1 of 2 groups that would receive either sham product or autologous platelet-rich plasma at the conclusion of cardiopulmonary bypass. All clinicians involved in the procedure were blinded to minimize any biases in transfusion practices. After surgery, the 2 groups were compared. Variables included perioperative blood loss, coagulation profiles, and transfusion requirements.

Results.—No significant difference was seen in transfusion requirements between the 2 groups in the first 24 hours or for the entire hospitalization period. The median of homologous units transfused during the first 24 hours was 10.5; the total median perioperative homologous transfusion requirements were 13 and 11.5 units for the platelet-rich plasma and sham groups, respectively. Minor changes in coagulation function were noted with collection and administration of platelet-rich plasma. As would be expected, the removal of platelets and plasma resulted in an increase in the prothrombin time and a decrease in the platelet count and fibrinogen in the autologous platelet-rich plasma group. No significant difference was seen in perioperative blood loss between the 2 groups.

Conclusion.—When both the cardiac surgeon and the anesthesiologist were blinded, platelet-rich plasma did not reduce blood loss or homologous transfusion requirements in patients undergoing repeat valvular surgery. Further blinded studies are recommended to define the efficacy of blood conservation therapies and conditions for optimal clinical response in patients undergoing other types of cardiac surgery.

▶ The growing number of options to reduce blood use in cardiac surgery make the determination of efficacy of any single procedure very difficult. The collection of autologous platelet-rich plasma is a candidate procedure that is time consuming and requires expensive technology, but its appeal based on the provision of fresh autologous platelets at the conclusion of surgery is strong. This study from the Mayo Clinic was carefully performed, including a sham collection and return control group. The results showed no change in transfusion patterns compared with control patients. The blinding of the physician team adds strength to the study design. Based on the findings of this study, the use of autologous platelet-rich plasma is difficult to recommend as an application in cardiac surgery.—P.M. Ness, M.D.

Adult Transfusion Practice

Rational Approach to Postoperative Transfusion in High-Risk Patients
Baxter BT, Minion DJ, McCance CL, Eskildsen JM, Heffele JJ, Lynch TG (Univ of Nebraska, Omaha; Omaha VA Med Ctr, Neb)
Am J Surg 166:720–724, 1993   116-95-6-24

Introduction.—Although it is well known that patients with impaired myocardial function require higher hemoglobin levels to maintain oxygen delivery during surgery, there are no current guidelines to determine when it is appropriate to transfuse surgical patients who have significant coronary artery disease. Therefore, the development of transfusion guidelines based on observed cardiac function in patients with significant coronary artery disease undergoing major vascular operations would be very valuable. The effects of preoperative volume loading on cardiac function, postoperative oxygen delivery, and hemoglobin levels necessary for adequate oxygen delivery in this high-risk population were assessed.

Methods.—For a 30-month period, all patients considered high risk because of a history of congestive heart failure, recent myocardial infarction, severe angina, or impaired ventricular function who were undergoing abdominal aortic aneurysm repair, bypass of aortoiliac disease, distal bypass, or carotid endarterectomy were treated using a standard protocol. There were 39 men in this series. Pulmonary artery wedge pressure was used to estimate left ventricular end-diastolic pressure and to develop a Starling curve for each patient before surgery. This curve was used to determine the pulmonary artery wedge pressure that would result in optimal cardiac function. This filling pressure was maintained during the operation and for the next 48–72 hours. Pulmonary artery wedge pressure, cardiac output (CO), hemoglobin levels, arterial oxygen saturation, and systemic vascular resistance were monitored. Oxygen delivery was then calculated.

Results.—The preoperative volume loading increased CO by 15% to 22%. The postoperative CO was unchanged, except for a decline in those patients undergoing Carotid endarterectomy. Systemic vascular resistance decreased in the patients with abdominal aortic aneurysm and aortoiliac disease. The postoperative oxygen delivery declined 25% to 31% because of a decrease in hemoglobin. Although postoperative oxygen delivery was marginal in one third of these patients, there was no compensating increase in CO.

Conclusion.—Preoperative optimization significantly improved CO during and after vascular surgery in this high-risk population. However, a postoperative decrease in hemoglobin resulted in a decrease in oxygen delivery, which the patients were unable to compensate for. The inability to increase oxygen delivery in these high-risk patients indicates that maintenance of adequate oxygen-carrying capacity through red cell transfusion remains important in this population. These findings provide a basis for the long-standing practice of maintaining hemoglobin levels of at least 10 g/dL in high-risk patients.

▶ This study represents a carefully performed analysis of oxygen delivery in patients at high risk for ischemic events. The purpose of the investigation was to optimize fluid balance and blood flow preoperatively and then to assess the need for postoperative transfusions based on these physiologic parameters. The study concluded that the old cutoff of 10 g of hemoglobin may be necessary for high-risk patients and that strict adherence to limited transfusion protocols may poorly serve some patients in whom ischemic events are more likely.—P.M. Ness, M.D.

Effectiveness of Perioperative Recombinant Human Erythropoietin in Elective Hip Replacement
Canadian Orthopedic Perioperative Erythropoietin Study Group (Ottawa Civic Hosp, Ont, Canada)
Lancet 341:1227–1232, 1993   116-95-6–25

Background.—Because of the risk of viral infection transmission, attempts are made to decrease the transfusion requirements of patients undergoing surgery. Whether recombinant human EPO decreases blood transfusion needs in patients having elective hip arthroplasty was determined.

Methods.—Two hundred eight patients were enrolled in the multicenter, double-blind, randomized, placebo-controlled trial. All patients received daily subcutaneous injections of EPO or placebo beginning 10 days before surgery. Then 78 patients, composing group 1, received placebo for 14 days; 77 patients in group 2 received EPO, 300 units/kg, to a maximum of 30,000 units, for 14 days; and 53 patients in group 3 received placebo on days 10 to 6 before surgery, with EPO administration for the next 9 days.

Findings.—A primary outcome event, defined as any transfusion or a hemoglobin concentration of less than 80 g/L, occurred in 46% of group 1 patients, 23% of group 2 patients, and 32% of group 3 patients. The mean numbers of transfusions in groups 1, 2, and 3 were 1.14, .52, and .7, respectively. The respective mean reticulocyte counts the day before the operation were 72, 327, and 170 × 10^9/L (Fig 6–3). Five patients in group 1, 8 in group 2, and 8 in group 3 had deep venous

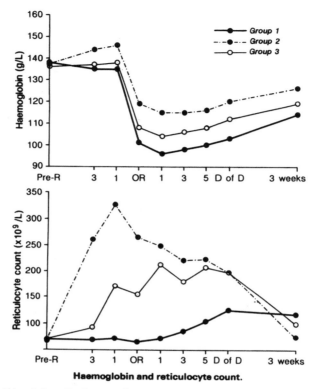

Haemoglobin and reticulocyte count.

Fig 6–3.—*Abbreviations: Pre-R,* prerandomization; *OR,* operation day; *D of D,* day of discharge. (Courtesy of the Canadian Orthopedic Perioperative Erythropoietin Study Group: *Lancet* 341:1227–1232, 1993.)

thrombi. Patients with a hemoglobin concentration of less than 135 g/L before randomization benefited most from EPO.

Conclusion.—In these patients undergoing elective hip arthroplasty, EPO administered for 14 days perioperatively decreased the need for blood transfusion. This treatment was also well tolerated.

▶ The use of perioperative EPO has been advocated to facilitate autologous blood donation, but the efficacy of this approach remains controversial. This paper studies the use of EPO in elective hip replacement in a double-blind fashion without autologous blood collection. The results suggest decreased transfusion requirements for patients undergoing primary hip surgery but little benefit for patients undergoing hip revision, who tend to have more perioperative bleeding. Maximal benefit was seen in patients with lower hematocrits on entry. Deep venous thrombosis was more common in treated patients, but there was no statistically significant difference. Additional confirmatory studies will be of interest to determine whether the costs of EPO can be justified in terms of the benefit to the patient of decreased transfusion requirements without additional complications from EPO therapy.—P.M. Ness, M.D.

Economic Impact of Inappropriate Blood Transfusions in Coronary Artery Bypass Graft Surgery
Goodnough LT, Soegiarso RW, Birkmeyer JD, Welch HG (Washington Univ, St Louis, Mo; Univ Hosps of Cleveland, Ohio; Dartmouth-Hitchcock Med Ctr, Hanover, NH)
Am J Med 94:509–514, 1993   116-95-6–26

Introduction.—Currently, nearly 12 million RBC units are administered to about 3½ million patients each year in the United States. Apart from the issues of blood inventory and safety, the costs of transfusion are expected to have an increasing impact on transfusion practices in the coming years.

Objective.—The costs of blood support were analyzed for patients having primary, elective coronary artery bypass graft surgery. Data were obtained for 30 consecutive adult patients at each of 18 tertiary care hospitals that participated in a national audit. Red blood cell transfusions were considered to have been inappropriate if administered to replace RBC volume losses of less than 15%.

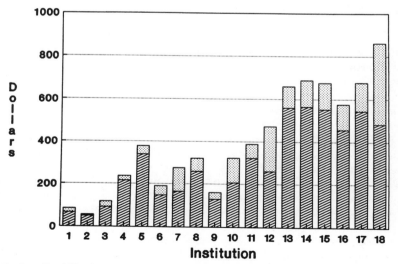

Fig 6–4.—Total blood costs and costs of inappropriate transfusions during 30 coronary artery bypass graft procedures at each of 18 institutions. Costs of transfusions given appropriately (*hatched bars*) and inappropriately (*stippled bars*) are indicated. (Courtesy of Goodnough LT, Soegiarso RW, Birkmeyer JD, et al: *Am J Med* 94:509–514, 1993.)

Findings.—Blood purchase costs at the participating institutions varied more than twofold, and the range of RBC units transfused varied more than 10-fold. The range of total blood components administered varied more than 40-fold. Twenty-seven percent of all blood units were transfused unnecessarily; individual hospital rates were as high as 43%. Forty-seven percent of platelet units, 32% of plasma units, and 15% of RBC units were administered inappropriately. The mean institutional cost per patient for all blood components transfused was $397, and the cost of inappropriately transfused units was $96 (Fig 6–4).

Conclusion.—Transfusion costs are a significant part of total costs for coronary artery bypass graft surgery. Costs could be significantly decreased by applying practice guidelines and by establishing quality improvement programs aimed at decreasing the number of transfusions administered inappropriately.

▶ The recent literature of transfusion medicine has documented the many adverse effects of transfusion. When blood is administered without meeting minimal medical requirements, substantial monetary costs can accrue and any adverse effects from these unjustified transfusions represent additional expenses to be borne by the health-care system. This study demonstrates wide variability in transfusion practices in centers supporting coronary artery bypass surgery and major discrepancies in the use of red cells and other blood components. The authors have presented convincing data indicating that quality assurance programs could play a useful role in this setting to decrease potential transfusion overuse.—P.M. Ness, M.D.

High-Dose Aprotinin Reduces Blood Loss in Patients Undergoing Total Hip Replacement Surgery
Janssens M, Joris J, David JL, Lemaire R, Lamy M (Univ Hosp, Liège, Belgium)
Anesthesiology 80:23–29, 1994   116-95-6–27

Background.—Reportedly, the use of aprotinin has successfully reduced blood loss during cardiac and hip replacement surgery. As yet, the mechanism responsible for this reduction of blood loss has not been fully elucidated. This randomized, controlled, double-blind study was conducted to confirm the beneficial effects of high-dose aprotinin on blood loss and on the use of blood products in patients undergoing total hip replacement surgery.

Patients and Methods.—Forty patients scheduled for total hip replacement surgery participated. They were randomly assigned to receive either aprotinin or normal saline. The anesthesia and surgical techniques were standardized, and a systematic deep venous thrombosis prophylaxis was used. Clotting and coagulation status were analyzed, and renal and hepatic function were assessed.

Results.—The total intraoperative and postoperative blood loss was decreased from 1,943 mL to 1,446 mL as a result of the use of aprotinin. The total amount of blood transfused per patient in the control group was 3.4 units compared with 1.8 units in the aprotinin group. There was a significant prolongation of the activated partial thromboplastin time after surgery as a result of aprotinin. However, the other coagulation test results did not differ between the 2 groups.

Conclusion.—The use of high-dose aprotinin during total hip replacement surgery decreases blood loss. In addition, aprotinin further decreases the amount of blood transfusions.

▶ Aprotinin is a fibrinolytic inhibitor that has been used in test tubes and patients. A number of trials have been performed in cardiac surgery to determine whether intraoperative blood loss and subsequent transfusions can be limited by the drug. The results have been mixed in this setting, although the drug has recently been approved by the Food and Drug Administration. This trial in orthopedic surgery appears to demonstrate decreased blood loss and transfusion requirements in carefully studied patients compared with controls. The increased activated partial thromboplastin time in treated patients is difficult to explain, suggesting that the mechanism of action of the drug to decrease blood loss is not really understood. How this drug therapy fits with other options (e.g., predeposit, intraoperative blood salvage, postoperative salvage) to limit blood loss and blood transfusions in the surgical setting remains to be determined.—P.M. Ness, M.D.

Association of Sickle Cell Disease, Priapism, Exchange Transfusion and Neurological Events: Aspen Syndrome

Siegel JF, Rich MA, Brock WA (Schneider Children's Hosp, New Hyde Park, NY)
J Urol 150:1480–1482, 1993   116-95-6–28

Background.—The incidence of priapism in patients with sickle cell anemia ranges from 6% in children to 42% in adults. The link between the occurrence of acute neurologic events and partial exchange transfusion to treat priapism in patients with sickle cell disease has only recently been recognized. A case report was presented.

Case Report.—Boy, 10 years, with homozygous sickle cell disease was admitted to the hospital with priapism of 20 hours' duration. His hemoglobin level was 6.3 g/dL with an Hb S level of 79.4%. He received 3 partial exchange transfusions, which increased his hemoglobin level to 13.5 g/dL with an Hb S level of 20.8%. Because the priapism persisted, surgical treatment was planned. During the next partial exchange transfusion to further lower his Hb S level, the boy complained of nausea and headache and the transfusion was stopped. Within 30 minutes of discontinuation, he became obtunded and nonresponsive, with left deviation of both eyes and right hemiparesis. Bradycardia and apnea requiring ventilatory support developed, and the patient had a tonic-clonic seizure. Penile detumescence occurred shortly thereafter. All neurologic deficits resolved within 48 hours.

Comments.—The association of sickle cell anemia, priapism, exchange transfusion, and neurologic events is a newly recognized syndrome with significant therapeutic implications. The acute neurologic events are thought to be related to cerebral ischemia, which may occur after an acute increase in total hemoglobin with a concomitant decrease in Hb S and the subsequent release of vasoactive substances during penile detumescence.

▶ This interesting case report suggests that neurologic events can be a complication of exchange transfusion therapy in sickle cell anemia patients being treated for priapism. The authors provide a literature review to suggest that their case is representative of what they have called the ASPEN syndrome. Although hematologists are probably well advised to look for neurologic complications in exchanged sickle cell patients who have had surgical manipulations for priapism, the designation of this patient as part of a unique syndrome is of questionable value for diagnosis or therapy.—P.M. Ness, M.D.

No Requirement for Cryoprecipitate or Platelet Transfusion During Liver Transplantation

Gerlach H, Rossaint R, Slama K, Streich R, Keitel M, Blumhardt G, Bechstein W, Lemmens P, Lohmann R, Neuhaus P (Free Univ, Berlin)
Transplant Proc 25:1813–1816, 1993   116-95-6–29

Background.—Extensive transfusion of blood components is a typical requirement during orthotopic liver transplantation. The procedure brings a number of complications, including those resulting from the infusion techniques themselves. A new management strategy was proposed whereby the infusion of balanced electrolyte solution is reduced to avoid hemodilution, aprotinin is administered at the beginning of surgery, and blood replacement is confined to packed RBCs and fresh frozen plasma.

Methods.—A total of 140 orthotopic liver transplants were performed on 128 adult patients. The first 10 patients were treated with antifibrinolytic drugs. The other 46 patients received aprotinin as an intravenous bolus injection in a dose of 500,000 units 3 times: at induction of anesthesia, immediately before anhepatic phase, and before revascularization of the liver graft. The transplantation was performed according to established surgical procedures. For reperfusion, the liver graft was flushed in situ with 500–800 mL of blood. The intraoperative volume substitution was limited to RBCs and fresh frozen plasma only.

Results.—Of the 140 patients undergoing orthotopic liver transplantation, 62 were extubated in the operating theater. Forty-one patients were extubated within 6 hours. In the 24-hour postoperative period, an average of 2.4 units of RBCs and 5.7 units of fresh frozen plasma had to be transfused. Twenty-two patients underwent relaparatomy as a result of bleeding complications. No adverse reactions to bovine aprotinin were seen, nor were any perioperative thrombembolic complications noted. A total of 112 patients are still alive and well, a survival rate of 87.5%. Two patients died, 1 of a fulminant septic infection with aspergillus, and the other of sudden cardiac failure with high filling pressures. One other patient experienced a lethal intracranial hemorrhage 11 months after surgery; at autopsy, the patient was seen to have local recurrence of central bile duct carcinoma.

Conclusion.—The perioperative strategy consisting of rigid avoidance of hemodilution, administration of $CaCl_2$ and the protease inhibitor aprotinin, and restriction of blood transfusion to packed RBCs and fresh frozen plasma was successful and brought no fatal hemorrhagic complications or enhanced transfusion requirements. In view of the risks and cost of blood products, this protocol may bring improved clinical results. Further studies are recommended to investigate the mechanism of hemostaseologic alterations during liver transplantation.

▶ Providing blood components for liver transplantation is a major problem for blood centers and transfusion services. Although the number of units used by the average patient has dropped as reflected in this article, the extreme use in occasional patients is always a concern. This article caught my attention for several reasons. First, the mean blood use was very low with the use of a protocol including avoidance of hemodilution, calcium supplements, and aprotinin. Second, the protocol did not use platelets, which are used in large quantities in many transplant centers.—P.M. Ness, M.D.

Cost-Effectiveness of White Cell-Reduction Filters in Treatment of Adult Acute Myelogenous Leukemia
Balducci L, Benson K, Lyman GH, Sanderson R, Fields K, Ballester OF, Elfenbein GJ (Univ of South Florida, Tampa)
Transfusion 33:665–670, 1993   116-95-6–30

Background.—Refractoriness to platelet transfusion may be caused by HLA alloimmunization that follows exposure to multiple blood components from different donors in patients treated for acute myelogenous leukemia (AML). To circumvent or prevent HLA alloimmunization, unfiltered or filtered pooled platelets may be used until alloimmunization develops, with crossmatch-compatible single-donor platelets used thereafter, or single-donor platelets may be used from the beginning of treatment. The cost and cost-effectiveness of these 3 strategies in the treatment of AML were compared.

Methods.—Data related to treatment, the risk of refractoriness, and costs was gathered from English language articles on transfusion medicine and from experience at 1 center. Software-based decision analysis included cost-effectiveness, sensitivity analysis, threshold evaluation, and Monte Carlo sensitivity analysis.

Outcome.—In patients without bone marrow transplantation (BMT), the cost was $12,557.14 for using unfiltered pooled platelets until alloimmunization and crossmatch-compatible single-donor platelets thereafter, $11,406.17 for using filtered pooled platelets until alloimmunization and crossmatch-compatible single-donor platelets thereafter, and $13,016.16 for using single-donor platelets from the beginning. In recipients of BMT, the cost was $14,002.72 for unfiltered pooled platelets, $12,281.89 for filtered pooled platelets, and $13,727.48 for single-donor platelets. The threshold in regard to risk of refractoriness to filtered pooled platelets was .3 for the first strategy and .27 for the second strategy without BMT and .28 for the first strategy and .4 for the second strategy with BMT. The Monte Carlo sensitivity analysis demonstrated the use of filtered blood components to be more cost-effective in 76% of patients.

Conclusion.—In the treatment of adult AML, unfiltered or filtered pooled platelets may be used until alloimmunization develops with crossmatch-compatible, single-donor platelets used thereafter, or single-donor platelets may be used from the beginning of treatment. The use of WBC reduction filters was the most cost-effective approach. Clinically, this means that WBC reduction in blood components is unlikely to result in increased cost. This decision analysis model may be useful in assessing the cost-effectiveness of any proposed practice change.

▶ This study attempts to justify the use of leukodepletion filters in patients with AML by determining the cost-effectiveness of their use compared with unfiltered random platelets and single-donor platelets. The authors abstracted data from other studies to apply to their statistical model and concluded that leukodepletion could be justified as more cost-effective than the other approaches. Obviously, their conclusions depend on the strength of their assumptions; because these assumptions for alloimmunization rates are based on historical controls, the potential for inaccuracy is introduced. Another concern is the use of patient charges rather than true costs, with the common problem of mixing costs and charges in the analysis. The most valid way to approach this issue is first to demonstrate the efficacy of various methods to reduce alloimmunization to platelets in similar patients. The Trial to Reduce Alloimmunization to Platelets (TRAP) is a multicentered funded by the National Institutes of Health study that is assessing the use of leukodepletion, reduced donor exposure, and ultraviolet irradiation to prevent alloimmunization. Until the data from this trial become available, the expense of leukodepletion will be difficult to justify on medical or economic grounds.—P.M. Ness, M.D.

Blood Component Supplementation During Massive Transfusion of AS-1 Red Cells in Trauma Patients

Faringer PD, Mullins RJ, Johnson RL, Trunkey DD (Oregon Health Sciences Univ, Portland)

J Trauma 34:481–487, 1993   116-95-6–31

Background.—Blood component transfusions have been advocated by the Office of Medical Applications of Research and the National Institutes of Health. Thus, most blood collected in the United States is now separated into a red cell product, with plasma and platelets further divided into specific components. At the immediate institution, the red cell products used for transfusions in trauma patients are AS-1 red cells that contain 100 mL of additive saline and less than 50 mL of donor plasma. During hemorrhage and massive transfusions of these cells, coagulation test results have frequently been critically abnormal. Coagulation component transfusions in trauma patients receiving more than 10 units of AS-1 red cells during the first 24 hours after injury were examined.

Patients and Methods.—Forty-four adult patients experiencing acute trauma during a 33-month period were identified. During massive transfusion of red cells, repeated blood coagulation tests were obtained to direct component treatment. To analyze blood component therapy, patients were divided into 4 groups, including those with blunt trauma without brain injury, those with penetrating trauma without brain injury, those with blunt trauma with brain injury, and those with penetrating brain injury.

Results.—Coagulopathy developed in 70% of patients. Similar coagulation anomalies were noted in patients with blunt or penetrating trauma during massive transfusions. At admission, abnormal coagulation test results were seen in more than 40% of the patients with exsanguinating hemorrhage from penetrating trauma or blunt trauma with an associated brain injury. In contrast, coagulopathy at admission was not seen in patients with blunt trauma but no associated brain injury. Patients received an average of 25 AS-1 red cell units, with a range of 10–77. In addition, patients were exposed to an average of 80 donors, with a range of 11–252. In 57% of patients, exsanguination and brain injuries constituted the primary causes of death.

Conclusion.—During massive transfusions with AS-1 red cells, profoundly abnormal coagulation tests are common. Repeated coagulation testing is encouraged.

▶ Most of the red cell transfusions administered in the United States are provided as additive red cells with minimal remaining platelets and coagulation factors. This paper reviewed the experience in a trauma center and found some intriguing results as well as some previously documented phenomena such as the common finding of coagulation abnormalities in the setting of acute head injury. Since the move to component therapy, the average trauma patient in this study received 25 units of red cells and blood components from an average of 80 donors. Although the safety of blood components has dramatically improved, with specific tests for HIV-1 and HIV-2 and antibody for hepatitis C virus, these patients are at significant risk for adverse transfusion effects. The authors recommend serial coagulation testing as a means of providing specific therapy, rather than prophylactic regimens that would likely increase donor exposures.—P.M. Ness, M.D.

Effects of Blood Transfusion on Oxygen Transport Variables in Severe Sepsis
Lorente JA, Landín L, De Pablo R, Renes E, Rodríguez-Díaz R, Liste D (Hosp Ramón y Cajal, Madrid; Hosp Universitario de Getafe, Madrid)
Crit Care Med 21:1312–1318, 1993   116-95-6–32

Purpose.—Previous studies have shown that sepsis is characterized by an abnormal oxygen delivery to oxygen uptake relationship. The effectiveness of increasing oxygen delivery with a packed red cell transfusion as a means of improving oxygen use in septic patients was evaluated in a prospective, randomized, interventional crossover study.

Methods.—Sixteen patients with severe sepsis and a hemoglobin concentration of less than 10 g/dL received, in random order, 800 mL of packed red cells transfused during 90 minutes and a dobutamine infusion at a dose of 10 µg/kg/min. Hemodynamic and oxygen transport variables were measured before and after each intervention. At least 20 minutes were allowed during dobutamine infusion to reach the steady state.

Results.—Dobutamine infusion increased the oxygen delivery by a mean of 48.5% and oxygen uptake by a mean of 21.7%. Blood transfusion increased the oxygen delivery by a mean of 21.4%, but the oxygen uptake did not change significantly.

Conclusion.—The failure of blood transfusion to increase the oxygen uptake in septic patients with an abnormal oxygen delivery to oxygen uptake relationship illustrates that oxygen uptake in these patients depends more on blood flow than on global oxygen delivery.

▶ This carefully performed clinical study suggests that hematocrit increments achieved by transfusions are less important in maintaining oxygen delivery than improvements in perfusion. The paper is another example of the use of clinical monitoring technology that may someday be available to guide clinicians in more appropriate transfusion management.—P.M. Ness, M.D.

Pediatric Transfusion Practice

Suppression of Erythropoiesis by Intrauterine Transfusions in Hemolytic Disease of the Newborn: Use of Erythropoietin to Treat the Late Anemia

Scaradavou A, Inglis S, Peterson P, Dunne J, Chervenak F, Bussel J (New York Hosp–Cornell Med Ctr, New York)
J Pediatr 123:279–284, 1993   116-95-6–33

Introduction.—Fetal isoimmune hemolytic disease is now treated with intrauterine transfusion (IUT). This has changed the clinical picture for these neonates. Although they are born with a normal hematocrit, they may have severe postnatal anemia without increased levels of EPO. Intrauterine transfusion may suppress erythropoiesis. The potential of EPO as a therapeutic agent for postnatal anemia was investigated in 4 infants who received multiple IUTs to treat fetal isoimmune hemolytic disease.

Treatment.—Patients with postnatal anemia after IUT were treated with 200 units of EPO per kg subcutaneously 3 times per week.

Results.—Despite severe anemia, bone marrow hypoplasia and low levels of EPO were documented in these infants. After 2–4 weeks of EPO treatment, reticulocytosis and increased hemoglobin values were detected. One patient had a recurrence of anemia after cessation of EPO therapy but responded to retreatment with EPO.

Conclusion.—The results of this small pilot study suggest that treatment with EPO may shorten the duration of postnatal anemia and decrease the requirement for transfusion in infants with Rh hemolytic disease. A controlled trial is under way to evaluate EPO in the treatment of hemolytic disease and postnatal anemia of the newborn.

▶ When therapy of hemolytic disease of the newborn is considered, the intrauterine phase and the peripartum period are clearly recognized as times when transfusion support is often required. However, it is less commonly recognized that late anemia can occur as a result of suppression of erythropoiesis by these earlier transfusions; many infants require transfusion support in the postnatal period. This report suggests that subcutaneous EPO injections can reduce the late anemia and subsequent requirements for transfusion. A controlled, clinical trial is about to be initiated.—P.M. Ness, M.D.

Comparison of Two Preservation Solutions for Erythrocyte Transfusions in Newborn Infants
Goodstein MH, Locke RG, Wlodarczyk D, Goldsmith LS, Rubenstein SD, Herman JH (Temple Univ, Philadelphia; American Red Cross Blood Service, Philadelphia)
J Pediatr 123:783–788, 1993   116-95-6–34

Purpose.—Anticoagulant solutions for packed RBCs that contain mannitol, adenine, and dextrose (AS-1) have several advantages over the citrate-phosphate-dextrose-adenine (CPDA-1) solutions. Because the safety of AS-1 in packed RBCs for very-low-birth-weight (VLBW) infants has not been established, CPDA-1–preserved packed RBCs are still used in the neonatal intensive care unit. The safety and efficacy of AS-1–preserved packed RBCs in VLBW infants were investigated.

Patients.—Sixteen premature infants with a mean birth weight of 863 g and a mean gestational age of 26 weeks were randomly allocated to receive small-volume transfusions with AS-1–preserved packed RBCs or CPDA-1–preserved packed RBCs. Eleven infants were on mechanical ventilation and 5 were receiving nasal continuous positive airway pressure. The mean age of the infants at the time of transfusion was 5 days.

Results.—After transfusion, the mean hemoglobin concentration was increased in both treatment groups, but the mean hemoglobin increase in infants receiving CPDA-1–preserved packed RBCs was .9 g/dL greater than that seen with AS-1–preserved packed RBCs. The difference was attributed to the higher hematocrit of red cells preserved with CPDA-1. Infants treated with the AS-1–preserved packed RBCs had improved glucose homeostasis compared with those treated with CPDA-1–preserved packed RBCs. This difference was attributed to the higher dextrose content of AS-1–preserved packed RBCs. There were no other significant differences in any of the measured parameters between the 2 groups.

Conclusion.—Packed RBCs preserved with AS-1 are as safe and effective as CPDA-1–preserved packed RBCs when used to increase the hemoglobin concentration in VLBW infants.

▶ When modifications to blood collection procedures are suggested, they are often introduced into adult transfusion practices before becoming accepted for neonatal transfusions. Neonatologists have been slow to adopt the additive anticoagulant preservative solutions that have become routine in adult medicine; they have been exercising appropriate caution because of concern that the constituents may have unknown risks for neonates. This study should reassure neonatologists that blood collected in CPDA-1 and AS-1 are equally safe and effective. Because both solutions contain adenine, a constituent that may be toxic in very high doses, this study will not necessarily convert skeptical neonatologists from the traditional citrate-phosphate-dextrose blood to the additive approach.—P.M. Ness, M.D.

A Randomized, Controlled Trial of Platelet Transfusions in Thrombocytopenic Premature Infants

Andrew M, Vegh P, Caco C, Kirpalani H, Jefferies A, Ohlsson A, Watts J, Saigal S, Milner R, Wang E (McMaster Univ, Hamilton, Ont, Canada; Hosp for Sick Children, Toronto; Women's College Hosp, Toronto; et al)
J Pediatr 123:285–291, 1993   116-95-6–35

Background.—In sick newborns, thrombocytopenia is the most common hemostatic abnormality. Whether the early use of platelet concentrates would decrease the incidence or extension of intracranial hemor-

Intracranial Hemorrhage

	Treated (n = 78)		Control (n = 74)	
	Initial	End	Initial	End
Grade 0	38	33	37	32
Grade I	19	18	23	22
Grade II	9	3	5	3
Grade III	5	13	4	10
Grade IV	7	11	5	4
PVL	0	0	0	3
Overall increase	22 (28.2%)		19 (25.7%)	

Abbreviation: PVL, periventricular leukomalacia.
(Courtesy of Andrew M, Vegh P, Caco C, et al: *J Pediatr* 123:285–291, 1993.)

rhage in such infants was determined in a multicenter, prospective, randomized, controlled study.

Patients and Methods.—Four Canadian tertiary neonatal care units participated. A total of 152 premature infants with a birth weight of 500–1,500 g, gestational age younger than 33 weeks, and platelet counts of less than 150×10^9/L during the first 72 hours of life were enrolled. Of these, 74 were randomly assigned to receive conventional therapy only, whereas the remaining 78 received conventional therapy and platelet concentrates at a dose of 10 mL/kg. Treated infants were permitted to receive as many as 3 infusions during the study, the aim being to maintain a platelet count of less than 150×10^9/L until day 7 of life. Secondary outcome measures included the effects on bleeding as reflected by the amount of blood product support administered and a shortened bleeding time.

Results.—During the study, platelet counts in treated infants remained significantly increased compared with those in the control group. New intracranial hemorrhages developed or an already existing hemorrhage became more extensive in 22 of the treated and 19 of the control infants (table). Both initial and follow-up ultrasonography revealed that a comparable number of infants had each grade of intracranial hemorrhage. Fresh frozen plasma and packed RBCs were administered to a similar number of infants. However, treated infants received less of both. In treated infants, the bleeding time was prolonged before the infusion of platelet concentrates but shortened after infusions were administered. After a subanalysis of control infants, it was found that the 21 with platelet counts of less than 60×10^9/L had received more fresh frozen plasma and packed RBCs on at least 1 occasion compared with those with counts greater than 60×10^9/L.

Conclusion.—Early infusion of platelet concentrates resulted in increased platelet counts and shortened bleeding times. However, the incidence or extent of intracranial hemorrhage was not decreased in these infants. It has been suggested that prophylactic platelet transfusions need not be administered to nonbleeding premature infants with counts of more than approximately $60 \times 10^9/L$.

▶ Many thrombocytopenic premature infants receive prophylactic platelet transfusions to prevent intracranial hemorrhage or to limit its extension; in some infants, a platelet count of 150,000/μL is the target of these transfusions. This controlled, randomized study showed that prophylactic transfusions did not limit the initiation or spread of intracranial hemorrhage, suggesting a more reasonable cutoff of 60,000/μL.—P.M. Ness, M.D.

Transfusion Therapy for Severe Anemia
Jayabose S, Tugal O, Ruddy R, Wuest D, Ciavarella D (New York Med College, Valhalla)
Am J Pediatr Hematol Oncol 15:324–327, 1993   116-95-6–36

Background.—Recommendations on transfusion of packed RBCs for children with severe anemia generally suggest a slow rate of transfusion or transfusion with intervals of several hours for cardiovascular stabilization. These recommendations have not been evaluated in clinical studies in children. A recent study in adults with severe anemia found no adverse hemodynamic or clinical effects from more rapid transfusion. The safety and efficacy of a new transfusion regimen, continuous transfusion therapy, in children with severe anemia were prospectively evaluated.

Transfusion Therapy.—Twenty-two children with severe anemia of gradual onset requiring transfusion of packed RBCs were enrolled in a prospective study of the regimen of continuous transfusion therapy. A continuous infusion of packed RBCs was administered through a peripheral vein at a rate of 2 cc/kg/hr until the desired volume was reached. The volume to be transfused was computed by the increase in hematocrit per 1 cc of packed RBCs/kg transfused. The children were closely monitored throughout the transfusion for any adverse hemodynamic or clinical effects.

Results.—The 22 children all had significant tachycardia on admission but had a decrease in heart rate by the completion of transfusion. The mean decline in the heart rate was 28% of the baseline heart rate. None of the children had an increase in heart rate or any physical signs of congestive heart failure during or after the transfusion. Four patients in the aplastic crisis of sickle cell anemia had the smallest increase in hematocrit. The other 18 children had a mean increase in the hematocrit of 1.04%/cc/kg of packed RBCs.

Conclusion.—The recommendation for a slow rate of transfusion of packed RBCs for children with severe anemia appears to be based on common practice and not on clinical evidence. Transfusion of packed RBCs at a steady rate of 2 cc/kg/hr was safe and effective in most study children with severe anemia. None of the children had any adverse hemodynamic or clinical effects during or after transfusion. The major advantage of the continuous infusion regimen is that the shorter time needed for the transfusion results in a shorter hospital stay.

▶ Many pediatric transfusion practices are based on treatments derived from adult practices that are often designed to avoid unusual adverse transfusion outcomes. In adult practice, it is common to transfuse red cells slowly to a patient with severe chronic anemia to avoid the problems of fluid overload. No rigorous studies of infusion practices have been performed in children with severe anemia. This paper describes a continuous transfusion protocol for infants and children that shortened the duration of transfusions without complications.—P.M. Ness, M.D.

Transplantation and Immunomodulation

Blood Transfusions and Prognosis in Colorectal Cancer

Busch ORC, Hop WCJ, Hoynck van Papendrecht MAW, Marquet RL, Jeekel J (Univ Hosp Rotterdam-Dijkzigt, The Netherlands; Erasmus Univ, Rotterdam, The Netherlands)

N Engl J Med 328:1372–1376, 1993   116-95-6–37

Background.—Blood transfusion seems to affect the prognosis of patients undergoing surgery for cancer adversely, although this has not been proven. A randomized, multicenter trial was done in patients with colorectal cancer to determine whether autologous blood transfusion decreases the rate of cancer recurrence and improves survival compared with allogeneic transfusion.

Methods.—Four hundred seventy-five patients were included; 236 patients received allogeneic transfusions, and 239 received autologous transfusions. Patients in the autologous-transfusion group donated 2 units of blood before their operation.

Findings.—The 4-year colorectal cancer-specific survival rates were 67% and 62% in the allogeneic and autologous transfusion groups, respectively. Of the 423 patients having curative surgery, 66% receiving allogeneic transfusion had no colorectal cancer recurrence at 4 years, compared with 63% in the autologous transfusion group (Fig 6–5). Recurrence risk was significantly higher in patients receiving blood transfusions of either type compared with patients not needing transfusions. Relative recurrence rates (2.1 and 1.8, respectively) were not significantly different.

Conclusion.—The use of autologous compared with allogeneic blood for transfusion in patients undergoing surgery for colorectal cancer does

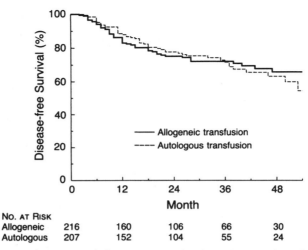

Fig 6–5.—Disease-free survival of all 423 patients with colorectal cancer who underwent curative surgery. The disease-free survival at 4 years was 66% in the allogeneic-transfusion group and 63% in the autologous-transfusion group ($P = .93$). The 95% confidence interval for the difference between these percentages (autologous minus allogeneic) ranged from -16% to $+10\%$. (Courtesy of Busch ORC, Hop WCJ, Hoynck van Papendrecht MAW, et al: N Engl J Med 328:1372–1376, 1993.)

not improve prognosis. Either type of transfusion is associated with poor prognosis, most likely because of the circumstances necessitating it.

▶ This is a long-awaited prospective investigation of the effect of blood transfusions on cancer recurrence. Previous retrospective analyses have produced many suggestive positive trials but a significant minority of negative studies as well. This study showed no difference in cancer recurrence in patients who were randomized to get autologous blood or bank blood. On the other hand, patients who got any blood had a poorer prognosis, probably due to clinical circumstances that necessitated transfusions as part of their surgical management. It would be difficult to perform a similar study in the United States that randomizes patients to receive bank blood without offering autologous options. The issue of medical severity of transfused vs. nontransfused patients will remain difficult to resolve. Many statistical methods for handling this problem do not satisfy skeptical clinicians, and the alternative of sham transfusions for patients who do not require them would be difficult for many researchers to support.—P.M. Ness, M.D.

Allogeneic Blood Transfusion-Induced Enhancement of Tumor Growth: Two Animal Models Showing Amelioration by Leukodepletion and Passive Transfer Using Spleen Cells
Blajchman MA, Bardossy L, Carmen R, Sastry A, Singal DP (McMaster Univ,

Hamilton, Ont, Canada; Miles Inc, Berkeley, Calif)
Blood 81:1880–1882, 1993   116-95-6–38

Background.—Allogeneic blood transfusion reportedly can have immunomodulating effects in those receiving blood products. The mechanisms involved are unknown, but patients having malignant disease may be adversely affected. A number of nonrandomized, mainly retrospective studies suggest that allogeneic blood transfusions may compromise the outcome in surgically treated patients with cancer. Such transfusions apparently may enhance the growth of primary tumors and increase the formation of metastatic pulmonary nodules in inbred mice.

Objective.—The effects of leukodepletion of allogeneic blood before transfusion were examined in both mice and rabbits to clarify how transfusions may promote tumor growth. In addition, whether the effect can be passively transferred by spleen cells from allogeneically transfused animals was determined.

Findings.—Leukodepletion studies using VX-2 tumor cells indicated that tumor growth is promoted by leukocytes in donor blood and that this effect is abolished by removing leukocytes before transfusing the blood. Numbers of metastatic pulmonary nodules were significantly more frequent in both mice and rabbits receiving whole blood than when leukodepletion, which was more than 99% efficient, was performed. Significantly more metastatic nodules were found in animals given spleen cells from allogeneically transfused animals than in those receiving cells from syngeneically transfused animals, or animals receiving leukodepleted allogeneic blood.

Conclusion.—It is likely that the tumor-promoting effect of transfusing allogeneic blood may be avoided by administering leukodepleted blood products to patients with malignant disease.

Experimental Animal Model of Refractoriness to Donor Platelets: The Effect of Plasma Removal and the Extent of White Cell Reduction on Allogeneic Alloimmunization

Bordin JO, Bardossy L, Blajchman MA (McMaster Univ, Hamilton, Ont, Canada; Canadian Red Cross Society, Hamilton, Ont, Canada)
Transfusion 33:798–801, 1993   116-95-6–39

Background.—A high percentage of multiply transfused patients with thrombocytopenic bleeding associated with bone marrow failure become refractory to random-donor platelets, limiting the platelets' effectiveness. The development of refractoriness to random-donor platelets has been causally associated with the WBCs. White blood cell reduction filters with variable efficiency effectively decrease the incidence of platelet alloimmunization. The threshold number of WBCs below which alloimmunization would no longer occur has not been determined. An an-

Platelet Survival and Refractory Rate in New Zealand White
Rabbits That Received WBC-Reduced Red Cell Suspensions or
Red Cell Suspensions Both WBC-Reduced and Plasma-Depleted

Transfused component	n	Mean ± SD platelet survival (hours) (95% CI*)	Refractory rate
WBC-reduced red cells	34	50.8 ± 18.2 (12.6-98.8 hours)	29.4%
WBC-reduced, plasma depleted red cells	12	54.9 ± 7.0 (43.8-70.1 hours)	0%

* *Abbreviation:* CI, confidence interval.
(Courtesy of Bordin JO, Bardossy L, Blajchman MA: *Transfusion* 33:798–801, 1993.)

imal model was used to examine the relative efficiency of second- and third-generation filters in decreasing the frequency of refractoriness to allogeneic platelets. The possible incremental benefit of removing supernatant plasma to prevent platelet refractoriness was also evaluated.

Methods.—California Black rabbits were used as blood donors with New Zealand White rabbits as transfusion recipients. After 8 weekly transfusions, the platelet survival time in each recipient animal was evaluated. The effect of second-generation vs. third-generation filters on WBC reduction was analyzed. Groups of animals also received transfusions with red cell suspensions that had been either WBC-reduced or both plasma-depleted and WBC-reduced.

Results.—The groups receiving second- or third-generation WBC-reduced blood showed no difference in the mean platelet survival and rate of refractoriness to allogeneic platelets. The rabbits that received WBC-reduced and plasma-depleted red cells had a significantly lower rate of allogeneic platelet refractoriness than those that received only WBC-reduced red cells (table).

Conclusion.—The combined use of plasma depletion and WBC reduction decreased the frequency of refractoriness produced by allogeneic blood transfusions more than the use of WBC reduction alone. The removal of supernatant plasma may be an important adjunct to WBC reduction in decreasing alloimmunization after allogeneic blood transfusion.

▶ The leading suspect in the search for the immunomodulatory source in blood transfusions is the allogeneic white cell. Because clinical studies in patients are so difficult, these researchers turned to animal models (mice and rabbits) to demonstrate that leukodepleted red cells did not prompt tumor growth in animals with malignant disease. Similar animal systems were also employed by the same investigators to study the effect of WBC contamination and the removal of plasma on alloimmunization after transfusions.—P.M. Ness, M.D.

Adverse Effects of Transfusion

The Infectious Risks of Transfusions in the United States: A Decision-Analytic Approach
Heymann SJ, Brewer TF (Harvard School of Public Health, Boston; Harvard Med School, Boston)
Am J Infect Control 21:174–182, 1993
116-95-6–40

Background.—Almost two thirds of the 20 million units of blood products transfused in the United States every year are packed RBCs. Transfusion is often lifesaving, but it carries several infectious and noninfectious risks despite universal screening and donor deferral. The greatest infectious risks are the development of AIDS as a result of transmission of HIV or of cirrhosis from the transmission of non-A, non-B hepatitis (NANBH) in blood products. A decision-analytic model was used to provide explicit quantitative guidelines to determine when the risk of death from all causes associated with transfusion exceeds the risk of death associated with anemia.

Model.—The decision-analytic model provided results in terms of a transfusion threshold. The transfusion threshold is the value for which a patient would find it equally desirable to have and to forego a transfusion. The transfusion threshold is stated in terms of risk of dying of anemia. The analysis determined the transfusion threshold on the basis of risk per unit of blood transfused. Sensitivity analyses were conducted on independent variables, including the rate of HIV seroconversion, the rate of acquiring AIDS, the rate of dying of AIDS, the risk of acquiring and dying of NANBH, and the usefulness of different outcomes.

Results.—In the United States, screening and donor deferral have made the risk of death from HIV, NANBH, and other infectious and noninfectious complications of transfusion extremely small. On the basis of reported transfusion complication rates and an independent worst-case calculation of the risk of AIDS and NANBH, transfusion with RBCs should be recommended if the chance of dying of anemia can be decreased by at least 1/1,100.

Conclusion.—The results of this decision-analytic model can be used to develop transfusion guidelines based on quantitative information. In the United States, the risk of infectious or noninfectious complications of transfusion are extremely small. Transfusion with RBCs is worthwhile and should be recommended if the chance of dying of anemia can be decreased by at least 1/1,100. In the United States, undertransfusion is a potential problem despite the relative safety of the blood supply. Conversely, overtransfusion for the reduction of morbidity should be avoided because the risk of mortality is small but does exist. This decision-analytic model may be useful in assessing the risk of death associated with transfusion of other blood products or in assessing risk from other potential or future contaminants of the blood supply.

▶ In the face of the widespread media attention to the infectious risks of transfusion, it is difficult to convince patients and their physicians that the risks of undertransfusion may be more substantial than the risks of acceptable transfusion. This paper employs a decision-analytic approach to prove that minimal diminution of the risk of dying of anemia outweighs the risk of transfusion-associated infection. Although many transfusion specialists realize this fact and are beginning to observe clinical states whereby undertransfusion may produce significant ischemic injury, the trend toward minimizing transfusion support will be difficult to counteract. In addition, accrediting agencies such as the Joint Commission on Accreditation of Healthcare Organizations are requiring hospitals to adopt transfusion criteria such as red cell transfusion guidelines that have not been substantiated with carefully performed current clinical studies using modern therapeutic approaches.—P.M. Ness, M.D.

Heterosexually Acquired Human Immunodeficiency Virus Infection and the United States Blood Supply: Considerations for Screening of Potential Blood Donors
Petersen LR, Doll LS, White CR, Johnson E, Williams A, and the HIV Blood Donor Study Group (Ctrs for Disease Control, Atlanta, Ga; American Natl Red Cross, Rockville, Md)
Transfusion 33:552–557, 1993   116-95-6–41

Background.—Surveillance data on AIDS show that the incidence of HIV infection from male homosexual contact and drug injection peaked during the mid-1980s. However, the incidence of HIV infection attributed to heterosexual contact continues to increase in the 1990s. This increase in heterosexual HIV infection has raised concerns about the safety of blood transfusions. Many HIV-1–seropositive blood donors do not know they are infected, and they would not be excluded as donors by current deferral criteria unless they or their partners were known to be HIV-positive.

Participants and Methods.—A 2-phase study was conducted at 20 blood centers. The first phase, involving 508 seropositive blood donors, was done from May of 1988 through August of 1989. The second phase was conducted from January of 1990 through May of 1991 and involved 472 donors. Blood samples from all donors were subjected to an enzyme immunosorbent assay, with repeatably reactive samples tested via the Western blot method. Similar questionnaires were used during both phases, except that items requiring additional information pertaining to heterosexual transmission risk were added during phase 2.

Results.—There was an overall decrease in HIV prevalence from phase 1 (.021) to phase 2 (.018). The HIV risk factors among HIV-1–seropositive donors were similar during both phases. Positive serologic tests for syphilis, hepatitis B core antibody, or hepatitis C antibody were found among 13% of male participants and 17% of female participants during phase 2. The median numbers of previous-year and lifetime sex partners were as follows: for men they were 2 and 30, respectively, and for women they were 1 and 7, respectively. Of those reporting heterosexual transmission risk, 31% of the men and 6% of the women also reported having had either syphilis or gonorrhea within 3 years of donation.

Conclusion.—The heterosexual transmission of HIV infection and its impact on the safety of blood transfusion are not worsening at this time. Therefore, deferring donations based on the number of sexual partners or history of sexually transmitted disease will have little benefit and will result in exclusion of a large number of donors who are not infected with HIV.

▶ Although HIV infection can definitely be acquired by heterosexual relationships, this study of HIV-positive blood donors conducted by the Centers for Disease Control does not show a major impact of heterosexual transmission on blood safety. It also shows that any attempt to use the number of sexual contacts as a means to defer high-risk blood donors will exclude many noninfectious donors and have little current impact on transfusion-associated AIDS cases.—P.M. Ness, M.D.

Trends in Transfusion-Associated Acquired Immune Deficiency Syndrome in the United States, 1982 Through 1991
Selik RM, Ward JW, Buehler JW (United States Dept of Health and Human Services, Atlanta, Ga)
Transfusion 33:890–893, 1993   116-95-6–42

Purpose.—Testing of donated blood for HIV antibody and changes in blood use practices have lessened the risk of transfusion-related HIV infection. However, AIDS continues to be diagnosed in blood transfusion recipients. The overall efficacy of measures to prevent HIV transmission by blood transfusion was investigated.

Methods.—The investigators analyzed trends in reported transfusion-associated AIDS, both by year of transfusion and by year of diagnosis through June of 1992. The analysis by year of diagnosis was stratified by age to define important age-related differences.

Results.—The year of transfusion analysis showed 56 cases in 1978, peaking at 714 cases in 1984. In 1985, when screening for HIV antibody was initiated, the number of cases decreased to 288. From 1986 through 1991, there were less than 20 reported cases per year. The investigators reinvestigated a sample of cases attributed to transfusions since 1985, and their findings suggested that only one fourth of those cases actually resulted from transfusion. By year of diagnosis, the number of cases increased from 14 in 1982 to 824 in 1987, remaining relatively stable at that level thereafter. Almost all reported cases diagnosed in 1991 were caused by transfusions administered before 1986. Stratification by age showed that after 1987, the number of cases diagnosed in individuals aged 65 years or older decreased dramatically, remained stable in those aged 45–64 years, and continued to increase in those aged 25–44 years. The median age of patients with reported transfusion-related AIDS declined from 59 in 1986 to 47 in 1991.

Conclusion.—Screening for HIV antibody and other blood use measures has almost completely eliminated transfusion-related transmission of HIV. However, many cases of infection were transmitted before screening began, and AIDS continues to be diagnosed among increasingly younger patients. The age-related differences are explained by the shorter mean interval between transfusion and AIDS diagnosis in older adults.

▶ This report provides a concise overview of the transfusion-associated AIDS epidemic in the United States from the perspective of cases reported to the Centers for Disease Control. Of particular note is the rapid decrease in reported cases from transfusions occurring after 1985 and the consistent low level of remaining reports. These trends suggest that the HIV donor screening protocols are highly effective, but rare cases of HIV transmission can occur from donors who are in the process of seroconverting but are seronegative at the time of donation.—P.M. Ness, M.D.

Photochemical Inactivation of Cell-Associated Human Immunodeficiency Virus in Platelet Concentrates

Lin L, Londe H, Hanson CV, Wiesehahn G, Isaacs S, Cimino G, Corash L (Steritech Inc, Concord, Calif; California Dept of Health Services, Berkeley; Univ of California, San Francisco; et al)
Blood 82:292–297, 1993   116-95-6-43

Background.—Although the rate of viral infection caused by blood transfusions is low, a small risk of transmission remains. Additionally, there is the continuing risk of new pathogens that may develop and spread through the donor population before screening tests can be developed. A potential solution to these problems would be the development of a decontamination strategy that would result in universal inactivation of all potential pathogens. Psoralens are DNA-binding compounds that bind DNA with high specificity in the presence of ultraviolet light (UVA), and may thus serve as wide-spectrum pathogen inactivators. The effects of this photochemical decontamination technique

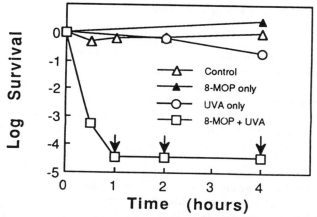

Fig 6–6.—Inactivation of cell-associated HIV-1 using 8-MOP. Infected H9 cells (2.5 × 10⁷) were seeded into platelet concentrates to yield a final infectious HIV-1 concentration of .5 × 10⁶ PFU/mL. Contaminated samples were treated with 8-MOP (300 µg/mL) and UVA (320 to 400 nm, 17 mW/cm²) for as long as 4 hours. Samples were obtained at 30 minutes, 1 hour, 2 hours, and 4 hours for measurement of residual HIV-1 infectivity. The HIV-1 infectivity is expressed as the $\log_{10}$ of residual fraction of infectious HIV-1. Treatment time is expressed in hours. *Arrows* indicate infectivity is below the detection limit of the MT-2 plaque assay (< 10 PFU/mL). (Courtesy of Lin L, Londe H, Hanson CV, et al: *Blood* 82:292–297, 1993.)

on cell-associated HIV-1 in platelet concentrates were examined, and a novel assay to monitor inactivation efficiency was developed.

Methods.—Human platelet concentrates were obtained within 1–2 days of donation and mixed with high-titer (approximately 10⁶ plaque-forming units/mL) cell-associated HIV-1 from H9 cells. The infected samples were treated with 300 µg of 8-methoxypsoralen (8-MOP) per mL and then by long-wave UVA at 17 mW/cm² for as long as 4 hours. Psoralen-DNA adduct formation was monitored by measuring the inhibition of polymerase chain reaction (PCR) amplification of an HLA-DQ-α fragment.

Results.—Sixty minutes of photochemical decontamination treatment (8-MOP 300 µg/mL, UVA 17 mW/cm²) resulted in the inactivation of .5 × 10⁶ plaque-forming units of cell-associated HIV-1 (Fig 6–6). Moreover, no virus was detectable by infectivity assay. Fifteen 8-MOP–DNA adducts per 1,000 bp were formed after 60 minutes, whereas no adducts were formed in the absence of UVA. When more than 8 psoralen-DNA adducts per 1,000 bp were present, PCR-mediated amplification of a 242-bp cellular DNA sequence was inhibited.

Conclusion.—High titers of cell-associated HIV-1 in platelet concentrates are inactivated by photochemical decontamination, and the number of 8-MOP–DNA adducts in nucleated cells is sufficient to inhibit amplification of DNA segments that encode for as few as 80 amino acids.

▶ A simple method to sterilize blood would be useful to reassure patients and physicians. While these approaches are being hotly pursued to eradicate viruses such as HIV, the side benefit to hematologists would be the eradication of bacteria that occasionally contaminate platelets and can cause septic platelet transfusion reactions. The potential toxicity of psoralens and the cost-effectiveness of the methodology will require study before implementation.—P.M. Ness, M.D.

Human T-Cell Leukemia Virus Type II Infection Frequently Goes Undetected in Contemporary US Blood Donors
Hjelle B, Wilson C, Cyrus S, Bradshaw P, Lo J, Schammel C, Wiltbank T, Alexander S (Univ of New Mexico, Albuquerque; United Blood Services, Albuquerque, NM; Blood Systems Inc, Scottsdale, Ariz; et al)
Blood 81:1641–1644, 1993   116-95-6-44

Introduction.—Blood centers in the United States screen for HTLV antibodies by using an enzyme-linked immunosorbent assay (ELISA) and then a Western blot in the case of a positive result. The tests are based on HTLV-I antigen and may not be sensitive to HTLV-II. To determine whether the current ELISA test used to screen blood donations is sensitive to serum antibodies to HTLV-II, the rate of HTLV infection in ELISA-negative donors was estimated.

Methods.—Two methods of estimating the HTLV infection rate in ELISA-negative donors were used. The donation histories of 60 ELISA-positive, Western blot–positive donors were retrospectively evaluated for previous ELISA-negative donations. Sera were also collected prospectively for a 2.5-month period from consecutive blood donors with a high-negative ELISA. Samples were analyzed with ELISA, Western blot, and polymerase chain reaction.

Findings.—The donation histories of 60 ELISA-positive and Western blot–positive donors at a single blood center were examined. Of these donors, 8 had made a total of 16 previous donations, giving a 21% rate of undetected anti-HTLV antibodies in this group. Among these 8 donors, 1 was infected with HTLV-I, and the rest were infected with HTLV-II. There was no clear demarcation between the previous negative responses of these donors and uninfected donors. When 178 high-negative ELISA sera were collected prospectively and tested by Western blot, 11 were positive. Ten of these positives were HTLV-II positive.

Conclusion.—The ELISA currently used to screen donated blood supplies for HTLV antibodies missed 43% of HTLV-II infections and 20% of HTLV-I infections in these groups of patients. Screening tests with greater sensitivity to HTLV-II are being developed.

▶ When blood banks introduced testing for HTLV-I in blood donors in the late 1980s, many practitioners did not realize that the tests would also detect HTLV-II. This overlap complicated donor counseling because HTLV-II is not known to be specifically associated with a disease process. On the other hand, HTLV-I is clearly associated with 2 disease patterns: adult T-cell leukemia and a neuropathy known as tropical spastic paraparesis. Several intriguing case reports have emerged that suggest an association of a chronic neuropathy with HTLV-II. If disease associations are confirmed, the detection of HTLV-II may become an important issue in blood screening. Because this paper suggests that many assay systems are not sufficiently sensitive to detect some cases of HTLV-II, a specific disease association would stimulate assay improvements to enhance recipient safety and donor counseling.—P.M. Ness, M.D.

Absence of Hepatitis B Virus DNA Detected by Polymerase Chain Reaction in Blood Donors Who Are Hepatitis B Surface Antigen Negative and Antibody to Hepatitis B Core Antigen Positive From a United States Population With a Low Prevalence of Hepatitis B Serologic Markers

Douglas DD, Taswell HF, Rakela J, Rabe D (Mayo Clinic and Mayo Found, Rochester, Minn)
Transfusion 33:212–216, 1993   116-95-6-45

Background.—A polymerase chain reaction (PCR) amplification technique found hepatitis B virus (HBV) DNA in 4% of blood donors negative for hepatitis B surface antigen (HBsAg) and positive for antibody to hepatitis B core antigens (anti-HBc). The population examined had a high prevalence of hepatitis B serologic markers. The prevalence of HBV DNA was assessed in a group of HBsAg-negative, anti-HBc–positive blood donors from a population with a low prevalence of hepatitis B serologic markers.

Methods and Findings.—A sensitive, nested PCR assay was used to assess 158 units of blood that was repeatedly reactive for anti-HBc. Blood was donated by 119 donors for allogenic (93 units) and autologous (65 units) use. No HBV DNA could be detected by PCR in the 39 units donated by 83 allogeneic donors or in the 65 units donated by 36 autologous donors.

Conclusion.—Anti-HBc testing is not an efficient means of screening for potential hepatitis infection. This test is associated with low specificity among those populations with a low prevalence of hepatitis B serologic markers.

Significance of Antibody to Hepatitis B Core Antigen in Blood Donors as Determined by Their Serologic Response to Hepatitis B Vaccine

Aoki SK, Finegold D, Kuramoto IK, Douville C, Richards C, Randell R, Fernando L, Holland PV, Zeldis JB (Univ of California, Davis, Sacramento)
Transfusion 33:362–367, 1993   116-95-6–46

Background.—Testing of blood donors for antibody to hepatitis B core antigen (anti-HBc) is a nonspecific means of decreasing the risk of transmission of the hepatitis C virus. Blood centers in the United States report that approximately 1.1% of repeat donors are reactive for anti-HBc in enzyme immunoassay (EIA). The results are apparently false positive in about 35% of these donors because they have no evidence of previous or current hepatitis B virus (HBV) infection. Large volumes of donated blood are unnecessarily discarded each year because of false positive anti-HBc reactions. To eliminate nonspecific, false positive reactions and still detect persons with HBV infections in the past, a more specific interpretation of an anti-HBc EIA-reactive result was tested. The interpretation was based on the donor sample-to-cutoff absorbance ratio.

Methods.—Fifty-eight volunteer blood donors who had been previously deferred as donors at least twice solely on the basis of reactive anti-HBc tests were vaccinated for hepatitis B. The serologic response to the vaccine was noted. Interpretation of the anti-HBc EIA-reactive result was based on the donor sample-to-cutoff absorbance ratio. An anamnestic response to vaccine indicated past infection with hepatitis B, whereas a primary response to vaccine indicated no past infection with hepatitis B.

Results.—Of 58 donors, 53 responded to HBV vaccination. Nine donors had anamnestic responses and 44 had primary responses (table). Two percent of the donors with historically weak anti-HBc had an an-

Blood Donor Responses to Hepatitis B Vaccine Compared With Strength of Prior Anti-HBc–Reactive Enzyme Immunoassays (EIAs)

Response to hepatitis B vaccine	Results of prior anti-HBc EIAs	
	Strong*†	Weak †
Anamnestic	8 (53%)	1 (2%)
Primary	6 (40%)	38 (88%)
None	1 (7%)	4 (9%)
Total	15 (100%)	43 (100%)

* Indicates donor sample-to-cutoff absorbance ratio of < .45.
† The groups "Weak" and "Strong" were not homogenous with respect to vaccine response (P < .005).
(Courtesy of Aoki SK, Finegold D, Kuramoto IK, et al: *Transfusion* 33:362–367, 1993.)

amnestic response compared with 53% of the donors with historically strong anti-HBc. Testing with anti-HBc using the microparticle EIA method also correlated well with hepatitis B vaccination results.

Conclusion.—A narrower interpretation of reactive anti-HBc EIA results based on the donor sample-to-cutoff absorbance ratio was tested. The more precise interpretation provided improved specificity as an indicator of past hepatitis B infection but resulted in a slight loss of sensitivity. This narrower interpretation may result in fewer deferrals for false positive anti-HBc tests. However, confirmation by HBV vaccination is expensive and time-consuming. Improved assay methods or a confirmation test for anti-HBc will decrease the number of blood donors unnecessarily deferred because of false positive results.

▶ Testing blood donors for anti-HBc has been the source of many problems for blood centers. It was instituted as a surrogate test for non-A, non-B hepatitis prior to the discovery and implementation of testing for antibody to hepatitis C virus. Some critics claim that it should have been used earlier as a screening test for donors at risk for HIV infection. Although it is occasionally positive as a sole marker of hepatitis B infection, more commonly a positive test in a blood donor indicates previous infection or a true false positive test. Despite efforts of assay manufacturers to develop more specific screening tests, a significant percentage of patients and donors with anti-HBc have irreproducible results or no evidence of previous infection.

The Aoki study (Abstract 116-95-6–46) is based on the theory that an individual with anti-HBc from a previous infection would react to hepatitis B antigen with a secondary or anamnestic response, whereas an individual with a false positive test result would react with a primary response. Their results provide a cumbersome method to handle an anti-HBc–positive individual because they show that most donors have previous infection. The Douglas study (Abstract 116-95-6–45) used PCR to determine whether core positive blood donors have evidence of HBV DNA and would thus be capable of transmitting hepatitis B; their results show that anti-HBc–positive donors in low-prevalence areas are not infectious. These studies confirm that anti-HBc testing is not particularly useful for subclinical hepatitis B in blood donors; the test is also difficult to interpret for the blood donor without a specific confirmatory test to assist in donor counseling.—P.M. Ness, M.D.

Evidence of Hepatitis in Patients Receiving Transfusions of Blood Components Containing Antibody to Hepatitis C

Aoki SK, Holland PV, Fernando LP, Kuramoto IK, Anderson S, Sazama K, Schoening V, Johnson P, Wilber JC, Fenner L, Alter HJ (Sacramento Med Found Blood Ctr and Ctr for Blood Research, Calif; Chiron Corp, Emeryville, Calif; NIH, Bethesda, Md)
Blood 82:1000–1005, 1993   116-95-6–47

Background.—The hepatitis C virus (HCV) is responsible for non-A, non-B hepatitis. The first Food and Drug Administration–approved test for HCV was the enzyme immunoassay EIA1. Blood banks began using it immediately in May of 1990. The rate of transmission of HCV by antibody for HCV (anti-HCV) EIA1-reactive blood components that were transfused just before the introduction of the new test was studied.

Patients and Methods.—There were 96 patient participants: 54 controls and 42 recipients of HCV EIA1–reactive, homologous blood components. Assays used included EIA1; a second-generation assay, EIA2; reverse-transcriptase–polymerase chain reaction (RT-PCR); and 4-antigen strip immunoblot assay (RIBA2). Each participant completed a 1-page questionnaire before enrolling in the study. Follow-up of the 42 patients was conducted at 3-, 6-, and 12-month intervals post-transfusion.

Results.—The EIA1 assay indicated that 10 of the 42 patients were anti-HCV reactive on follow-up. The assay EIA2 indicated that 12 were anti-HCV reactive. The RT-PCR test detected HCV RNA in 5 seronegative recipients. Overall, HCV infection was found in the blood of 17 of 42 patients. The 54 patients in the control group remained EIA1-nonreactive and RT-PCR–negative for 1 year. Only 1 patient became EIA2 reactive. Of the recipients of the anti-HCV reactive blood transfusions (those reactive to both the EIA2 and RIBA2), 14 had evidence of HCV infection compared with only 3 of the 27 recipients of EIA1-reactive and RIBA2-nonreactive blood.

Conclusion.—Blood components found reactive by both the EIA1 and RIBA2 may transmit HCV with a frequency greater than 90%, whereas those reactive for anti-HCV EIA1 may have transmitted HCV only 40% of the time.

▶ This retrospective study shows that transfusing blood from donors with positive tests for anti-HCV has a high likelihood of causing seroconversion in the blood recipient. If the donor was positive for anti-HCV, the rate of seroconversion was 40%; when the anti-HCV positive donor also had a positive recombinant immunoblot assay, the rate increased to 90%. These results verify the value of anti-HCV screening and the many false positive tests that occurred with earlier versions of anti-HCV testing in blood donors.—P.M. Ness, M.D.

Search for Intrafamilial Transmission of Hepatitis C Virus in Hemophilia Patients

Brackmann SA, Gerritzen A, Oldenburg J, Brackmann H-H, Schneweis KE (Univ of Bonn, Germany)
Blood 81:1077–1082, 1993   116-95-6–48

Objective.—Because little is known about the risk of hepatitis C virus (HCV) infection in contacts of infected patients with hemophilia, the risk was compared with that of acquiring hepatitis B virus, hepatitis A virus, and HIV infections in relatives of patients with hemophilia positive for anti-HCV antibody. The index group included 141 patients with hemophilia A, hemophilia B, or von Willebrand's disease who had been positive for anti-HCV on several occasions, using first- and second-generation anti-HCV enzyme immunoassays.

Findings.—All but 4 of 228 household contacts of the index patients were negative by both assays, whereas 1 was positive by both methods. Three contacts had positive results from the first-generation assay and negative results from the second-generation assay. Twelve percent of nonsexual household contacts and 13% of sex partners were positive for antibody to hepatitis B-core antigen (anti-HBc). Contacts of index patients with chronic hepatitis B were most often positive for anti-HBc. Contacts participating in controlled self-treatment did not have an increased rate of hepatitis B virus infection compared with controls. Of 44 sex partners of index patients, 5 (11%) were positive for anti-HIV, matching the age-adjusted rate for the general population.

Implications.—Even sexual contact with HCV-infected patients with hemophilia within households does not increase the risk of HCV infection. In addition, controlled self-treatment is not an added risk factor for HCV or hepatitis B virus infection.

▶ Although hepatitis C is a common infection, as witnessed by the detection of anti-HCV in approximately .5% of otherwise healthy blood donors, its mode of spread is confusing. It can be spread sexually, but a number of studies have shown that high-risk groups for sexually transmitted diseases have much lower rates of anti-HCV than anti-HIV or anti-hepatitis B virus. This study looked at families of patients with hemophilia to determine how much intrafamilial transmission occurred in these apparently high-risk families. Whereas family members with sexual contacts had similar rates of hepatitis B virus infection to nonsexual household contacts, very few household contacts had anti-HCV. Additionally, there was no evidence of spread of HCV in households where the patient was undergoing intravenous self-treatment. These studies make counseling family members of patients infected with hepatitis C very difficult.—P.M. Ness, M.D.

Transmission of Hepatitis A to Patients With Hemophilia by Factor VIII Concentrates Treated With Organic Solvent and Detergent to Inactivate Viruses

Mannucci PM, Gdovin S, Gringeri A, Colombo M, Mele A, Schinaia N, Ciavarella N, Emerson SU, Purcell RH, and the Italian Collaborative Group (Univ of Milan, Italy; NIH, Bethesda, Md; Univ of Maryland, College Park; et al)
Ann Intern Med 120:1–7, 1994   116-95-6–49

Background.—Hepatitis A virus (HAV) is rarely transmitted through blood transfusion because no chronic carrier state exists. However, a large outbreak of hepatitis A in patients with hemophilia was recently reported in several Italian centers. In the 2 months before diagnosis, all patients had received a large-pool factor VIII concentrate produced by a manufacturer that used a solvent-detergent–based method of inactivating blood-borne viruses. Since that time, 88 similar cases of HAV transmission through infected blood have been reported in Europe. Whether the factor VIII preparations were associated with HAV infection was investigated.

Methods.—The first 29 patients having hemophilia and jaundice diagnosed who later had HAV were matched with controls with hemophilia but no jaundice. The participants responded to a questionnaire concerning the 2-month period before the onset of jaundice. Included was information about exposure to lots of factor VIII concentrate and the virucidal methods used to treat them, contact with others with jaundice, travel abroad, and consumption of raw shellfish. Measurements were taken of HAV sequences sought by polymerase chain reaction in lots of factor VIII and in serial serum samples from 2 patients who had contracted hepatitis. Amplification by polymerase chain reaction was also carried out on complementary DNA transcribed with reverse transcriptase from matched sets of factor VIII and recipient serum samples, and the nucleotide sequence of amplified HAV genome was determined.

Results.—No significant difference was seen between patients and controls regarding travel to high-risk hepatitis countries, consumption of raw shellfish, or contact with others with jaundice. Patients with hepatitis were more likely than controls to have received a factor VIII concentrate treated with a solvent-detergent mixture and to have had larger infusions of the concentrate during the presumed HAV incubation period. Viral sequences of hepatitis A were seen in 5 of 12 tested lots of factor VIII. Genomic sequences of HAV obtained for 2 matched sets of factor VIII and recipient serum samples were identical within each set but different for the 2 sets.

Conclusion.—Hepatitis A was transmitted to these patients through factor VIII concentrate treated by a solvent-detergent virucidal method that does not effectively inactivate nonenveloped viruses. Although vaccination of susceptible patients against HAV is recommended, other blood-borne, nonenveloped viruses for which vaccines are not yet available can pose similar risks to this patient population.

▶ Factor VIII concentrates manufactured from plasma donors use large pools of plasma derived from thousands of donations, thus enhancing the chance that a contaminated unit will be included. Viral inactivation methods have lessened the risk of contracting many infectious agents through heat inactivation or the use of various organic solvents. The solvent-detergent approach is very effective against lipid-enveloped viruses such as hepatitis B and C or HIV, the most feared pathogens. On the other hand, other viruses such as HAV and parvovirus B19 do not possess an envelope; therefore, the solvent-detergent approach would not be effective. This report demonstrates the failure of the solvent-detergent method to prevent hepatitis A transmission by factor VIII concentrates. More important, it prompts concern about similar problems that could occur with fresh frozen plasma treated with solvent-detergent methods. The technology to provide solvent-detergent fresh frozen plasma may soon be licensed in an effort to ensure complete eradication of HIV and hepatitis B and C. To be able to use this technology, the plasma from single donors will be pooled before solvent-detergent treatment. This pooling step raises the concern that minimal reductions in the risk of HIV, hepatitis B and hepatitis C virus may be balanced by the increased risk of infection with a nonenveloped virus.—P.M. Ness, M.D.

The Impact of Blood Transfusion on the Occurrence of Pneumonitis in Primary Cytomegalovirus Infection After Liver Transplantation

Mañez R, Kusne S, Martin M, Linden P, Irish W, Torre-Cisneros J, Kramer D, Ho M, Starzl TE (Univ of Pittsburgh, Pa)
Transfusion 33:594–597, 1993   116-95-6–50

Background.—For patients undergoing liver transplantation, cytomegalovirus (CMV) is the most frequent post-transplant infection. There are 2 types of post-transplant infections: primary infection, which occurs when a CMV-seronegative transplant recipient becomes infected with CMV, or secondary infection, which results from activation of a latent CMV strain or infection of a new strain in CMV-seropositive transplant recipients. The symptoms of primary CMV infection are often more severe. The effect of the transfusion of CMV-seropositive blood on the occurrence of primary CMV infection after liver transplant was evaluated.

Patients and Methods.—Twenty-nine patients participated. Of these, 14 patients in group A received a graft from a CMV-seropositive donor, and 15 patients in group B received a CMV-seronegative graft.

Results.—Cytomegalovirus infection developed in 11 of the group A patients and 2 of the group B patients. Pneumonitis resulting from the primary CMV infection occurred among 5 of the group A patients. No significant difference was noted between the number of patients in either group A or B who did or did not have CMV disease develop and the number of units of seropositive blood each received. However, the group A patients who contracted CMV pneumonitis had received a higher total number of blood units than other patients who contracted other CMV infections.

Conclusion.—The total number of blood units and the total numbers of CMV-seropositive blood units transfused had no effect on the incidence of primary CMV infection after liver transplantation. However, the number of units transfused had an impact on the severity of infection in the recipients of a CMV-seropositive allograft.

▶ Cytomegalovirus infection is a serious problem in the setting of liver transplantation. The sources of CMV infection are threefold: the donor organ, the blood transfusions, and reactivation of the patient's previous CMV infection. Devising recommendations for CMV prevention is difficult because the large quantities of blood required cannot be typically met with seronegative blood and because in many cases, the donor liver is not tested but is subsequently found to be positive. This paper confirms that the graft is commonly the source of CMV primary infection. In those patients who received a seropositive graft, the total number of transfused units seemed to be a more important predictor of CMV disease than the number of seropositive units transfused. We currently try to provide CMV-seronegative or leukodepleted blood for recipients of CMV-seronegative liver transplantation, regardless of the CMV status of the donor, which is often unknown.—P.M. Ness, M.D.

Detection of Parvovirus B19 in Donated Blood: A Model System for Screening by Polymerase Chain Reaction
McOmish F, Yap PL, Jordan A, Hart H, Cohen BJ, Simmonds P (Royal Infirmary, Edinburgh, Scotland; Protein Fractionation Centre, Edinburgh, Scotland; Central Public Health Lab, London; et al)
J Clin Microbiol 31:323–328, 1993   116-95-6–51

Background.—Human parvovirus B19, usually spread through the respiratory route, can also be spread by parenteral transmission in blood transfusion products made from plasma pools containing blood donated during the viremic stages of B19 infection. A very sensitive, rapid technique for routinely screening large numbers of donated blood units for B19 infection was investigated.

Methods and Findings.—The new method involves polymerase chain reaction (PCR). In a 3-month trial, B19 DNA was identified in 6 of 20,000 consecutive units of blood (.03%) in levels ranging from 2.4×10^4 to 5×10^{10} copies of viral DNA per mL. In the interval between donation and recall, seroconversion for B19-specific IgM and IgG occurred, and circulating B19 DNA disappeared in 4 of the 5 implicated donors who could be recalled. B19 DNA was found in 18 of 27 batches of non–heat-treated factor VIII and IX concentrate made from donated plasma not screened for B19 DNA. Dry heat treatment decreased detectable B19 from factor VIII concentrates but did not always eliminate it, which is consistent with recent observations that current techniques for virus inactivation in blood product manufacture are not sufficient to eliminate B19 infection completely.

Conclusion.—These PCR screening methods could be routinely used to prevent B19 transmission in blood and blood products and the iatrogenic transmission of infection. Polymerase chain reaction screening may also be used for detecting and excluding a range of other transmission-related viruses for which current serologic methods are only partly effective.

▶ Although there are no current recommendations that we should screen donor blood for evidence of parvovirus infection, this methodology should be of interest as an example of a system that may be applicable for this virus or other candidate viruses in the future.—P.M. Ness, M.D.

Transfusion-Associated Graft-*Versus*-Host Disease Caused by Leukocyte-Filtered Stored Blood

Hayashi H, Nishiuchi T, Tamura H, Takeda K (Osaka Natl Hosp, Japan)
Anesthesiology 79:1419–1421, 1993   116-95-6–52

Background.—Although the incidence of transfusion-associated graft-vs.-host disease is low, its mortality is high. The disease usually results from viable or immunocompetent lymphocytes from fresh transfused blood products. Rarely is it seen after transfusion of stored blood. The best means of prevention is τ-irradiation of blood before transfusion or the elimination of lymphocytes by filtering. The first case of transfusion-associated graft-vs.-host disease seen after transfusion of nonirradiated, stored (7-day-old) packed red cells despite leukocyte filtering was reported.

Case Report.—Man, 72, underwent coronary artery bypass graft surgery and valve replacement. The patient was transfused with 2 units of nonirradiated leukocyte-filtered packed RBCs that had been stored for 7 days. Five units of fresh frozen plasma were added to control bleeding. Six days after surgery, a persistent fever developed, although the patient's hemodynamic state was stable. On the ninth day, a skin rash developed, and 2 days later the aspartate aminotransferase and alanine aminotransferase levels increased significantly to 485 and 761 units/L, respectively, whereas his platelet count decreased. A skin biopsy specimen later showed necrotic keratinocytes with eosinophilic cytoplasm, the vacuolar degeneration of basal cells, and a lymphocytic infiltrate, all signs of transfusion-associated graft-vs.-host disease. Treatment with methylprednisolone and G-CSF was ineffective, and the patient died of coagulopathy, sepsis, and multiple-organ failure 16 days after surgery.

Discussion.—Transfusion with fresh blood products is a known risk factor for transfusion-associated graft-vs.-host disease. In contrast, stored blood products have, in the past, been considered much safer, because they contain fewer viable lymphocytes. However, as this case demonstrates, transfusion-associated graft-vs.-host disease can and does result after transfusion of stored blood products, and the only valid means of preventing it is by routine τ-irradiation of all blood products. Because there is currently no effective treatment for this disease, every effort should be made to minimize the transfusion of donated blood.

▶ This case report proves a point that would have been very difficult to establish with a controlled clinical trial. Transfusion-associated graft-vs.-host disease is an uncommon event, most likely caused by allogeneic white cells that engraft in a susceptible host. Irradiation of blood will prevent this complication but irradiation equipment is expensive and not always immediately available. These facts have prompted the question of whether leukodepletion by filtration would be equivalent to irradiation of blood to prevent graft-vs.-host disease. This case report demonstrates a filtration failure, suggesting that an expensive comprehensive trial is not worth performing.—P.M. Ness, M.D.

Call Mosby Document Express at **1 (800) 55-MOSBY** to obtain copies of the original source documents of articles featured or referenced in the YEAR BOOK series.

Subject Index*

A

Abdominal
pain after etoposide in Hodgkin's
disease, 95: 250
surgery, general, with
low-molecular-weight heparin,
phlebographic deep vein
thrombosis after, 95: 189
trauma, autotransfusion of
culture-positive blood in, 94: 372
ABL-BCR (see BCR-ABL)
ABO
-incompatible bone marrow transplants,
hemolysis of transfused group O
RBCs in, 94: 359
-incompatible liver transplants,
immunohematologic complications
of, 94: 392
minor-mismatch causing immune
hemolytic anemia after renal
transplant, 95: 15
Abortion
habitual
factor XII deficiency and, 94: 134
fibrinolytic balance and lupus
anticoagulant and, 94: 157
ABVD chemotherapy (see Chemotherapy,
ABVD)
Academic
sequelae of acute lymphoblastic
leukemia treated in infancy,
94: 316
N-Acetylglucosamine
incorporation in biosynthesis of GPI
anchor, specific defects in
paroxysmal nocturnal
hemoglobinuria, 95: 20
Acid-base
changes after massive transfusions,
94: 380
Acipimox
effects on lipid pattern and plasma
fibrinogen in type 2 diabetics,
94: 174
Acquired immunodeficiency syndrome (see
AIDS)
Acremonium
infections after bone marrow transplant,
95: 354
AcSKDP
stem cell inhibition by, 94: 73
Actin
reorganization in chemotactic
factor-activated leukocytes,
mechanisms for, 95: 68

Actinomycin D
after MDR1 gene treatment (in mice),
94: 320
Acyclovir
-resistant herpes simplex infections after
marrow transplantation, foscarnet
for, 94: 339
Adenosine
diphosphate-induced platelet α-granule
release, effect of aspirin on,
95: 113
Adhesion
leukocyte adhesion deficiency type 2
causing recurrent severe infections,
94: 103
neutrophil, effects of G-CSF and
GM-CSF on, 94: 105
Adolescents
Hodgkin's disease treatment in, cardiac
disease after, 95: 240
Adriamycin (see Doxorubicin)
Age
agranulocytosis and, clozapine-induced,
95: 75
-dependent effect on level of factor IX,
95: 147
effect on HIV-induced lymphocyte
changes in congenital clotting
disorders, 94: 148
-related increase of pepsinogens in
transfusion donors, effect of
Helicobacter pylori infection on,
94: 350
Agen test
in pulmonary embolism, suspected,
95: 177
Aging
anticoagulant response to warfarin and,
94: 192
Agranulocytosis
clozapine-induced, 95: 73
AIDS
(See also HIV)
bone marrow in, gelatinous, 94: 116
Kaposi's sarcoma in, and cytokine
production, 94: 114
-related non-Hodgkin's lymphoma,
chemotherapy in, 95: 263
transfusion-associated, in U.S., 95: 409,
411
Albumin
-globulin ratio in recurrent stroke,
95: 179
Alglucerase
in Gaucher disease type 1, 95: 43
Alkalinization

---

* All entries refer to the year and page number(s) for data appearing in this and the
previous edition of the YEAR BOOK.

heparin-induced thrombocytopenia,
95: 128

Fcγ
fragments, infusion for acute immune
thrombocytopenic purpura, in
children, 95: 124

Febrile
children with sickle cell disease,
outpatient ceftriaxone in, 95: 22
neutropenic conditions after
mitoxantrone/etoposide before
marrow transplant in relapsed
Hodgkin's disease, 94: 245
neutrophilic dermatosis, acute, during
G-CSF therapy, 94: 91

Femoral
head osteonecrosis in sickle cell disease,
hip arthroplasty for, 94: 35

Fetus
-globin-gene expression of β-globin
disorders, butyrate stimulation of,
94: 42
liver, bipotential precursors of B cells
and macrophages in (in mice),
94: 68
loss (*see* Pregnancy, loss)
RhD type, prenatal determination by
DNA amplification, 95: 370
stem cells, hematopoietic, liver-derived,
homing to bone marrow, 94: 67
thrombocytopenia, 95: 126
transplantation of adult human marrow
cells into (in sheep), 94: 66

Fever
GM-CSF causing, 94: 92
in hemophagocytic syndrome, reactive,
94: 108
Q, anticardiolipin antibodies and
dependence of serum cofactor in,
95: 167
in retinoic acid syndrome in acute
promyelocytic leukemia, 94: 293

Fibrillation
atrial, low-dose warfarin in, 95: 192

Fibrin
polymers, plasma crosslinked, 94: 202

Fibrinogen
alpha-chain sites, role in platelet
aggregation, 94: 121
in arterial disease, peripheral, 95: 178
as cardiovascular risk factor, 94: 175
in children, 95: 182
Dusart, 95: 228
gamma-chain
carboxy-terminal residues in, and
platelet aggregation, 94: 123
sites, role in platelet aggregation,
94: 121

genotype and risk of peripheral
atherosclerosis, 94: 176
levels
in angina pectoris and myocardial
infarction, 94: 201
in diabetics, type 2, effects of
bezafibrate and acipimox on,
94: 174
effect of anesthesia on, 95: 227
relation to personal history of prevalent
hypertension, diabetes, stroke,
intermittent claudication, coronary
heart disease, and family history,
95: 183
as risk factor for cardiovascular events
after stroke, 94: 168
in stroke, recurrent, 95: 179

Fibrinogenolysis
tissue plasminogen activator-induced,
effect of α₂-antiplasmin
supplementation on (in rabbit),
95: 219

Fibrinolysis
effects of anesthetic regimens on,
95: 227
in hemodialysis patients, effect of EPO
therapy and withdrawal on, 95: 5

Fibrinolytic
balance and repeated spontaneous fetal
loss, 94: 157
proteins in myocardial infarction and
angina pectoris, 94: 201
shutdown, postoperative, and plasma
levels of type 1 plasminogen
activator inhibitor, 94: 171
system, effects of anabolic steroids on,
95: 142

Fibrinopeptide A
increase in patients with systemic lupus
erythematosus and anticardiolipin
antibodies, 95: 168
urinary, in peripheral arterial disease,
95: 178

Fibroblast
growth factor, basic, effect on
proliferation of megakaryocyte
progenitor cells, 95: 48

Fibronectin
matrix in marrow fibrosis of hairy cell
leukemia, 95: 281

Fibrosis
marrow, in hairy cell leukemia, cause of,
95: 281
portal, and marrow transplantation in
adult thalassemia, 94: 43

Fibrous

Author Index

A

Abboud CN, 346
Abels RI, 378
Abildgaard CF, 144
Ablin AR, 317
Abshire TC, 149
Addonizio LJ, 259
Agnelli G, 175
Ahlbom A, 309
Ahmann G, 277
Ahn DK, 381
Albo VC, 317
Alexander JB, 226
Alexander S, 414
Alexanian R, 279
Allen PK, 236
Alter BP, 28
Alter HJ, 417
Alving BM, 161
Alvir JMJ, 73
Aly MH, 17
Amadori S, 269, 331
Amess JAL, 311
Anandakumar C, 173
Anderson DC, 69
Anderson DR, 199
Anderson GF, 360
Anderson J, 246
Anderson JE, 344
Anderson JR, 348
Anderson KC, 349
Anderson MJ, 24
Anderson S, 417
Anderson SM, 32
Andersson BS, 290
Andersson M, 291
Andreeff M, 286, 318
Andrew M, 402
Anguenot T, 214
Anklesaria P, 64
Anquist K, 196
Ansell JE, 142
Antico VF, 262
Antin JH, 340, 349
Aoki SK, 416, 417
Appelbaum FR, 276, 333, 344, 366
Archimbaud E, 298, 306, 307
Arduino C, 53
Aricó M, 244
Arkin S, 144
Arlien-Søborg P, 212
Armenti FR, 133
Armitage JO, 343, 348
Arter A, 148
Arthur DD, 289
Asfour A, 376
Ash RC, 341, 349
Åstedt B, 223
Aster RH, 123
Astori C, 254
Attal M, 347
AuBuchon JP, 382

Auer G, 298
Aul C, 292
Auzanneau G, 307
Avanzi GC, 53
Avvisati G, 269, 306
Azuma H, 220

B

Babyn PS, 27
Backstrom L, 326
Bader SB, 245
Badger CC, 276
Bailly P, 367, 368
Balducci L, 397
Ballester OF, 397
Banaji M, 352
Bao W, 182
Barbui T, 159
Barcos M, 246, 301
Bardossy L, 406, 407
Barlogie B, 279
Barnard D, 332
Barnett MJ, 266
Barr ML, 259
Barr TA, 350
Bartch G, 349
Barzegar S, 141
Basile F, 118
Bass EB, 360
Bassand J-P, 214
Bastion Y, 307
Bates S, 270
Bauer KA, 141
Bauer TL, 133
Bauters F, 307
Baxter BT, 390
Baynes RD, 11
Beamer N, 179
Beard CJ, 253
Bearman SI, 353
Bechensteen AG, 8
Bechstein W, 396
Beck GJ, 226
Bednarczyk EM, 356
Behm FG, 324
Belanger C, 318
Belanger R, 351
Belch JJF, 5
Beljaards RC, 257
Bell W, 108
Ben-Bassat I, 106
Bene MC, 357
Benjamin D, 332
Bennett J, 301, 302
Bennett PR, 370
Bensinger WI, 344, 366
Benson D, 363
Benson K, 397
Beran M, 284, 285, 286, 319
Berckmans RJ, 177
Berenson GS, 182
Bergelin RO, 215

Bergström K, 209
Berliner N, 58
Berman E, 318
Bernard P, 335
Bernard Y, 214
Bernasconi C, 254
Bernstein ID, 276
Berntorp E, 191
Berti E, 257
Bertino J, 318
Bessler M, 20
Beynen FMK, 389
Bhagat SKM, 235
Bierling P, 120, 122
Bierman PJ, 348
Biesma DH, 379
Billadeau D, 277
Billett AL, 334
Binder T, 268
Biondi A, 306
Birkmeyer JD, 382, 393
Bixby T, 349
Blajchman MA, 406, 407
Blanchard CG, 263
Blanchette V, 123
Bleyer WA, 317
Bloomfield CD, 246, 289
Bloy C, 368
Blume KG, 333, 350
Blumhardt G, 396
Boccalon H, 194
Bödewadt-Radzun S, 283
Boileau J, 351
Boiron J-M, 335
Boisclair MD, 169
Bolan CD, 161
Bolgiano DC, 363
Bolwell BJ, 349
Bona R, 167
Bonan JL, 113
Boneu B, 194
Bonfils S, 194
Bonnet M-C, 124
Bonny Y, 351
Bontempi N, 244
Bordigoni P, 357
Bordin JO, 407
Boschetti E, 175
Bottoms S, 170
Bounameaux H, 189
Bouras Y, 214
Boveri E, 254
Bovill EG, 136
Bowen D, 307
Boyarsky A, 17
Boyett J, 326
Boysen G, 212
Brackmann H-H, 418
Brackmann SA, 418
Bradshaw P, 414
Brandjes DPM, 177
Brandmaier R, 268
Brant R, 196
Braverman IM, 273

495